THE COMPLETE CANCER CLEANSE

A Proven Program to Detoxify and Renew Body, Mind, and Spirit

Cherie Calbom, M.S.
Fr. John Calbom, M.A. • Michael Mahaffey, P.C.

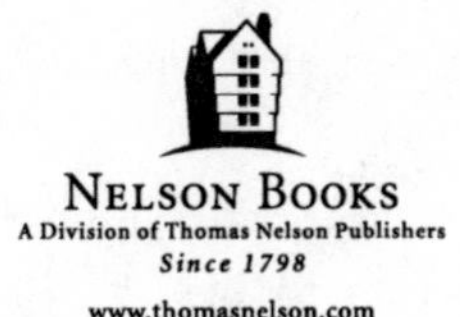

Nelson Books
A Division of Thomas Nelson Publishers
Since 1798
www.thomasnelson.com

Published in Nashville, Tennessee, by Thomas Nelson, Inc.

Nelson Books may be purchased in bulk for educational, business, fund-raising, or sales promotional use. For information, please e-mail SpecialMarkets@ThomasNelson.com.

Library of Congress Cataloging-in-Publication Data

Calbom, Cherie.

The complete cancer cleanse : a proven program to detoxify and renew body, mind, and spirit / Cherie Calbom, John Calbom, Michael Mahaffey.

p. cm.

Includes bibliographical references.

ISBN 978-0-7852-6295-4 (hbk.)

ISBN-10: 0-7852-8863-5 (tpc)

ISBN-13: 978-0-7852-8863-3 (tpc)

1. Cancer--Alternative treatment. 2. Detoxification (Health) I. Calbom, John. II. Mahaffey, Michael, P.C. III. Title.

RC271.A62 C34 2003

616.99'406—dc22

2003015478

Printed in the United States of America

06 07 08 09 RRD 5 4 3 2 1

CONTENTS

PART ONE:
The Complete Detoxification Program

PART TWO:
A Renewal of Your Body, Your Mind, and Your Spirit

CONTENTS

PART ONE

The Complete Detoxification Program

1

A THREE-PART STRATEGY FOR HEALING

Love's strength, stands in love's sacrifice,
and he who suffers most, has most to gain.
—AUTHOR UNKNOWN

Cancer is still the great mystery disease. We all pray that we'll never get it, yet here we are. When first diagnosed, we search for answers to a myriad of questions: What is cancer? What caused it? What are my treatment options? Will I die? Cancer diagnosis is shocking enough to send us into a state of terror, like being thrown into the strong currents of a rushing river. We want answers, and we want them *now*.

Answers are essential: the better informed we are about our disease, the greater the odds of overcoming it. The history of cancer incidence in the West, and particularly the United States, speaks volumes. Prior to this century, cancer was rare and afflicted only a small percentage of the population. Stanislas Tanchou, a French pioneering scientist in the field of vital statistics in the 1830s, tabulated Paris mortality rates; he reported that cancer deaths comprised about 2 percent of the total number of deaths at that time. At the turn of the century, the cancer death rate in the United States was calculated at about 4 percent of the population.[1]

Current cancer statistics are sobering:

- Cancer is the cause of one in five deaths in the United States
- Cancer will affect one in three people in the United States
- Over 1.2 million cases of invasive cancer are diagnosed each year.

- An additional 1.5 million cases of noninvasive cancer will be diagnosed yearly.
- More than five hundred thousand people will die from cancer each year.
- Children ages three to fourteen years die of cancer more than any other disease.
- The total cost of cancer care and mortality is over 15 percent of all health-care costs, exceeding more than 110 billion dollars.

Statistics do not show that we are making progress in prevention or treatment of cancer. Indeed the facts show the opposite—we are losing the war. The number of new cases of nearly every form of cancer has increased annually over the last century.[2] From 1930 to the present, despite all our therapies and technology, cancer incidence has continued to increase.

WHAT IS CANCER?

Cancer is not a disease of modern man. For more than four thousand years it has afflicted human beings. In fact, ancient Egyptian and Greek medical tracts describe cancerous conditions. Writings about Cosmos and Damian, healing physicians of the third century, recount the unusual healing of deacon Justinian's cancerous leg.

Hippocrates described the illness, calling it *karkinos,* meaning the crab. Historical writings describe tumor growths as having a central area with channels that spread out like arms into surrounding tissue. Ancient observers thought these growths looked like a crab; therefore, it's logical that the Latin word for crab is *cancer.*

By simple definition cancer is a malignant growth or growths and the illnesses caused by those growths. It all starts in a cell. That cell (or group of cells) escapes homeostatic control (equilibrium of the internal environment), reproduces at will, and shows abnormal growth patterns. Also known as neoplasms (meaning new growth), these growths compete with normal cells for energy and nutrition, and are to some degree autonomous. "New growth" is not an accurate description of most cancers, however, because it often takes from five to twenty years for a tumor to develop from the first mutated cells to a tumor mass.

Cancer cells lose the more specialized functions characteristic of normal cells while at the same time acquiring increased growth function. This increase results in an invasion of the surrounding tissue and the formation of secondary growths at a distance—known as metastasis. Their metabolism is different from that of a normal cell; something happens to alter these cells chemically. Professor Otto Warburg, two-time Nobel Prize–winner in medicine, was the first to suggest that cancer cells are anaerobic, meaning that they function in the absence of free oxygen. He discovered that oxygen in cancer cells was replaced by an energy–yielding mechanism known as glycolysis, which means that the cancer cells feed on the fermentation of glucose (sugar).[3]

Cancer has two characteristics that make it life threatening: it invades tissue and spreads to vital organs where it may compress, obstruct, or destroy vital functions. As cancerous tumors attach themselves to organs, tissues become oxygen starved. Cancer cells appear to take priority over normal cells in acquiring amino acids and nutrients; thus the tumor grows while the rest of the body experiences deficiency and often wasting.

The development of cancer is considered to be a two-stage process. During the initiation stage there is a transformation of a cell, causing it to change (mutate) in some manner, due to the interaction of such factors as chemicals, radiation, viruses, or injury. The transformation occurs rapidly, but the transformed cell or cells may be dormant for a long time until activated by a promoting agent(s). During the promotion stage, many substances, even noncarcinogens such as hormones, can play a part in the rapid cell division characteristic of cancer. In this promotion stage, the tumor forms, unless the mutated cells are destroyed by the immune defense system or through treatment.[4]

John and Cherie Calbom believe their schnauzer, MacKenzie, had a tumor that was an example of this two-stage development process. When he was diagnosed with a malignant tumor in his right-front paw, they couldn't figure out why he would get cancer. After all, he'd had the very best of everything: organic food, vitamins, purified water, fresh air, daily walks, a stress-free life, and oodles of love and attention. But with a little thought, it began to make some sense. When he was about ten months old, he jumped off their second-story deck—a scampering squirrel was simply too much temptation. Gathering him up, Cherie examined four bloody paws—nothing broken, they learned, just very bruised. Daily walks in the neighborhood that summer proved to be problematic. Neighbors sprayed their lawns with chemicals, and often MacKenzie got sick upon returning from their strolls. Perhaps the injury followed by the lawn chemicals initiated cell mutations in his toe, and nine years later, other factors finally promoted a tumor. Today, minus only one toe, he's completely well, thanks to their holistic vet and his nontraditional canine cancer-care program.

YOUR AUTHORS' PERSPECTIVES ON THIS DISEASE

Each of your authors brings a different perspective to a study of cancer. Cherie is a nutritionist who has studied the relationship between cancer and nutrition for the last sixteen years. She is well-known in the United States as the "Juice Lady" for her work with juicing and health and for the numerous books she has written, such as *Juicing for Life.* Her husband, Father John Calbom, is an Orthodox priest who is also a psychotherapist and a behavioral medicine specialist. And Michael Mahaffey is a cancer survivor who is the cofounder of Cedar Springs Renewal Center. Getting cancer changed the direction of his life, and as a result, he has dedicated his time, money, and efforts to helping other cancer patients survive and discover how to live each day to the fullest.

In this first chapter they'd like to give you a glimpse of how they became so involved with this disease.

CHERIE'S STORY

One blustery March day in Iowa, our family gathered in the church "to pay our last respects," as my aunt said. All of us who loved my mother sat in silence, stunned by grief. "A lovely life snuffed out far too soon," someone said in passing. My grandmother nodded.

That was the day the music died forever; her music, that is. The piano keys she once played for hours a day lay as cold as her fingers. The funeral service passed like a short winter snow flurry, and then, as sleepwalkers unaroused, we headed for the altar. I could barely see over the edge of the casket. My knees became weak, and I didn't think I could breathe when I saw her face, motionless and white. A lady leaned down and told me she was in heaven. I only knew my mother was dead. At six, I had no idea what breast cancer was, but it had killed her.

This was my defining moment—one that shaped my life. From that time on I wanted to know what cancer was, what caused it, how it could be prevented, and how it could be cured. Years later it was no mystery that I felt compelled to respond to an ad in our university bulletin regarding a small grant to research nutrition and cancer. I was awarded the money, which supported an intense medical and scientific literature search. This project also became my master's thesis at Bastyr University, titled "Nutrition as an Adjunct to Cancer Treatment." The Center for Alternative Cancer Research, the sponsors of the grant, liked my project and printed it as a book titled *Nutrition and Cancer: Is Nutrition the Missing Piece in the Cancer Treatment Puzzle?*

That project is what led me to write Part One of *The Complete Cancer Cleanse*. But before I tell you what this book can offer you on your journey to complete health and healing, I want to tell you about what cleansing has done for me in my own recovery from illness.

It was 1978 and I was single, twenty-something, and working in Hollywood for Pat Boone. Life was exciting! Debby Boone's "You Light up My Life" was a big hit, and the Boone office was a flurry of activity. I had a chance to meet scores of singers, songwriters, and TV personalities. One was Kathie Lee Johnson (now Gifford). I spent a Thanksgiving Day in her home, and she arranged a blind date for me with TV singer Tom Netherton. That was just one of many exciting party and event invitations that came my way because of my job.

In the midst of the fun, I started feeling tired—too tired to do much more than lie on the couch after work. Then I began turning down invitations because I was so fatigued, and I spent most of my weekends sleeping. When I got the flu, it never seemed to end. I was perennially lethargic and suffered continuously from a low-grade fever and swollen glands. My muscles and joints ached, and I didn't sleep restfully through the night. I had a devastating case of what we now know is chronic fatigue syndrome and fibromyalgia; but at that time, doctors didn't have a clue as to what was going on in my body. Imagine my chagrin when it was suggested that I was depressed and should see a psychiatrist. Depressed! Life had been anything but depressing. The only thing I was depressed about was my health, and the fact that no one seemed to be able to help me.

Finally, I had to quit my job and move to my father's home in Colorado Springs—too sick to work and unable to afford my apartment. I visited a holistic doctor who tested me for food allergies, and I left his office with a list of offending foods longer than my arm. It seemed like I had nothing left to eat but tree bark and lettuce.

Not finding any promising answers from the medical profession, I finally turned to health food stores. I talked with employees and searched the bookshelves, where I did find answers. There was something *I could do* to change my health. I discovered I was eating all the wrong things—enough junk to kill a healthy young gorilla, as I say in my book *The Juice Lady's Guide to Juicing for Health*. My body needed nutrients to heal and gain energy. I had never particularly cared for vegetables, salads, or whole grains, but they were the foods I needed to eat to get well. From my reading, I also learned about the healing benefits of fresh juice and the restorative power of juice fasting. Two health-care professionals pointed out that my body was toxic. It needed to be cleansed from all the toxicity I'd collected over the years.

New knowledge in hand, and armed with my first juicer, I designed my own program, starting with a kick-off, five-day juice fast made up of mostly vegetable juices. For the remainder of the summer, I turned to vegan foods and fresh juice I made daily, along with periodic juice fasts. Instead of getting better, though, I felt worse. My body was experiencing what is known as a *healing crisis*. My father thought I was going to kill myself with this program, but I assured him nothing could be better for me than vegetables, whole grains, and vegetable juices. And besides, before I started my program, I had felt like I was dying anyway, so what did I have to lose?

On the fifth day of my kick-off juice fast, I experienced a miracle: my body expelled a tumor about the size of a golf ball. It had its own blood supply of small blue veins and was obviously "starved" by my fast. My body expelled it through my colon. I have no idea if this tumor was benign or malignant; one doctor said it was probably a polyp (benign). I will never know for certain what it was, because I didn't think to take it to someone for examination, but I was so thankful it was gone. Then, midway through my cleanse program, I tried a gallbladder flush at the recommendation of my holistic health-care provider. My body expelled dozens of pea-sized, green-colored gallstones as a result.

I continued my self-designed program for three months, never cheating with even one unhealthy morsel. One day I awoke early, feeling like jogging (a first!). I had energy to spare and wished I could give some away to those in need. Even as a child, I couldn't remember feeling this good. That day was my turning point. From then on, I felt *vibrant, healthy,* and *strong*—three words I'd never used to describe myself.

Frequently, people ask me why I got as sick as I did at such an early age. After all, I didn't smoke, habitually drink alcohol, or take drugs, so what was it? I did love junk food, fast food, and sweets. But then so do a lot of other young people, and they don't get sick. I believe my mother had the beginning stages of cancer when I was conceived, which probably set the stage for my weakened immune system. I inherited my mother's poor eating habits (a love of sweets and dislike of vegetables), and on an emotional level, I leaned toward her propensity for stuffing negative emotions, rather than expressing or releasing them. Add to that the eye-stinging Los Angeles smog, and a picture begins to form of a toxic internal environment I had created unknowingly.

I owe my good health today to the holistic approach I've taken—periodic juice fasts, whole foods, lots of vegetables, freshly made juice every day, nutritional supplements, filtered water, pure air, exercise, and some very intense work through the years on physical, mental, and emotional cleansing, prayer, and inner healing. When it came to cleansing the soul, I had some significant emotional baggage to discard. Pockets of pain and toxic emotions congested my soul like the stones in my gallbladder. Parts of my wounded soul and "breaks in being," as they're called, needed healing. There were tears to release and letters of forgiveness to write. All these processes worked together for my complete recovery from illness and the restoration of my health and wholeness.

It is for your restoration and wholeness that I have written the first eight chapters on cleansing the body because I know firsthand what cleansing can do to facilitate healing. And I also know what it is like to search for answers and find none, to look for help unsuccessfully. Early in my career as a nutritionist, I resolved to help save the lives of mothers, fathers, children, friends, and family members from the grief of losing someone they love to cancer, and to offer help and hope to those who are fighting to live and overcome their disease.

Like many health professionals, I've seen firsthand how important it is to eat nutritiously and detoxify the body. In fact I'm convinced that these factors should be a significant part of everyone's cancer treatment and prevention program, no matter what other treatments are chosen. The key words in The Complete Cancer Cleanse Program are *detoxification*—of the body, mind, and spirit—and *renewal.*

It is to that end that I have designed this program around the many aspects of cleansing the body, with specific programs for the four primary organs of elimination—the liver, intestines, kidneys, and lungs—and the four supporting channels of elimination—the gallbladder, the lymphatic system, the dermal system (the skin), and the blood. All these channels of detoxification need to be fed superior nutrition and cleansed from toxicity to experience healing, restoration, and prevention of disease. I will present a complete Live Foods/Whole Foods Diet Plan and give you the "superhero" healing foods that will support your recovery. Then I will help you renew your body through the necessary nutrients from A to Zinc, which will build your immune system and restore nutritional balance and vitality.

At times throughout this book I will refer to Chinese or Oriental Medicine, because the East offers the West complementary medical and nutritional wisdom that has withstood the test of time. In days of yore, and to some degree still at present, there has been a belief that Oriental Medicine does not have scientific support on which to base its philosophy and, therefore, is not valid. A lack of understanding of this medical tradition seems to lie at the core of these discussions.

A five-thousand-year-old practice of medicine and classifications of foods has proven over time its effectiveness in many areas of treatment, and now many Western scientists and doctors are sharing their scientific, medical, and research knowledge with the East—and in turn are learning about traditional Oriental herbal and dietary remedies. For those concerned about differing religious beliefs, it is important to differentiate

Eastern medicine from Eastern religions and glean from the medical wisdom of the centuries.

Next, my husband, John, will tell you how cancer has influenced his life.

JOHN'S STORY

In the summer of 1995, I was seated on a plane, flying from Pennsylvania, where Cherie and I had moved so I could attend an Eastern Orthodox Seminary, to Seattle, with many questions playing over and over in my mind. How could my father have had a stroke? He looked like a screen star—curly, light brown hair with hardly a strand of gray, very few wrinkles, and a healthy looking, trim physique. He'd retired at fifty, sold his law practice, and for the next twenty years lived for the game of golf. He was one of those die-hards—even out in the snows of late fall on crisp Moses Lake, Washington, mornings for the sheer love of the game. Each winter, he and my stepmom religiously drove off to Palm Desert for a couple of months, where golf was king. Life was fairly stress-free for my father. So what went wrong?

As the hours ticked away in flight, I thought about my work at St. Luke Medical Center with the cancer patients who had come to us for help. Husbands, wives, fathers, moms, children—all concerned, sometimes desperate to help themselves or the one they loved. I'd never been on the other side of the desk; no one in my immediate family had ever been seriously ill—until now.

By the time I reached the hospital, my father could not talk. For six weeks, it was a silent journey of watching and waiting, as he lay in a coma most of the time. And then he died. He'd entered the hospital with severe abdominal pain, but very much alive, and he never walked back out.

I was outraged! Was this malpractice? I demanded answers. Further investigation revealed colon cancer, which had generated a blood clot that had caused the stroke. Our family was stunned. How could such a healthy looking man, with no signs or symptoms of ill health, have had life-threatening colon cancer?

Cherie and I tried to answer that question by reviewing his lifestyle, which did reveal several possible factors. Dad loved meat and grilled outdoors often during the summer. He also enjoyed the recommended two alcoholic drinks per day that are popularly touted for heart disease prevention. From Cherie's research, we learned that both of these items contribute to colon cancer.

Golf courses are heavily sprayed with chemicals to keep them beautiful and pest free, but that's not so good for the humans who come into contact with these chemicals every day they play golf. Dad also could get quite uptight in stressful situations; perhaps the biggest stressor preceding his death was building his new house on the lake. If only I could have talked to him—could have known that these things might take his life—I might have turned his health around with a few simple interventions. But then none of us would ever have guessed that anything about his health needed turning around.

Like Cherie, the loss of someone I love has impacted my life; this thief called cancer stole a person dear to me. Because of this loss, coupled with my interest and education in psychology and theology, I have focused on how to prevent and heal cancer from an emotional, mental, and spiritual perspective.

I began my education in theology and quickly realized that to help people in their personal and spiritual growth, I needed to better understand human nature. That led me to get my master's degree in psychology, and then to bring the two fields of study together. I trained in biofeedback and worked in behavioral medicine at St. Luke Medical Center. From my behavioral medicine work I learned the importance of listening to the messages our body sends to us as a key to what is going on inside, not only physically, but in the mind, will, emotions, and spirit.

This work has led me to write Chapters Nine, Ten, and Eleven. Part of the detoxification program in The Complete Cancer Cleanse is cleansing your mind and your emotions as you incorporate spiritual cleansing strategies. Toxic thoughts and emotions are as destructive to your body as polluted air and water or adulterated food. My prayer is that you can put the information in these chapters to work in your life to cleanse and heal your total being.

In Part Two, our friend and associate, Michael Mahaffey, will walk you through his PurposeFull Living plan, the journey he took when he was diagnosed with acute leukemia over twenty years ago. Here's Michael to tell you about his fight with cancer.

MICHAEL'S STORY

In February of 1983, foggy, fuzzy vision and total lack of physical energy finally sent me to an appointment with my doctor, Dr. Tom Dolkas. He hadn't seen me in his office for such a long time that he used the opportunity to draw blood and perform a brief physical exam. He was unable to get me to sit still for more than that. Eleven hours later, he called the ranch.

"Michael, I want to come to your place to talk," he said.

"Tom, my ranch is twenty-five miles from town and not easy to find in the dark. Whatever it is, just tell me now."

I really wasn't listening as he rambled off four or five possible diagnoses, ranging from herpes to acute leukemia. But then I began to hear the urgency in his voice. "I've scheduled an appointment for you at an oncologist's at 8:00 AM." He concluded, "I want you to have a bone-marrow test."

Assuring myself that it was no big deal, I told him I'd be there and hung up the phone. Shortly after I went to bed, Kathleen, my wife, joined me. Her attempt at reassurance created little comfort for the worry that was beginning to enter my mind, and sleep was elusive. When I finally dozed off, it was a restless slumber, filled with a lot of tossing and turning and confusing dreams.

During the night, and completely unbidden, the conversation with Tom replayed many times over in my mind. What did he see in the blood tests? Maybe it was good news? I had already stopped drinking . . . maybe that was a clue? Probably had to do with my weight. I tipped the scales at 275 pounds and carried a drinking gut out in front of me. I was really under a lot of business stress . . . maybe it was nerves? I accused myself of being paranoid. I knew I was trying to figure things out so that I could be in control of this situation. I was upset that Tom knew something about me that I didn't. I began to get anxious. I didn't have time to be ill. I needed to know what was going on. In reality, I knew as little about herpes as I did about leukemia.

The next day both Kathy and I were locked into our own private thoughts as we sped to the appointment.

At 8:00 AM we entered the oncologist's office and were greeted by his staff, laughing and joking with one another. It was easy to be carried along by their mood. My only anxiety that morning was about taking time away from business. I just wanted to get the testing over with so I could get back to work.

After we were ushered to an examining room, the oncologist abruptly entered and immediately began explaining what he was going to do to me. Without any preliminary discussion, he intoned, "I am going to drill into your pelvis and aspirate marrow from your hipbone. Then I'll view the sample under a microscope and render my findings. At the same time, a sample will be sent to the lab for testing. It should only take a couple of hours."

Not much of a bedside manner. I didn't like what he said, and I certainly didn't like how he said it.

The doctor was already applying a local anesthetic to my right hip when I muttered, "Just do it."

Kathy grimaced along with me as he burrowed a long, corkscrew-like needle directly into the bone. I'll admit to clenching my teeth and holding my breath for the ten long seconds it took to suck the marrow from my bone up through the aspirator. When he was done, the doctor left the room without saying a word. Kathy and I were silent, too, as the nurse told us that we would need to return later for the results, after the test specimen returned from the lab.

Kathy and I went directly to my office, where we made some attempt at small talk, pretending that it was just a normal day. I made a few calls, looked over some proposals. But by mid-morning, when the lab called us, we had both grown very edgy.

"Bad news," the lab tech said. "We need to get another blood test from you. We kinda goofed on the one the doctor drew. He needs another draw so he can base his judgment on both the bone marrow sample and your blood test."

I took a quick drive over to the lab, and then we spent more time just waiting. Finally, it was time to return for the test results. Just after noon, we were back in the oncologist's office. In marked contrast to that morning's gaiety, the office was now quiet. The staff was talking in whispers as we sat in the waiting room, leafing through year-old *Life* magazines, and, for the first time in many months, we sat squeezing each other's hands.

Finally we were led into the oncologist's private office, which seemed dark and confining. Clusters of medical journals and reference books were tucked into every nook and cranny, even stacked on the floor. When he entered, he didn't immediately acknowledge us, but went to shut the blinds even more. It felt as though he was turning the shade to keep someone from seeing in, not to keep the sun's glare out.

This morning I had wanted to like him, but now I didn't even try. I just knew that he was going to give us bad news. For long minutes more we quietly waited, and then he pronounced his verdict. Staring absently at Kathy, he mumbled a few words, then—seeming to gather courage—he began. "The results are positive," he said.

Without drawing a breath, he continued monotonically, "You have acute myelogenous leukemia, one of the most deadly forms of blood cancer that strikes older adults. The leukemia cells are dividing at a very high rate, interfering with the production of red blood cells, white blood cells, and platelets. To be frank, the malignant cells are overrunning your immune-response system, and my prognosis is that you have just thirty, maybe up to forty-five, days to live."

Numb as I was, the doctor's sterile, impersonal report managed to reach my brain.

"You can live out your life without treatment. Or you can submit to chemotherapy, which, though it's devastating to the body, could extend your life ninety days. If you're fortunate enough to go into remission, you might live six months—eighteen if you're really lucky."

Time out! my mind screamed. *I'm only forty-two years old, and this guy is telling me I only have one month to live, maybe ninety days. And that's if I'm lucky!*

I wanted to beat him up, overturn his desk, scatter his precious books and journals, make him say it was all a bad dream. I grabbed for Kathy's hand and she for mine. Our tears started flowing as the oncologist continued his mechanical recitation of the side effects of chemotherapy.

Somehow managing to find words, but speaking in a small voice like a child lost in her own nightmare, Kathy asked, "If Michael goes through a program of chemotherapy, he'll be okay. Is that what you're saying?"

"Regrettably, no," he responded. "Michael stands a very slight chance of surviving. Chemotherapy can prolong his life, but . . ."

That was all I could handle. I couldn't listen to him anymore. The doctor continued talking as I went deep within myself.

I was experiencing a fear like no other fear I had felt in my life. Frantically, I wondered how my kids could make it without a dad, how my family would get by financially. As I thought of Kathy, I turned toward her. She was trembling, maybe in a state of shock, and desperately trying to handle this for both of us. The doctor was responding to another of Kathy's questions as my consciousness returned to his darkened dungeon of an office.

"We're getting out of here!" I commanded, pulling Kathy out of her seat.

"Michael, you are in a very serious condition and deteriorating quickly," the oncologist protested. "You need to make some very important decisions, and you need to make them now."

I had made a decision. I needed to get back to my world. I wanted to get in my car, my canyon, my ranch, my office, on the phone making money—to familiar territory where I would be in control. The diagnosis had stolen my power, and my only thought was to get out of there and get back in command of my life.

Outside the office, and in my fear-filled anger, I crashed awkwardly into Kathy, but we managed to climb into my car. For an instant I felt relieved by the simple act of sliding behind the wheel.

"Buckle up; we're going home!" I barked to Kathy.

The curve of the seat gripped my body. It felt comfortable; this was my world. The feeling of control surely would return to me now.

The top was off the Porsche and the sun was bright and warm. As I turned the key in its ignition, I noticed 453,000 miles on the odometer. I had owned this car for nine years, and we had traveled all those miles together. How many more would we travel?

With Kathy mute beside me, we sped through the canyon at speeds reaching ninety miles an hour. I tried to believe that power and control were being restored to me as we moved along. It was only a temporary feeling, but absolutely welcome and much needed at that moment.

As we drove the final straightaway to the ranch, tears returned to stream down our cheeks. I asked myself, *Where has the time gone? What do I have to show for my life?*

Now this crisis of cancer was pulling the strings tight around what remained. Thirty days to live offered me few possibilities, with nothing to grab on to and no place to negotiate from. I sensed I could not talk my way through this. I was trapped. It didn't matter what I had, who I thought I was, or what I had done. Ironically, my survival up to now had been based on not being controlled by anyone or anything. Now, the cancer had control.

And that was the beginning of my struggle with cancer. Believe it or not, twenty years later I am still alive. In those in-between years I went through a process of renewing my soul and spirit and discovering the purpose for my life. I will tell you how and why this journey led to my recovery in Part Two.

We end this chapter with a final, encouraging word from all of us.

A FINAL WORD FROM ALL THE AUTHORS

We believe that everything has a purpose. It was out of our struggles that we have been able to design the programs in this book for your benefit. Elizabeth Kubler-Ross said, "Know that everything in life has a purpose. There are no mistakes, no coincidences, all events are blessings given to us to learn from." It is our desire that you learn from the challenges in your life, and grow in and through them. There is *great hope!* You have an opportunity to get well, to live disease free, and to complete the purpose for which you were born. We pray for your speedy recovery, fortitude to choose life, and complete healing and wholeness.

2

FACTS ABOUT CANCER AND CLEANSING

Detoxification is the missing link in American nutrition and Western medical care.

—ELSON HAAS, M.D., *The Detox Diet*

Cancer is a degenerative disease from which millions of people are suffering. The World Health Organization and the American Medical Association state that the United States is currently in the worst epidemic of chronic and degenerative diseases that mankind has ever known. The exact cause of cancer is unknown, and it is generally believed that there is no single universal cause, because many factors usually contribute to cancer development.

We do know that degenerative diseases are most often caused by lifestyle, with the number one offender being diet. Looking at the average American's lifestyle and food choices, it is no wonder cancer is increasing yearly. We eat too much fat, too much sugar, too much junk food, drink too much alcohol, and ingest too many chemicals in the form of preservatives, pesticides, and additives. Our air, soil, and water are filled with toxins. We're bombarded with free radicals (toxic reactive molecules).

Our lives are packed with stress. Our thoughts and emotions are often negative and self-defeating, and we find little time to care for our bodies and souls. Many of these factors contribute to a weakening of the body's defense system—our combat cells. With a less efficient immune system, mutated cells can evade normal surveillance and spread at will.

Often something happens to certain genes inside a cell to make them change. Mutations in these genes can turn them into *oncogenes* (*onco-* means tumor). These genes stay "turned on" all the time, signaling cells to keep dividing at an abnormal rate. The cells continue to reproduce abnormal copies, thus causing the tumor to grow. What turns these cells into oncogenes can be any number of carcinogenic (cancer-producing) substances.

Sir Percival Pott made the first observation of a carcinogenic agent in 1776. He associated the frequent appearance of cancer in the scrotums of chimney sweeps with the vast amount of soot and coal tar found on their clothing and bodies.[1] Since that time, many substances, both synthetic and naturally occurring, have been determined to be carcinogenic. Toxins that enter the body from the environment are known as exotoxins, and these agents can act as either initiators or promoters of mutated genes. Certain chemical carcinogens have a high propensity for causing mutations, such as aniline dye derivatives, asbestos, tars, and nicotine.

A slight change in the chemical structure of a noncarcinogenic substance can convert it to a carcinogen; some chemicals, though not considered to be carcinogenic alone, may become cancer causing when combined with other chemicals. And certain compounds are converted into carcinogens by the body. Most destructive of all are the carcinogenic substances that pour into our atmosphere without needing to be converted or combined with other chemicals.

There is widespread acceptance that 80 to 90 percent of all cancers in Western nations are attributable to environmental factors.[2] Within this category, there is a host of cancer-causing substances such as industrial chemicals, pesticides, ionizing radiation, free radicals, food additives, high-fat and high-sugar foods, refined foods, and adulterated foods. We are bombarded with these toxic, congesting, and damaging substances as never before in history. From the air we breathe to the water we drink and the food we eat, to our modern technology and "creature comforts," we are exposed daily to a host of carcinogenic agents.

Contrary to popular belief, the genetically inherited component of human cancer is relatively small. Much more important are toxins, especially exotoxins, nutrient deficiencies, and poor food choices. Exotoxins consist of chemicals, heavy metals, electromagnetic pollution, ELF (extremely low frequency) pollution, adulterated foods, synthetic fibers, and secondary toxic suppressors. If we were to talk with a group of cancer-researching detectives, we'd probably get a list of causative factors that looked something like this:

Exposure to chemicals from:
Industrial pollution
Cigarette, pipe, and cigar smoke
Automobile, bus, train, and airplane exhaust
Solvents, glues, and paints used in office and home interiors (formaldehyde, toluene, and benzene)
Personal care products: cosmetics, hair spray, and shampoo
Pesticides, herbicides, fungicides, and chemical fertilizers
Exposure to heavy metals from:
Tobacco smoke: nickel, lead, cadmium, and arsenic
Cookware: stainless steel, nickel, and aluminum
Jewelry: inexpensive earring wires or posts and other jewelry made of nickel or gold-plated jewelry with a nickel base
Hydrogenated fats and oils: nickel
Refined foods: nickel
Dentistry: porcelain crowns and restorative materials: nickel; amalgam fillings: mercury
Tap water: lead, cadmium, and aluminum
Exposure to electromagnetic pollution from:
Airplanes
X-rays
Excessive exposure to the sun
Nuclear power plants
Exposure to ELF (extremely low frequency) pollution from:
Microwave ovens
Cell phones
Electric blankets

Electric alarm clocks and clock radios

Metal innerspring mattresses

Water beds with heaters

Televisions, lamps, and computers (even if turned off)

Ionization-type smoke and carbon monoxide detectors

The foods we eat, ingesting too many:

Hormones and antibiotics in animal products

Pesticide-sprayed foods

Preservatives in food

High-fat foods and trans fatty acids (toxic fats)

Animal products and not enough vegetables, fruit, and whole grains

High-sugar foods

Caffeine-containing products

Processed and refined foods

Drugs: prescription and recreational, including alcohol

Exposure to synthetic fibers and materials:

NOTE: People often get sick, and some develop cancer, after moving into a new home, especially the very young (babies are most susceptible), pets, and the physically weak, because of all the chemicals they encounter, which are found in:

Carpeting, glue, and dyes

Carpet pads made of plastic, foam rubber, or latex

Wallpaper

Draperies

Fabrics and cotton sheets (often treated with formaldehyde to make them "wrinkle free")

Particle board

Exposure to secondary toxic suppressors:

Parasites, fungi, and yeasts (Candida is an overgrowth of yeast in your body that can easily become systemic)

Viruses and bacteria

Allergens (hay fever and food allergies)

In addition to all the exotoxins in our environment, our body produces toxins through normal daily functions, which are known as *endotoxins.* If we ate the purest food, drank the cleanest water, breathed the freshest air, and lived in a totally nontoxic environment, our body would still generate toxins that would need to be eliminated. Even under ideal conditions, we need to eliminate by-products (wastes) of our own cellular and biochemical activities. Normally, our body can process these self-generated toxins and a certain amount of external toxins without a problem, but when an excessive amount of toxins is added to this load through our water, the air we breathe, the food we eat, and the soil our food is grown in, our system becomes overwhelmed. Without adequate nutrients that are key in detoxification, toxins build up in the body.

One of the most destructive internal toxins is the free radical, which we generate through the normal process of metabolism; we also inhale, absorb, and ingest them. This renegade "bad guy" is a small molecule lacking an electron, and it hurtles through tissue looking for an electron to steal to complete the electron pairing. This stealing spree wounds cell membranes and can damage DNA. When an electron has been stolen, the "victim" molecule is transformed into another free radical, causing a chain reaction and more wounded cells. If these free radicals are not neutralized and eliminated, they irritate, inflame, and damage cells, thus contributing to chronic disease. Free radical damage has been implicated in cancer, aging, and many other diseases.

Endotoxins are also generated from undigested food and are produced as a by-product of microbes such as bacteria, yeasts, parasites, and fungi. When undigested food interacts with bacteria, yeasts, or fungi, it can putrefy, producing alcohol or ammonia. The by-products of these microbes, which are usually found in highest concentration in the colon, are called intestinal toxemia. If these toxins are absorbed into the bloodstream, they affect both our physical and mental health. The liver is able to detoxify a certain amount of these toxins, but when they reach a critical level, the liver becomes overwhelmed, and toxic material enters the bloodstream.

Toxins also can be created by destructive thoughts and emotional stress, such as:

- Stuffing emotions

- Harboring toxic emotions; suppressing feelings
- Holding trauma in the body's tissues
- Unforgiveness: holding on to resentment, bitterness, or hatred

Dr. Candace Pert, chief of brain biochemistry at the National Institute of Mental Health, has observed that signals emitted by the brain are profoundly influenced by the emotional and physical state of an individual. For example, excessive amounts of norepinephrine have been found in people who exhibit hostile attitudes. The presence of this chemical, associated with the arousal of the sympathetic nervous system, has been linked to damage of the lining of the coronary arteries and elevated blood pressure.[3] (See Chapter Nine for more information.)

When we accumulate more toxins than we can eliminate, overload occurs. The level of overload in our bodies depends on the amount, frequency, or potency of the toxins. If the body is overwhelmed and can no longer keep up with the work of neutralizing and eliminating the mess we've accumulated, waste materials build up as they do at a garbage dump. We may become like one of Dr. Don Colbert's patients who declared, "My body is more polluted than a toxic waste dump! If my body was a piece of earth, it would be too toxic for my neighbors to live next to!"[4]

Although not exhaustive, the list is clear in one respect: most cancers are caused by the environment in which we live and by the choices we make daily. In our efforts to produce more, obtain more, and enjoy more, we are literally poisoning ourselves to death. In their book *The Cancer Battle Plan,* Anne and David Frähm say, "Cancer is not as some people think, 'a thunderbolt of fate, striking at random with no cure or cause.' There is a cause-and-effect relationship between the environment we've created—the lifestyles we've chosen—and the health problems we're experiencing as a country. When it comes to identifying the chief cause of cancer, we have met the enemy and he is us!"[5]

WHAT IS DETOXIFICATION?

Detoxification is defined as the process of removing toxic substances or transforming them into something harmless. *Cleansing* denotes freeing a person from something unwelcome. (These terms are used interchangeably throughout this book.) Detoxification is a normal process of eliminating wastes and toxins from the colon, liver, kidneys, gallbladder, lungs, skin, lymph, and blood. This is one of the body's most basic functions and happens without a thought, like the beating of the heart. However, in our polluted world, the body's systems and organs, which were once functioning in a less-polluted world and capable of clearing out unwanted substances, are now completely overloaded. This means toxins remain in our tissues, clog our organs, poison our blood, and weaken our immune system.

"Detoxing simply means de-junking your body," say Morley and Wilde in their book *Detox*.[6] Some people call this process a spring-cleaning; others, a major tune-up. Whatever we call it, this is one of the most therapeutic measures we can take. With all the junk our body picks up from convenience foods and the pollution that pours into the earth, we just can't push the poisons out fast enough. Heavy metals, antibiotics, hormones, anesthetics, drug residues, pesticides, industrial chemicals, and solvents all get trapped within the body. Every system is affected. "Toxins can damage the body in an insidious and cumulative way," say Murray and Pizzorno in the *Encyclopedia of Natural Medicine*. "Once the detoxification system becomes overloaded, toxic *metabolites* (products of metabolism) accumulate. The accumulation of toxins can wreak havoc on our normal metabolic processes."[7]

In the early 1960s, wildlife biologist Rachel Carson wrote about what she discovered was pouring into our environment at an alarming rate. "Poisons!" she said. "Biologically potent chemicals indiscriminately [used] in the hands of persons wholly ignorant of their potential for harm." A friend of hers in Massachusetts sent her a letter painfully describing a mosquito control campaign near her home that had resulted in a mass death of songbirds. Legs drawn up to their chests, beaks gaping open, in a posture of horrifying convulsion, these birds lay scattered around her DDT-contaminated birdbath. This letter prompted Carson to embark on a comprehensive investigation of pesticides. In her classic, best-selling book *Silent Spring*, she documents a series of problems attributable to pesticides—from blindness in fish to blood disorders in humans.[8]

According to an Environmental Protection Agency report, more than 1,672,127,735 pounds of toxic chemicals were released into our air in 1993.[9] Many of these chemicals contain heavy metals such as lead, mercury, cadmium, arsenic, aluminum, and nickel. These metals tend to accumulate in the brain, kidneys, immune system, and many other parts of the body where they can profoundly affect normal functions. It is conservatively estimated that up to 25 percent of the U.S. population suffers from heavy metal poisoning.[10] The greatest share of heavy metal intoxication is due to industry. For example, lead from industrial sources and leaded petrol have contributed to over 600,000 tons of lead in the atmosphere.

Heavy metals are just one of the myriad of toxic substances we're bombarded with all the time. Linda Page, N.D., Ph.D. in her book *Detoxification* says,

> More than two million synthetic substances are known, 25,000 are added each year, and over 30,000 are produced on a commercial scale. Only a tiny fraction are ever tested for toxicity. The molecular structure of many chemical carcinogens interacts with human DNA, so long-term exposure may result in . . . genetic alterations. Hormone-disrupting pesticides and pollutants are linked to [ovarian, prostate, and] breast cancer. The World Health Organization implicates environmental chemicals in 60 to 80 percent of all cancers.[11]

When immune activity is compromised, immune cells, such as the natural killer cells that are responsible for destroying cancer cells, are unable to do their job properly. A compromised immune system is often a key factor in immune-compromised diseases such as cancer.

Ponder this for a moment: What if we continuously put new wax on an old linoleum floor, but never washed and stripped it? Think about the dirt buildup. Can you imagine what would collect, especially in the corners? What if we spilled chemicals on the floor and left them? What kind of molecular changes would take place in tile if we never cleaned up the spill?

Our body is more important than our floor, yet most of us never clean it on the inside. Toxic buildup collects in the largest proportion in our systems of elimination and detoxification. Consequently, our blood is not cleansed properly as it flows through the liver (filter system). Our colon (part of the elimination system) builds up putrefaction, and as a result, nutrients are not absorbed well and poisons are reabsorbed into our bloodstream. The kidneys (part of the elimination system) become overwhelmed, attempting to excrete toxic-laden urea. But it isn't just the elimination system that is affected; toxins also are stored in fat cells and bone, they collect in tissues and tissue spaces, and they clog our lymphatic system. On and on it goes! Yet, there is hope.

THE HEALING POWER OF A CLEANSING PROGRAM

Cleansing our body, soul, and spirit can help to clear out all the burdensome mess we've collected over the years. In his book *A Journey Toward Wholeness,* Dr. Kenneth Bakken recounts the story of Helen, who was diagnosed with advanced ovarian cancer. Tests revealed a tumor the size of a volleyball and metastases to the liver and other parts of the abdomen. Physicians told her that even if she survived surgery, which they doubted, she would probably not live more than a few weeks. A week after surgery, a weak, very emaciated, but very much alive Helen arrived at Dr. Bakken's office. She was determined to get well again. There was much more for her to accomplish in this life, she said, and she knew that she would be healthy again, somehow. She said she had uncovered the reason for her illness and had taken full responsibility for her condition; she was willing to make the necessary changes in her life.

Helen actively embraced her disease and learned from it. She changed her diet, began a fitness program, and spent several hours each day in meditation and prayer. Continually, she visualized herself surrounded by healing light. She asked God for help and received support and encouragement from family and friends.

Dr. Bakken did little medically except to strengthen her immune system with "biologic response modifiers," such as interferon, and to facilitate lifestyle interventions. After six months, all Helen's tests showed normal—blood work including the helper T-cell to suppressor-cell lymphocyte ratio, the chest X-ray, the CT scan, and the tumor markers. The real work and healing had been Helen's—physically, emotionally, and spiritually.[12]

Just as Helen addressed all areas of her life and made necessary changes, we too can take full responsibility for our health and turn our situation around. Professor Arnold Ehret says, "Not the disease, but the body is to be healed. It must be cleansed, freed from waste and foreign matter, from mucous and toxemia accumulated from childhood."[13] Though cleansing and detoxification are not new concepts, it is obvious that we need to apply this ancient wisdom now more than ever.

A Jewish sect known as the Essenes, who lived around the time of Christ, taught about fasting, cleansing, and eating nutritiously to cleanse the body as part of the sacred teachings. Many ancient religions scheduled cycles of fasting throughout the calendar year, and some of our most ancient cultures practiced fasting and colon cleansing with herbs and cleansing foods. Today, we are exposed to more toxic compounds in a year than someone in the first century would encounter in his or her lifetime. If people more than twenty centuries ago realized a need for cleansing, what can we say about our need? In an extremely toxic modern society, our ability to detoxify unhealthy substances is of critical importance to our overall health and imperative to our recovery from disease.

Benefits from Detox:

- Improvement in immune function
- Neutralization and elimination of free radicals and other toxins
- Assistance in destroying cancer cells while feeding healthy cells
- Clearing of mucous, congestion, and fermentation in the digestive tract
- Blood purification
- Cleansing of the palate: cravings for sugar, salt, fatty foods, junk foods, alcohol, and nicotine should lessen or disappear

Cleansing the major filter systems, which include the gastrointestinal, urinary, respiratory, lymphatic, and dermal systems, along with transforming harmful substances like free radicals into neutral metabolites, is of vital importance to our recovery from disease. Detoxification gives our body a chance to clear away all the congesting, irritating, inflaming, and damaging waste materials we've accumulated for years. Cleansing is an important component in our fight against cancer. When the body does not have to deal with lots of toxic waste on a daily basis, it can focus intently on attacking and destroying cancer cells, clearing out mucous and congestion, repairing the body, and restoring health.

WHERE SHOULD WE CLEANSE?

It is recommended that a person begin his or her cleansing program at home or at a place where rest and focus on the program are possible. If you are working, starting on a Friday is a good idea. Being tempted by coworkers to eat and drink substances that are not on the detoxification program may be too much to overcome otherwise. If family or household members also pose a problem with temptations or challenges to your decision to cleanse, it may be helpful to get away for a week or more to kick off your program. Even if other people don't pose a challenge, getting away for a while can be restful, stress-free, and healing.

Beginning one's program at a center designed for cleansing can be one of the most beneficial of all choices. There you can relax, not worry about preparing the right foods, and take advantage of therapies like colonics and massage. You can also learn a lot about cleansing and detoxification from classes offered at these centers, as well as from fellow sojourners. Being with supportive counselors, teachers, and cocleansers can also be very comforting.

Preparing for the Cleanse:

- Schedule the time necessary for the cleanse
- Prepare your spirit, soul (mind, will, and emotions), and body for this new experience
- Shop for all the necessary equipment, foods, and supplements before beginning
- Set your mind to stick with the program
- Be gentle with yourself when you aren't perfect

Several centers offer raw-foods diets, juice fasting or liquid diets, and cleansing programs: Michael Mahaffey's Cedar Springs Renewal Center (Sedro Woolley, Washington), Health*Quarters* (Colorado Springs, Colorado), Optimum Health Institute (San Diego and Austin, Texas), and

Sanoviv Medical Institute (Baja, California) offer a complete raw-foods cleanse program. For more information on these and other centers, see pages 321–22.

To completely devote yourself to cleansing and recovery, you may want to take a leave of absence from work, if that is possible. For many people, getting well is a full-time job in itself. If work leave is not possible, it's comforting to know that many people have completely recovered from cancer while maintaining a full-time job.

WHO SHOULD CLEANSE?

The answer is simple! Everybody should cleanse—and especially everyone with cancer. Can you imagine never changing the oil filter in your car? I can do more than imagine: I experienced just that! Young, naïve, and twenty-something, I was very unaware of mechanical requirements. I bought a used Volkswagen and just drove and drove that car without ever considering that I should change the oil and filter. One day the car died—literally stopped cold on the freeway. What a lesson! The liver, the major filter system in our body, is like the oil filter in our car. It filters blood, and all our blood must pass through the liver. When this organ gets clogged up, like an auto's oil filter overdue for changing, our blood will be contaminated and toxic. The more clogged our liver becomes, the more toxic our entire body.

When we have cancer, there's no question about cleansing. This important aspect of healing isn't a matter of "should," it's a matter of "how soon?" In his book *Cleanse & Purify Thyself,* Richard Anderson, N.D., says that if we have cancer, absolutely, we need cleansing.[14] Many health professionals concur that anyone who is ill should cleanse body as well as soul. "Sickness and degenerative disease are usually . . . nature's way of telling you that your body is toxic and needs to be cleansed," says Don Colbert, M.D.[15]

> **It seems clear that if a cancer warrior is going to have any hope of ultimately conquering cancer and winning back health, a very aggressive process needs to be undertaken to reverse the chronic degeneration of the body of which cancer is a symptom. It all comes down to changing the body's toxic chemistry through the metabolic processes of detoxification and diet—and the sooner the better.[16]**
>
> —ANNE AND DAVID FRÄHM, ***The Cancer Battle Plan***

WHAT TO EXPECT WHEN WE CLEANSE

The body has an inherent desire for perfect health. We have the ability to "earn our way back" to a whole state, no matter how poor our health is now. While the end result will be the absence of illness, greater vitality, and more energy, it is very common to feel worse before feeling better. As toxins are released and parasites and candida (overgrowth of yeast) die off, waste products pour into the system. When they are released faster than the body can eliminate them, we can experience symptoms such as fever, chills, nausea, diarrhea, cramps, headaches, skin eruptions, sleep disturbances, increased thirst, loss of appetite, fatigue, irritability, ear infection, head or chest cold, and flu-like symptoms. (If these symptoms continue for several weeks, however, see your health-care professional.) Sounds fun, doesn't it? This elimination phenomenon is often referred to as the "healing crisis" or the Herxheimer Reaction. Though the healing crisis may not be much fun, it's usually short-lived, and the results are more than fun—they're life changing![17]

Our personal history is carried in our body like rings around a tree, telling its story of illness, excess, abuse, or injury. These past experiences of trauma, injury, illness, or hurt that did not heal—whether physical, emotional, or mental—must be cleansed. The reactions to the detoxification can feel similar to the original illness, disease, or emotional trauma, but usually manifest in a milder form. For example, if one suffered a great deal with sinus infections as a child, a healing crisis may involve a sinus infection or two as residues from the original infections are eliminated.

There may be good days and not-so-good days that are all part of the ups and downs of the cleansing and healing process. All the systems of the body are working together to eliminate the waste and prepare the body for regeneration. Old cells are being expelled and replaced with new cells. "Sometimes the pain and symptoms during the healing crisis are more intense than that of the chronic disease, but it is temporary and necessary," says one health educator.[18] There is an important distinction, however: the purifying process is in motion and the body is in a healing state.

The healing crisis will often bring up personal issues. We may experience a surfacing of old wounds, both physical and emotional. Though we may have forgotten about illnesses, diseases, injuries, or emotional issues from the past, we are often reminded so that we can heal unfinished business.

A healing crisis usually lasts from one to three days, but if the body's energy level is low, it could last up to a week or more. One healing crisis is usually not enough for a complete cleanse and reversal of disease. A person in a chronic disease state may need to go through cycles of healing crises, with each one improving the state of health in some way. The body can experience an energy boost between cycles of elimination, until the toxins start dumping into the bloodstream again. Often the crisis comes after one feels especially well and quite energized, setting the stage for the next level of elimination. This process seems to go in cycles for a lot of people: energetic, terrific days, followed by periods of healing crisis symptoms.[19] Hang in there, though; it's well worth it. I know firsthand.

When I embarked on my first cleanse years ago in an attempt to recover from chronic fatigue syndrome and fibromyalgia, I felt worse than I had before. I was weak and tired often, with what seemed like a never-ending case of the flu. I experienced diarrhea, headaches, and dizziness, but I decided no matter how badly I felt, I wasn't going to give up my program. With a lot of fortitude I hung in there and it paid off. The morning I woke up with so much energy I wanted to go jogging, I knew it was worth it all. I'm so thankful I didn't let my healing crisis symptoms or my father's concerns dissuade me from my path to health.

In order to recover from disease, one should expect healing crises and work with the body, rather than trying to avoid the process because of unpleasant symptoms or bailing out too quickly because of tiring of the foods or the work required to get well. The detoxification process is likened to peeling layers off an onion. It has taken time to develop a chronically diseased state, and it will take time to eliminate waste buildup "one layer at a time," thereby restoring health to the body.

If the body is especially weakened or overwhelmed by the disease and/or by chemotherapy, radiation, or surgery, one should go slowly and make sure the elimination is gradual. Choose the "easy cleanse" phase of the cleanse program found throughout this book. Add raw vegetables slowly, if you haven't eaten them much in the past. And don't attempt an extended juice fast unless under supervision. The most important point to remember is: don't stop the cleansing process no matter how intense the symptoms. The cleanse program can be modified to meet your needs at any time. Most importantly, be sure to eat from the foods recommended in Chapter Five and avoid harmful foods and substances. By choosing foods and substances that add to the toxic load of the body, we stop our body from cleansing; then we have to start all over again. A very helpful strategy in the cleansing process is to support the body in every way possible.

How to Support the Cleansing Process:

- Drink plenty of purified water. Water helps flush toxins from the body. It's also important for healthy bodily functions. Drink eight to ten glasses of water daily. Make sure the water you drink is pure—free of chlorine, fluoride, chemicals, and bacteria. A good water purifier is an excellent investment in your healing process.
- Freshly made vegetable juices offer an abundance of antioxidants and minerals. Antioxidants in particular bind to free radicals and neutralize them. Juices are also rich in enzymes.
- Avoid all foods and substances such as caffeine and alcohol that would add a toxic burden on your body. For an extensive list of foods to avoid, see pp. 125–26.
- Develop your own list of comfort foods that are good for you—from a cup of hot herbal tea or healthy soup to creamy nut dips—whatever is healthy and works for you.
- Choose ways to comfort yourself other than food. Most of us have a list of comfort foods from our childhood that bring back warm, nurturing memories, but many of these foods are not nurturing for our bodies. We can learn to comfort and nurture our souls in ways other than eating. (See pp. 264–69 for ideas.)
- Make sure your elimination is good. If you are constipated or just not keeping up with the elimination process, you will experience more intense detox symptoms. Take flax fiber to keep the colon moving as needed. Eat lots of vegetables and other high-fiber foods, such as whole grains and legumes, and drink plenty of purified water.
- Colon cleansing in the form of enemas and colonics is very important during a detox process. Toxins build up quickly during cleansing, and it's important to eliminate them as efficiently as possible.
- Support your liver. Eat an abundance of liver-friendly foods and take liver-support nutrients—vitamins, enzymes, and herbs (see Chapter Seven).
- Breathe deeply. Toxins are expelled from the lungs, so holding your breath, which many of us do without realizing it, is counterproductive to cleansing. Stretch classes, where we are encouraged to breathe deeply, can be quite beneficial. Walking in fresh air and breathing deeply is of great benefit.

- Spend time outside in the fresh air every day. Oxygen is important. Remember, cancer cells are anaerobic (they live in the absence of oxygen). Most homes and buildings are sources of concentrated pollutants; therefore, get outside as often as possible, and soak up some sunshine. It's good for your body, soul, and spirit, and it provides vitamin D. Invest in a good air-filter system to clear toxins from your home.
- Rest. Now is the time to treat yourself to short naps (or long ones), leisurely baths, walks in the park, afternoons with a good book, and an exciting daydream or two. Vacations are really terrific support. Try one of the health retreats mentioned in the Resource Guide (see pp. 321–23). Your body is working hard to get rid of toxins, cancer cells, dead cells, and other wastes. This is the time to rest and support its marvelous work.
- Sleep, and sleep well. Powerful healing hormones are released while you sleep. It's time to feel good about getting a few extra hours of sleep—no guilt allowed.
- Keep a positive mental attitude. This is a health challenge you *can* overcome. Optimum Health Institute calls such challenges "health opportunities." Whenever you're tempted to think the worst, intercept that thought and interject a positive response. The often-quoted proverb is true: "A joyful heart is good medicine" (Prov. 17:22 NASB).

WHERE DO WE GO FROM HERE?

It is assuring to know that many people have lived through nearly every type of cancer and hopeless prognosis. They've fought back, and they've overcome. Michael will tell you of his journey to recovery and a new mission in life in Chapters Twelve through Fourteen. Taking action, and in particular cleansing the body, soul, and spirit of all toxicity, is one of the most positive steps a person can take toward complete recovery. In the next chapter you will learn about the various organs and systems of the body and how cleansing them can greatly facilitate your healing process.

3

THE DETOXIFICATION CHANNELS

We sometimes reach too quickly for a sedative for our nerves, when it is our liver that needs help.

—Sidney MacDonald Baker, M.D., *Detoxification & Healing*

Have you ever seen a river that's been blocked by a big log hung up on a rock? Nearly everything floating downstream collects at that point—sticks, branches, old tires, a boot, an old shoe, articles of clothing, plastic containers, pop cans, food packaging, and other debris. What an ugly mess! The same sort of thing can happen within our own body. Debris such as drug residues, heavy metals, environmental chemicals, pesticides, food additives, saturated animal fat, sugar, yeasts, fungi, parasites, and a host of other wastes can pile up in our system like riverbank junk. When we don't periodically cleanse our body, wastes accumulate in our channels of elimination, making us sick and preventing us from getting well.

This chapter will examine the functions of our four primary channels of elimination—the liver, intestines, kidneys, and lungs—and the four supporting channels—the gallbladder, skin, lymphatic system, and blood. Through our primary organs of detoxification (the liver, the intestines, the kidneys, and the lungs), we expel toxins. The body can either eliminate them by excreting them in the urine and feces or breath, or it can neutralize them. The gallbladder, lymphatic system, dermal system (skin), and blood are supporting channels in the detoxification process. As we cleanse our body, it is vitally important to keep all of these channels of elimination open and free flowing, like an unstoppable river. If you are taking chemotherapy drugs, which are highly toxic and challenging to eliminate, it is even more important to cleanse and support the liver as well as all other channels of elimination, in order to get well and live cancer free.

In his book *Dr. Jensen's Guide to Better Bowel Care,* author Bernard Jensen says, "I have found that taking care of the . . . main elimination systems is the most important thing we can do to gain and maintain health. Neither all the medicines nor all the therapies in the world will help much or provide any lasting relief if these systems are not functioning well."[1]

Let's begin with a look at the detoxification channels of the four primary organs of detoxification: the liver, the intestines, the kidneys, and the lungs.

THE PRIMARY ORGANS OF DETOXIFICATION

THE LIVER

The first primary channel of elimination is the liver. The liver is the key organ of the body's sanitation system, responsible for the greatest percentage of our detoxification. It is the largest internal organ, even larger than the brain, weighing between three and four pounds. Protected by the ribs, it is positioned on the right side under the diaphragm, occupying part of the abdomen. This is the busiest organ we have. About three pints of blood pass through the liver every minute, which is supplied by two separate sources: the hepatic artery and the portal vein. From the hepatic artery, the liver obtains oxygenated blood, and from the portal vein it receives deoxygenated blood containing newly absorbed nutrients. Liver cells extract nutrients, oxygen, toxic substances, and wastes from the blood. The toxins are either stored in the liver or neutralized (disassembled).

When the liver is unable to eliminate most of the wastes, carcinogens, and toxic substances, it becomes overwhelmed. Then, like river logs lodged on rocks, toxins accumulate. The body may attempt to maintain physical integrity by organizing a cleansing process, with symptoms such as a cold, flu, rash, diarrhea, or acne. If the body's attempt to cleanse is

The Primary and Supporting Channels of Detoxification

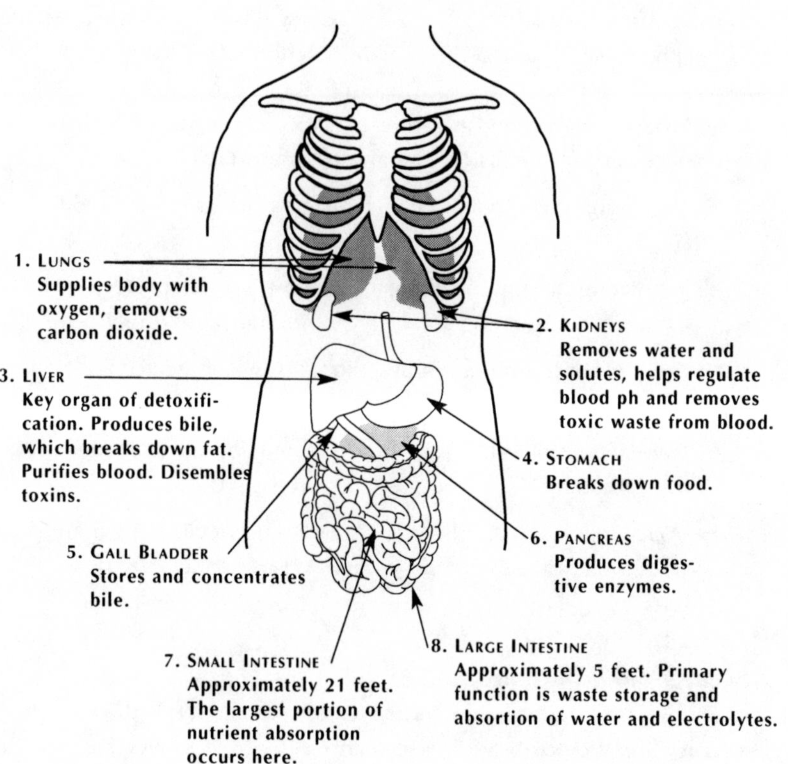

halted with over-the-counter or prescription drugs or some other means of suppression, the toxins are driven deeper within. As numerous attempts at cleansing are suppressed, the organs become weaker and weaker until we develop perennial fatigue, and eventually diseases such as chronic fatigue syndrome, autoimmune diseases, or cancer. The late Dr. Bernard Jensen observed that "in nearly every disease we find an improperly functioning liver and gallbladder."[2]

The liver performs hundreds of jobs every day that are crucial to life and health. Some of its most important functions include:

- Producing a yellowish-green substance called bile, which is necessary for emulsion and absorption of fats
- Regulating carbohydrate metabolism, which controls blood sugar
- Regulating protein metabolism, which produces proteins that transport substances such as fat, hormones, and drugs
- Making sex-hormone binding globulin, which makes and breaks down hormones
- Detoxifying internal toxins (endotoxins) and environmental toxins (exotoxins)
- Collecting waste: the liver contains Kupffer cells, which are part of the immune system; they are the "trash collectors" of the liver

The Liver's Role in Detoxification

Though the liver has many functions, its primary job is that of detoxification. Today detoxification is not an easy job. Our liver has to deal with toxic material never before encountered in history. Water treatment (chlorine and fluoride); industrial chemicals; chemical spraying, such as crop dusting and mosquito spraying; prescription drugs; pesticides; food additives; household chemicals; too much fat, sugar, salt, and alcohol; and microbes, such as parasites and fungi, can influence our liver every day. Constant abuse of the liver causes a host of health problems. Research shows that people chronically exposed to chemical toxins, such as pesticides, herbicides, fungicides, food additives, solvents, formaldehyde, drugs, and alcohol, have increased rates of cancer.[3]

Richard Anderson, N.D., says, "We cannot be healthy or recover from illness without a strong, clean, well-functioning liver. The life, health, and vitality of every single organ, gland, and cell are absolutely dependent upon the liver." He also notes that if heavy metals are in the liver, it cannot be completely healed. The metabolic function of the liver will be depressed, and it will become weaker and weaker unless it is cleansed.[4]

It is amazing what our livers can detoxify. On a daily basis the liver is able to process a multiplicity of noxious substances. But the detoxification process begins to break down when there aren't sufficient nutrients to assist the liver in detoxifying chemicals, heavy metals, and other toxins. And it is no wonder that Americans are experiencing nutrient deficiencies with all the junk food, overprocessed items, and chemically preserved products we eat.

Many detoxification processes depend on a generous supply of nutrients. For example, elimination of fat-soluble toxins, such as the heavy metals lead and mercury, is dependent on glutathione (a tripeptide composed of three amino acids). When we are exposed to increased levels of heavy metals and other toxins, and glutathione is used up faster than it can be produced or absorbed from our diet, we become susceptible to toxin-induced diseases, such as cancer. Glutathione is found in great measure in fruits and vegetables. Statistics of two different studies show that only 23 percent to 32 percent of the population in the United States eats even the minimum of five servings of fruits and vegetables each day, and less than 10 percent regularly consume citrus and cruciferous vegetables (broccoli, brussels sprouts, cauliflower, cabbage, kale).[5] Another example is sulfur-containing compounds that join two substances together such as drugs, food additives, hormones, and toxins from intestinal bacteria with sulfur-containing compounds—a process known as sulfation. When our diet is deficient in sulfur-containing foods, such as garlic, onions, and broccoli, or low in the amino acids methionine and cysteine—steroid hormones (estrogen and thyroid hormones), drug residues, and other toxins can build up to damaging levels. And methylation, which is joining methyl groups to toxins, can be impaired when the diet is deficient in choline, vitamin B_{12}, and folic acid.[6]

Michael Murray, N.D., and Joseph Pizzorno, N.D., have completed extensive research on detoxification and have demonstrated exceptional understanding of the detoxification pathways of the liver. In their book *Encyclopedia of Natural Medicine* they have elucidated a number of key roles the liver plays in detoxification.[7]

1. The Liver Filters and Purifies the Blood

One of the most important functions the liver performs is filtering the blood, as I mentioned earlier, and the liver is also in charge of blood storage; it is while in storage that the blood is processed and purified. Blood coming from the intestines needs the most processing, because it is filled with toxins such as bacteria, fungi, and partially digested proteins. When the liver is working properly, most of the bacteria and other toxins will be neutralized and secreted in a water-soluble form into the blood so they can be excreted via the kidneys or into the bile to be eliminated by the colon. When the liver is stagnant, blood purification will be less efficient, leading to a release of toxins back into the bloodstream.

Long-term liver stagnation produces excess heat, which is fueled by overconsumption of toxins such as alcohol, food additives, prescription drugs, pesticides, and high-fat foods (fried foods, meats, cheese, and eggs). According to the Chinese, liver heat, called *gan ho*, causes "fire to rise" and leads to dizziness, headaches, poor sleep patterns, agitation, irritability, moodiness, aggressive behavior, and anger. Resentment and repressed emotions are also often associated with a stagnant liver.

The liver's busiest time is between 1:00 AM and 3:00 AM. If we frequently wake up during these hours, chances are that we have a faulty detoxification system. Sleeplessness during the wee hours could indicate a liver that is "fired up" and in dire need of support and cleansing.[8]

Spaces in the liver known as sinusoids are vitally important for liver cleansing and nourishment. The sinusoids are lined with a variety of specialized cells, among which are the Kupffer cells. These cells are mobile and look a bit like miniature octopuses as they move about cleaning the blood and lymphatic fluid inside the sinusoids. Kupffer cells are our heroes! They surround and gobble up dead cells, cancer cells, viruses, yeasts, parasites, bacteria, chemicals, partially digested proteins, and harmful foreign particles. Once a Kupffer cell has ingested its victim, it munches it up with enzymes. If the Kupffer cells are overworked for too long, they can become overwhelmed, and the liver will no longer be able to keep the blood and lymphatic fluid clean.

Impure blood and lymph is a contributing factor in a host of illnesses and diseases. As toxins overload our system, we begin to notice symptoms such as allergies, headaches, or chronic fatigue, and as it worsens, degenerative conditions such as autoimmune diseases and cancer develop.[9]

2. The Liver Secretes Bile That Transports Cholesterol and Fat-Soluble Toxins

Next to filtering the blood, the second most important detoxification process of the liver is bile secretion and synthesis (a process of forming complex compounds). About one quart of bile is manufactured by the liver daily, which serves as a transporter of toxic substances that are then eliminated through the colon. Bile consists of bile salts, bilirubin, hormones, cholesterol, lecithin, and electrolytes. Additionally, bile will contain toxins that have been neutralized and rendered safe for elimination. Good quality bile is important to good health and is reflected in walnut-brown-colored stools. Bile promotes peristalsis—waves of involuntary muscle contractions that transport waste matter through the intestines; therefore bile is very important in preventing constipation.

The liver stores toxins in its fat cells. The more toxins it stores, the more the liver's efficiency is compromised, and bile flow is decreased. The liver can become constipated just like the colon. When the liver is congested, excretion of bile is inhibited, and a person will be increasingly prone to constipation. As toxins linger in the gut too long, bacteria can alter them in ways that are even more harmful to the body, and they can be reabsorbed back into the bloodstream, where they'll do more damage the second time around.[10]

The Chinese say the liver "cries" when it is in trouble.[11] It can become so overwhelmed with toxins that it cannot do an efficient job of neutralizing them for the bile. Consequently, bile becomes toxic, which can irritate the bile ducts, gallbladder, and intestines. This can lead to major health problems and ultimately to the development of cancer in the organs involved.

3. The Liver Disassembles Toxins with Enzymes in a Two-Step Process

A complex system of enzymes that are made in liver cells transforms fat-soluble chemicals into water-soluble substances so they can be excreted via the kidneys and colon. This detoxification process is carried out in two steps known as Phase I and Phase II.

Phase I of the enzymatic detoxification process involves activation of a series of enzymes known as cytochrome P450. This system is made up of about one hundred enzymes that break down (hydrolyze) toxins that are absorbed from the intestinal tract such as drugs, hormones, alcohol, nicotine, caffeine, and chemicals from food, air, soil, and water. Hydrolysis is a process that makes a fat-soluble toxin into a water-soluble product, an important step in detoxification and excretion. It's like snipping off a damaged bead from a necklace and sewing on a new bead (a hydrogen atom) to replace the defective, or in this case, toxic one.

When cytochrome P450 does not convert a toxin into a more water-soluble form, the toxin turns into an active intermediate, which is a more chemically reactive form. "'Sticky' is a better image," says Sidney M. Baker, M.D., in his book *Detoxification & Healing*. He likens the process to rubbing a balloon on a sweater. A sticky toxin is not something you want hanging around in your chemistry. It's more dangerous than it was before, producing free radicals as the toxins are transformed.

It is the job of the Phase II enzymes to metabolize these products (process them biochemically). Phase II enzymes are like garbage trucks that pick up the trash. As soon as the activated toxins or leftover molecules are stuck to carrier molecules, they are deactivated and made into a more soluble form in the water of our blood or bile—a process called conjugation.[12]

Problems can occur when Phase I is very active and Phase II is slow or inactive. Toxins build up. This is when we can see severe reactions to environmental toxins (exotoxins). When a person is exposed to low levels of toxins over a long period of time or to large amounts of toxins, an imbalance between Phase I and Phase II occurs. In this case, the majority of the nutrients are utilized for neutralizing toxins in Phase I. Consequently, there is a shortage of key nutrients for Phase II detoxification, and the "sticky trash" piles up. People with less efficient cytochrome P450 systems are more susceptible to cancer. This was exemplified in a study of chemical plant workers in Turin, Italy, who had a remarkably high rate of bladder cancer; tests found that the workers with the poorest detoxification systems were the ones in which this cancer had developed.[13]

Care and Support for Liver Detoxification

The authors of *How to Prevent and Treat Cancer with Natural Medicine* say, "The first step in supporting detoxification is to supply the body with the necessary building blocks for the manufacture of detoxification enzymes." Nutrients such as proteins, vitamins, and minerals are essential ingredients for making enzymes and their partners, the coenzymes (molecules that help the enzymes do their job).[14]

A number of nutrients and foods are key to supporting the detoxification work of the liver, many of which are reviewed in the *Encyclopedia of Natural Medicine.* Without these liver helpers, scores of important detoxification processes in the liver would not take place. For example, glutathione is the most important antioxidant for neutralizing free radicals generated by Phase I detoxification. Indole-3-carbinol, found in cruciferous vegetables (broccoli, cauliflower, cabbage, brussels sprouts, and kale), is an important plant chemical that stimulates both Phase I and Phase II detoxification enzymes. And a deficiency of magnesium can cause Phase II detoxification to slow down, causing a buildup of toxic intermediates.[15]

While many of the following nutrients are discussed in Chapter Seven, they are reviewed in this section specifically for their role in liver detoxification. For a review of general recommended dosages for each nutrient, a comprehensive guide is the *Encyclopedia of Nutritional Supplements.*[16] For supplemental dosages tailored for your individual needs, it is wise to seek the advice of a holistic health professional trained to make the appropriate recommendations.

Nutritional Factors for the Liver

Copper is required as a cofactor for certain cytochrome P450 enzymes to function, and is a necessary component in Phase I detoxification. A cofactor with the enzyme superoxide dismutase, copper is utilized in breaking down the free radical superoxide. Recommended copper-rich foods include almonds, hazelnuts, walnuts, pecans, split peas, carrots, garlic, ginger root, and turnips.

Magnesium is necessary for Phase I and Phase II detoxification. A deficiency can cause Phase II detoxification to slow down, allowing a buildup of toxic intermediates. Avoid magnesium oxide, gluconate, sulfate, and chloride as these forms are not well utilized by the body. Look for supplements that contain magnesium citrate, aspartate, malate, succinate, or fumarate. Recommended magnesium-rich foods include almonds, hazelnuts, walnuts, pecans, beets and beet greens, spinach, Swiss chard, collard greens, sweet corn, avocado, parsley, sunflower seeds, dandelion greens, garlic, fresh green peas, sweet potato, broccoli, cauliflower, carrot, celery, and asparagus.

Zinc functions in more enzymatic reactions than any of the other minerals and is needed for Phase I detoxification. The best forms of zinc are picolinate, acetate, citrate, glycerate, and monomethionine. Recommended zinc-rich foods include ginger root, pecans, split peas, oats, lima beans, almonds, walnuts, buckwheat, hazelnuts, green peas, turnips, parsley, garlic, carrots, black beans, corn, cauliflower, spinach, and cabbage.

Folic acid is involved in methylation (joining methyl groups to toxins for detoxification). Its most available form is folinic acid, which is better absorbed than folic acid. Recommended folic-acid rich foods include beans, lentils, split peas, walnuts, hazelnuts, almonds, spinach, broccoli, barley, brussels sprouts, oatmeal, cabbage, avocado, green beans, corn, and coconut.

Vitamin C is involved in both Phase I and Phase II detoxification. It has many roles, from helping the body manufacture glutathione to assisting in a detoxification process known as acetylation (detoxifying sulfa drugs and antibiotics). Vitamin C is best absorbed when combined with bioflavonoids that are present in half to equal amounts of the vitamin C. It should be taken as buffered vitamin C if you are overly acidic. Recommended vitamin C–rich foods include red chili peppers, red and green sweet peppers, kale, parsley, collards, broccoli, brussels sprouts, mustard greens, watercress, cauliflower, red cabbage, strawberries, papaya, spinach, lemon, turnips, mangos, asparagus, Swiss chard, green onions, and okra.

Some foods are also liver cleansing and supporting. These may overlap somewhat with the nutritional factors, but I mention them again because of their benefits to the liver.

Liver-Cleansing Foods

Cruciferous vegetables (cabbage, cauliflower, broccoli, Brussels spouts, and kale) are rich in the anticancer chemical indole-3-carbinol. This phytonutrient is an active stimulant of detoxifying enzymes in both Phase I and Phase II detoxification in the liver as well as the colon.

Sulfur-containing foods such as red peppers, garlic, onions, broccoli, and brussels sprouts assist in sulfation—the joining of sulfur-containing compounds with toxins.

Beets are known to be a powerful liver-cleansing vegetable. For the liver-gallbladder cleansing Beet Salad, see page 147, and for the liver-cleansing Beet Juice Express, see page 136.

Liver-support foods include artichoke, peas, parsnips, pumpkin, sweet potatoes, squash, yams, beans, broccoli, brussels sprouts, cabbage, carrots, cauliflower, celery, chives, cucumber, eggplant, garlic, kale, kohlrabi, mustard greens, okra, onion, and parsley.

Herbs

Some herbs can also assist the liver in its life-giving function.

Bupleurum root helps increase circulation to the liver. According to some health practitioners, it is also helpful in removing negative emotions that may be "stuck in the tissues," such as anger, grief, depression, and moodiness.

Curcumin, the yellow compound in turmeric, slows down Phase I detoxification while stimulating Phase II—a very good thing to prevent a pileup of toxic intermediates.

Dandelion has been shown to enhance the flow of bile, improve liver congestion, and reduce bile duct inflammation. Dandelion has a direct effect on the liver, causing an increase in bile production and flow to the gallbladder. It contains many nutrients and compounds that may improve liver function.[17]

Milk thistle contains the flavonoids silybinin, silydianin, and silychristin that have powerful antioxidant activity. Silybinin (makes up approximately 60 to 70 percent of silymarin) has been identified as the main active ingredient. Silymarin binds toxic free iron, protects cell membranes from free radical-induced damage, and blocks the uptake of toxins. It is also a potent free radical scavenger.[18] Silymarin has been shown to enhance liver detoxification by preventing the depletion of glutathione, which is linked to the liver's ability to detoxify.[19]

Liver-Cleanse Inhibitors

Many foods and substances are congesting or harmful for the liver, such as alcohol, drugs, caffeine, and nicotine; high-fat foods such as fried foods, meats, and cheese; and adulterated (molecular changes) foods such as margarine, hydrogenated oils, and aspartame. They interfere with the liver-cleansing process. For a complete list of the foods to avoid, see Chapter Five.

Let me give you one specific note here: avoid grapefruit. This citrus fruit has a component—naringin, a flavonoid (a phytochemical)—that has been shown in recent studies to inhibit a subunit of cytochrome P450 (CYP3A) enzymes. This is not a positive step when one is attempting to cleanse the liver and rid the body of stored-up toxins. However, studies indicate that grapefruit flavonoids may have anti-estrogenic properties, and thereby may be anticarcinogenic, which is a positive step. Therefore, when the cleansing process is completed and health is restored, grapefruit may be added back into the diet, provided you are not on medications where grapefruit is contraindicated. During the cleansing process, it is advisable to avoid this fruit.[20]

Toxic emotions. According to health educator Dr. Bernard Jensen, the liver is adversely influenced by negative emotions to a greater degree than any of other digestive organs. His observations about the liver concur with Chinese medicine dating back thousands of years—namely, that anger results in stoppage of bile flow, or liver stagnation, resulting in *fermenting and heat.* Also, if a person is overcome by a strong feeling of loathing, "the bile duct contracts and inhibits bile flow." Conversely, joy produces moderate increases in bile flow.[21] The old maxim is true: *we are what we eat; we are what we think, feel, and believe.*

THE INTESTINES

The second primary channel of elimination is the intestines. The small and large intestines comprise approximately twenty-six feet of intestinal tract, about the length of a tennis court. The small intestine is made up of three segments: duodenum, jejunum, and ileum. Mineral absorption takes place in the duodenum (the first foot of the small intestine). Water-soluble vitamins, carbohydrates, and proteins are absorbed in the eight-foot long jejunum; and the ileum, the remaining twelve-foot section, absorbs fat-soluble vitamins, cholesterol, fat, and bile salts. The last five-foot portion of the intestine through which food passes is the large intestine, also known as the colon. The colon is made up of three segments: ascending, transverse, and descending. Chyme, the thick fluid mass of partially digested food and gastric secretions, enters the ascending colon through the ileocecal valve. As it moves on across the transverse colon, liquid and nutrients are extracted, and the stool is formed into a semisolid state. Gradually it becomes firmer as it approaches the descending colon. About two-thirds of the stool is water, undigested fiber, and food products, and one-third is living and dead bacteria. This mixture enters the lowest portion of the bowel, which is the sigmoid colon, and empties into the rectum for excretion.

The Intestines' Role in Detoxification

Decades of studying the bowel and years of experience teaching patients about bowel cleansing enabled Dr. Bernard Jensen to help countless numbers of people balance their systems and restore their health. In his book *Dr. Jensen's Guide to Better Bowel Care,* Dr. Jensen presented a compelling argument for keeping this organ of elimination detoxified and functioning at its peak. Much of the material I present in this section reflects his insights on intestinal detoxification.[22]

The bowel has great importance among the organs of elimination. Just as a city's garbage collection is vital to its health, the body's waste disposal system is vital to our health. Imagine the problems and disease that would result in the breakdown of a city's trash collection. The same kind of thing happens on a small scale in our body when we don't eliminate waste efficiently.

The bowel's job is to take all the waste and toxic materials, which have been emptied into its long tube, and prepare them for elimination. Various movements process the chyme and push it through the small intestine—a process known as peristalsis. Within eight to ten hours of being consumed, food enters the large intestine (colon) for the final phase of digestion and elimination. The colon swarms with billions of microscopic organisms that play a major role in digestion. Friendly bacteria synthesize some vitamins and break down remaining proteins. Numerous toxic byproducts of this bacterial action are created. These substances are toxic, so this is why a bowel movement at least every eight to twelve hours is critical to good health.[23]

When there is insufficient fiber in the diet, the result is a stool that is very difficult to push through the intestines. The more time it takes for the feces to move along the intestinal tract, the more water will be absorbed and the harder the feces become, which makes them difficult to eliminate. As a person continues to eat a poor diet, the feces will remain in the gut longer and longer. Consequently, friendly intestinal flora (good bacteria) will be taken over by harmful bacteria. These putrefactive bacteria produce harmful chemicals—poisons, to be exact. The environment of the gut becomes somewhat like that of a stagnant pond—foul smelling and toxic. The stronger the odor of our stools and intestinal gas, the greater the indication of fermentation and putrefaction in our bowel.

One of the substances formed by proteolytic (protein digesting) bacteria is ammonia. It is the liver's job to convert ammonia into urea so the kidneys can excrete it. But if the liver is not functioning efficiently, ammonia may circulate in the blood. Confusion, fatigue, or drowsiness may be symptoms of excess ammonia, a result of protein metabolic wastes. It is believed that ammonia may be a contributing factor to cell mutations. The solution is to cleanse the liver so that it is efficient in converting ammonia to urea.

Other byproducts of a compromised intestine are clostridium perfringens enterotoxins: a toxin specific to the cells of the intestinal lining; hydrogen sulfide: a very toxic substance; tyramine: a putrefactive product of tyrosine; and many other toxins too numerous to mention. All of these toxic byproducts affect the health of our intestinal tract. Instead of enabling the bowels to complete their intended function of elimination, a poor diet and the resulting toxic byproducts contribute to toxins being released into our bloodstream. For example, hydrogen sulfide irritates the intestinal lining and causes intestinal toxins to more easily penetrate the intestinal wall. In this case, toxins are absorbed back into the bloodstream where they irritate and inflame other tissues. Autointoxication culminates when the body absorbs too much of its own toxic waste.

When the intestinal tract is continuously exposed to toxic compounds such as drugs, heavy metals, chemicals, and microbes, the intestine will create mucous substances to protect itself, and these substances can build up on the intestinal wall. This *putrefactive debris*, composed primarily of glycoproteins called mucin, prevents the proper assimilation of nutrients and contributes to toxins entering the bloodstream. The debris also promotes the growth of certain bacteria and offers a desirable environment for various parasites. Studies have shown that intestinal mucins are frequently altered to promote epethelial cell changes, which can lead to cancer.[24] If you have any doubt as to the validity of this assertion, you need look no further than the graphic pictures in the back section of *Dr. Jensen's Guide to Better Bowel Care*.

The intestinal tract feeds every cell, tissue, and organ in our body. When it is contaminated, the rest of the body will reflect that toxic state. A toxic bowel means we will have toxic blood and lymphatic fluid. This toxic situation will affect us right down to our DNA. It is imperative to cleanse the entire intestinal tract—and to cleanse it frequently. We can't afford a backup of waste in our system.

A car provides a good analogy of this. If we should decide to flush the radiator, but the opening where the fluids drain out is clogged, old fluids will back up when new fluids are poured in, and the job will turn into a mess. It's the same with our body. Unless the channels of elimination are open, we will not be able to efficiently expel wastes and carcinogenic substances. A toxic mess will build up in our body, and our healing process will be thwarted; our illness exacerbated.

Care and Support for Intestinal Detoxification

In Chapter Six I offer the intestinal cleanse program I have used for a number of years to cleanse my intestinal tract. In this section I highlight key nutrients that support intestinal detoxification, along with the emotions that are particularly harmful to the intestines.

Nutritional Factors

Calcium and magnesium. These minerals are necessary for muscle contraction and are important for good bowel tone and activity. Recommended foods rich in calcium are kale, collard greens, almonds, dandelion greens, watercress, sunflower and sesame seeds, beet greens, broccoli, and spinach. Recommended foods rich in magnesium are hazelnuts, pecans, walnuts, millet, beet greens, coconut, spinach, Swiss chard, collard greens, corn, avocado, parsley, and sunflower seeds.

Herbs

A number of herbs have been found to soften and break up the encrusted putrefactive material. Richard Anderson, N.D., discovered these herbs, thanks to a Native American friend who showed him how to use them effectively for intestinal cleansing. I have used this herbal formula for many years with great success in my own bowel-cleansing program. These herbs include barberry bark, cascara sagrada bark, fennel seed, ginger root, golden seal, lobelia leaf, myrrh gum, peppermint leaf, plantain leaf, red raspberry leaf, turkey rhubarb leaf, and sheep sorrel leaf. The second formula I use to strengthen the body and assist in breaking up the mucoid plaque includes alfalfa leaf, dandelion root, atlantic kelp, rose hips, shavegrass, yellow dock root, chickweed leaf, hawthorne berry, Irish moss, licorice root, and marshmallow root.[25] (NOTE: I don't recommend that you mix your own formula, since these herbs are not combined in equal amounts. See Products and Information.)

Foods

Apple juice. Apple juice has an abundance of soluble fiber (pectins), which holds moisture. For some people, apple juice has a slightly laxative effect. Freshly made apple juice is best, or if using commercial, choose unfiltered and unprocessed, and organic whenever possible. Keep in mind that apple juice is acidic.

As you use these nutritional factors to support your intestinal cleanse, beware of harmful nutritional factors such as saturated animal fats, trans fats, sugar, alcohol, refined foods, pesticides, preservatives, and fake foods. Finally, beware of harmful emotions.

Harmful Emotions

In ancient times the bowel was referred to as "the seat of emotions." Our emotions and our mental state have a profound effect on the bowel.

Peristalsis can be triggered or halted by emotions such as fear, worry, anxiety, anger, melancholy, or grief.

The Colon Flush

The therapeutic benefits of enemas have been known for centuries. Dr. Jensen says, "We know that Grandma always took care of the bowel. She would use enemas to clear a congested bowel." That was true for me. My grandmother's answer for nearly every illness was to flush the colon, and it often worked wonders. We lost this beneficial practice in the twentieth century with the introduction of antibiotics—the wonder drugs that supposedly would cure everything. Indeed, few scientific papers that address the subject of intestinal toxemia have been published since 1950. But scientific research or not—we know that keeping the bowel clean is paramount to staying healthy. Cleansing the bowel when ill is a key to our recovery. According to Jensen, "We cannot put clean, pure food into a dirty body and expect good results."[26]

THE KIDNEYS

The kidneys, a reddish pair of organs that resemble kidney beans in shape, are so important in our elimination system that we have been provided with two of them, even though we can function with just one. The kidneys are found just above the waist, between the parietal peritoneum (membrane that lines the abdominal cavity) and the posterior wall of the abdomen; they are about four to five inches long.

The Kidneys' Role in Detoxification

The major work of the urinary system is done by the nephrons (functional units of the kidneys). The other parts of the system are primarily passageways and storage areas. Nephrons carry out three major functions: they control blood concentration and volume by removing water and solutes (substances dissolved in another substance); they help regulate blood pH; and they remove toxic wastes from the blood.

The metabolism of nutrients results in the production of waste, including carbon dioxide. Protein breakdown produces toxic nitrogenous wastes such as ammonia and urea, which is greatly increased with the consumption of animal products. In addition, many of the essential ions such as sodium, chloride, sulfate, phosphate, and hydrogen tend to accumulate in excess of the body's needs. These excess nutrients and toxic materials must be eliminated, and the kidneys must deal with the overload and excrete it via the urine.[27]

The kidneys have significant work to accomplish under good conditions. But most Americans have overtaxed their kidneys, which suffer from the consequences of the Standard American Diet (SAD), just as the bowel and liver suffer. When the bowel becomes overwhelmed with toxins, the kidneys are forced to handle the excess burden. Refined sugar and too many sweet foods, sodium chloride (table salt), too much protein (animal products), alcohol, and processed foods are all harmful to the kidneys. Heavy metals, especially lead, mercury, and aluminum, are extremely hard on these organs.

Care and Support for the Kidneys

When we cleanse our body, it is important to support the kidneys because they must process more toxic substances than is customary. A number of herbs are helpful in strengthening and tonifying the kidneys. They help increase urine flow, reduce inflammation, and also can help remove uric acid and other crystal formations.

Here is a list of these strengthening herbs, nutritional factors, and kidney-nurturing foods:

Herbs and Nutritional Factors

Kidney support herbs are gravel root, juniper berries, uva ursi, burdock root, hydrangea root, parsley, marshmallow root, ginger root, and lobelia leaf. In proper combination, these herbs are very supportive for the kidneys. (See Products and Information on page 324 for recommendations.)

Nettles is a kidney tonic, and also thickens hair and enriches the blood. You can take nettles as a tea or herbal supplement.

Magnesium citrate, the most beneficial form of magnesium supplement, reduces urinary saturation of stone-forming calcium salts because it forms complexes with calcium. It also slows down crystalline growth of calcium salts.

Kidney-nurturing foods are cranberry, millet, barley, tofu, string beans, black beans, mung beans, mung sprouts, kidney beans and most other beans, kuzu root, watermelon and other melons, blackberry, mulberry, blueberry, huckleberry, water chestnut, wheat germ, potato, seaweeds, spirulina, chlorella, and black sesame seeds.[28]

Include these factors in your diet as you avoid the factors that are harmful to the kidneys.

Harmful Factors

Factors that deplete kidney vitality include toxins in air, food, water, and soil; intoxicants, such as alcohol, marijuana, cocaine, coffee, and tobacco; too much sweet-flavored food (sugars of all kind); too much protein (animal products); and heavy metals such as mercury, lead, and aluminum.

Toxic emotions. Fear can be deeply rooted in the kidneys. We are often unconscious of major areas of fear and insecurity, and especially how they are impacting our body. Excessive fear, beyond the healthy emotion that protects us, can foster a general insecurity about life. This injures the kidneys. Some of us experience the reverse—weak kidneys can foster fearful feelings, which can block us from loving experiences. Stressed, fear-ridden kidneys fail to remove excess water, which according to Chinese medicine "extinguishes the heart spirit" and its normal expressions of love and joy. The antidote is to renew the kidneys and adrenal glands by addressing deficiencies of body and soul.

THE LUNGS

The fourth primary channel of elimination is the lungs. The lungs are paired, cone-shaped organs that lie in the thoracic cavity. The heart and other structures in the mass of tissue between the lungs separate them from each other. They extend to a point about one inch above the clavicles and lie against the ribs. The right lung is thicker and broader than the left. It is also somewhat shorter than the left because the diaphragm is shorter on the right side to accommodate the liver, which lies below. The nose, pharynx, larynx, trachea, bronchi, and lungs comprise the respiratory system.

The Lungs' Role in Detoxification

The purpose of the lungs is to supply the body with oxygen and remove the carbon dioxide that is produced by cellular activities. Breathing is the process by which carbon dioxide is exchanged for oxygen. Some of the toxic waste processed by the body is expelled as a gas through the lungs.

Care and Support for the Lungs

Our lungs are on the front line for intake of airborne toxic chemicals, viruses, and allergens. There are several things we can do to support the detoxification role of the lungs. The full program for cleansing and supporting the lungs can be found in Chapter Six.

Cleansing Breath

Breathing is an important component to health and healing, but most of us don't breathe correctly. We tend to fill only our upper chest because we don't use our diaphragm. This is known as shallow breathing, and it contributes to fatigue and tension. Why not stop for a moment right now and take a deep, cleansing breath? Use your diaphragm to fill up the belly and the upper chest, hold for a count of two, and then expel the air.

Take deep, cleansing breaths often throughout the day. If you find yourself holding your breath, which many of us do during tense times, practice letting go. Then take several deep, cleansing breaths to purify the lungs. Oriental medicine says long, deep breathing can facilitate the cleansing of toxic emotions and confused, muddled thinking.

Include deep breathing in your cleanse as you avoid the factors that are harmful to the lungs.

Emotional Toxins

According to Chinese medicine, grief is the emotion that is most often associated with the lungs. When grief is resolved and expressed, internal health is strengthened. Repressed grief contributes to long-term contraction in the lungs, which interferes with distribution of nutrients and life force. Ultimately, the lungs become congested with undistributed matter. Those who have weak lungs may attempt to stifle their sadness, never completely letting go of their loss. These people may become very ill with respiratory conditions after a loss of someone or something they held dear. According to the Chinese, nearly everyone with lung problems has unresolved sadness or grief that inevitably must be cleared in order to heal and experience good health. By sharing sorrowful feelings with others and releasing our grief, we can heal those areas where deep illness could develop or currently resides.[29] (See Chapter Nine.)

THE SUPPORTING CHANNELS OF DETOXIFICATION

In addition to the four primary channels of elimination—the liver, the intestines, the kidneys, and the lungs—our bodies have four supporting organs of detoxification—the gallbladder, the skin, the lymphatic system, and the blood.

THE GALLBLADDER

The first supporting organ of elimination is the gallbladder. The gallbladder is a small pear-shaped sac about three to four inches long that sits in a groove on the lower side of the liver. The gallbladder's function is to store and concentrate bile, which is made in the liver, until it is needed in the small intestine. Besides emulsifying fat, bile helps lubricate the intestines and gives the familiar brown color to stools. In the gallbladder, water and minerals are absorbed from the bile, and it becomes darker in color. This produces the walnut-brown color—a sign of good quality bile; stools that are light colored reflect insufficient bile.

The Gallbladder's Role in Detoxification

One of the primary routes of eliminating toxins is through the bile. Bile is concentrated in the gallbladder and becomes a carrier substance by which many toxins are expelled from the body.

Care and Support for Gallbladder Detoxification

Because good quality bile is so important in the elimination of toxins, it is vitally important that we care for the gallbladder and support its function. We know from research that a high-calorie, high-protein, high-fat diet contributes to gallstones, and to what is known as *sand* or *mud* (gallbladder congestion). In comparing autopsies from countries such as France, India, Japan, Portugal, South Africa, Sweden, and Uganda, it was found that a low-calorie, low-protein, low-fat diet along with increased vegetable intake was associated with a low incidence of gallstones.[30]

Many people do not show the typical signs of gallstones or other gallbladder congestion in that they have no abdominal pain, yet there may be stones, sand, or mud. Signals of gallbladder congestion other than abdominal pain are backaches, belching, bloating, coated tongue, constipation, dark complexion or pasty complexion, dizziness, heartburn, fatty food intolerance, fullness between meals, headaches, tension in the back part of the shoulder under the neck, high blood pressure, nausea, bitter taste in the mouth, jaundice, slow pulse, strong appetites, or a quick, irritable temper.[31] In *Healing with Whole Foods*, Paul Pritchford says, "Most chronically ill people need gallbladder cleansing before recovery is complete."[32]

You may have only a few symptoms of gallbladder congestion and still have gallstones or other congestion. I never dreamed I had so much as one stone. I was thirty-one, slim, and had only a few of the digestive symptoms noted above, so imagine my surprise when a health-care practitioner pressed on the liver/gallbladder point on my foot and I nearly flew out of the chair. He said this indicated gallstones and suggested a gallbladder flush. To my complete astonishment, dozens of stones about the size of large green peas, some appearing greenish purple, were expelled from my body in the flush. Subsequently, my digestive symptoms disappeared. I believe the gallbladder flush was one of the important cleansing processes that contributed to my complete healing from chronic fatigue syndrome and fibromyalgia.

The complete Gallbladder Cleansing Program can be found in Chapter Six, but a number of key gallbladder-support foods and supplements are highlighted in this section.

Gallbladder-Friendly Fiber, Juices, and Foods

Fiber. Toxins will remain in the liver longer when the excretion of bile is inhibited, a condition known as cholestasis. In the intestines, bile and toxins are absorbed by dietary fiber and discharged. When the diet is deficient in fiber, toxins and bile are reabsorbed into the system. We can increase fiber in our diet by daily increasing our vegetable, legume, and whole grain servings. I also recommend taking flax fiber. (Barleans makes an organic flax fiber, which can be found at most health food stores.)

Olive oil and apple juice or lemon juice. The gallbladder flush I have used effectively incorporates olive oil and apple juice or lemon juice. There are a number of variations to this program, but basically they produce the same results. Until recently, this program has been pessimistically viewed, debated, or dismissed, but a very exciting observation about this gallbladder cleanse was published in the prestigious medical journal *Lancet* in December 1999. It is the case report of a female with a history of gallstones who took one liter of apple juice every day for a week, and on the seventh day drank one cup of olive oil before going to bed. The next morning she collected the gallstones from her stool and took them to a university hospital where they were determined to be fatty stones.[33] The complete outline of this olive oil and juice program can be found in Chapter Six.

Gallbladder-friendly foods. Pears, apples, parsnips, radishes, seaweed, lemons, limes, and the spice turmeric help to hasten the removal of gallstones and other congestion. In addition, drink chamomile tea each day and take two tablespoons of cod liver oil.

Gallbladder Supplements

Lecithin. A low concentration of lecithin in the bile may contribute to gallstones. A study published in *Lancet* found that lecithin was effective in dissolving or reducing stones.[34] Taking just 100 milligrams of lecithin three times a day will increase concentration in the bile.

Iron, vitamin C, and vitamin E deficiencies have been shown to contribute to gallstones. An iron-deficient diet appears to alter hepatic (liver) enzyme function, which increases gallbladder bile cholesterol and promotes crystal formation.[35] Get plenty of iron-rich foods such as pumpkin seeds, sunflower seeds, millet, almonds, parsley, Jerusalem artichokes, beets and beet greens, Swiss chard, dandelion greens, and green peas. Vitamin C greatly enhances the uptake of iron so include plenty of the following with your iron-rich foods: red, yellow, and green sweet peppers, kale, parsley, collard greens, broccoli, mustard greens, watercress, cauliflower, red cabbage, and spinach. To prevent vitamin E deficiency, make sure you include generous servings of sunflower seeds, almonds, spinach, oatmeal, asparagus, brown rice, pecans, carrots, and peas.

Lipotropic nutrients. Lipotropic factors are those that speed up the removal of fat or decrease fat deposits in the liver. These agents include choline, methionine, betaine, folic acid, and vitamin B_{12}.

Milk thistle. Research indicates that milk thistle may dissolve gallstones by increasing the solubility of the bile.[36]

Include these supplements in your cleanse, and be careful to avoid sugar. Besides contributing to an acidic pH in the body, which is conducive to cancer growth, sugar also contributes to gallstones and billiary tract cancer.[37]

THE SKIN

The second supporting channel of elimination is the skin. Considered a secondary organ of elimination, the skin is the largest of the elimination organs, a backup for the other organs of detoxification. The skin is considered an organ because it consists of tissues structurally joined together to perform specific activities. For the average adult, it occupies a surface area of approximately three thousand square inches. The skin has about six major functions: it maintains body temperature; protects the body from bacterial invasion, toxins, dehydration, and UV rays; perceives stimuli; excretes wastes, water, salt, and organic compounds; synthesizes vitamin D; and bolsters immunity.

The Skin's Role in Detoxification

Due to its large surface area, the skin can expel significant amounts of cellular wastes, which are eliminated through the sweat glands and mucous secretions. The condition of the skin reflects the condition of everything beneath it. When the other organs of elimination such as the liver and colon are overloaded, the skin must pick up a larger-than-normal portion of the waste to eliminate. It will sweat them out or throw them off with rashes, pimples, boils, acne, or abscesses. Often during a cleansing program, skin eruptions such as these will appear as the body attempts to get rid of toxins. As the toxins clear from the body, the skin clears up as well.

Care and Support for the Skin

Drink plenty of purified water to assist your body in elimination and incorporate dry skin brushing daily. These two simple techniques are particularly helpful for the skin's detoxification process. A complete skin cleanse program is in Chapter Six. The skin also mirrors our emotional state. See The Emotional Cleanse Program in Chapter Nine.

THE LYMPHATIC SYSTEM

The third supporting organ is the lymphatic system. The lymphatic system consists of fluid called lymph, vessels that transfer lymph (lymphatics), and a number of structures and organs that contain lymphatic tissue, which include the lymph nodes that filter lymph, the thymus gland, the tonsils, and the spleen. Lymphatic ducts drain lymph from the body and empty it into the jugular vein. Lymphatic tissue contains white blood cells (lymphocytes, neutrophils, eosinophils, basophils, monocytes, and macrophages—cells that filter the lymph) that protect the body from foreign cells, microbes, and cancer cells.

The Lymphatic System's Role in Detoxification

The lymphatic system is a supporting channel of elimination. It picks up intracellular waste and dumps it in the bloodstream, which delivers the waste to the organs of elimination for processing. Immune cells in the lymphatic tissue get rid of harmful bacteria and unwanted cells, such as cancer cells, by making contact with these substances, engulfing, and destroying them. Liver health is a key to the lymphatic system's health. The lymph can become stagnant, just as the liver can stagnate. Therefore, it is important to cleanse the liver along with the lymphatic system.

Care and Support for the Lymphatic System

Exercise greatly benefits the lymphatic system. Unlike the blood, the lymph has no pump to push it through its vessels; therefore, it depends on movement of our extremities, our muscles, and our respiratory system to force the lymph through the body. Exercise is imperative in cleansing the lymphatics and massage is quite helpful.

Diaphragmatic breathing. Deep breathing is very beneficial in helping move the lymph through the vessels. Use your diaphragm to fill your belly and upper chest with air, hold for a count of two, and expel the air. Do this several times a day. Remember to breathe deeply throughout the day, and be sure not to hold your breath when you're tense.

Skin brushing. Just brushing your skin with a natural bristle brush two minutes a day will help to move the lymph through the vessels. Before you shower, brush in a circular motion, starting with the feet and legs and moving up the body. This will stimulate, strengthen, and tone the lymphatic system.

Lymphatic drainage massage. This particular, light-touch massage is very helpful in moving lymph through the body.

THE BLOOD

The fourth supporting channel of elimination is the blood. The blood is an important channel in the detoxification process. It has been called the body's "river of life" because it transports oxygen, hormones, and nutrients to the trillions of cells in the body and carries wastes to the organs of elimination. Blood regulates pH, body temperature, and the water content of cells.

The Blood's Role in Detoxification

Our blood carries carbon dioxide to our lungs, and waste products from our cells and lymphatic system to our liver, kidneys, lungs, and sweat glands to be expelled. Our blood also protects us from toxins and foreign invaders through special combat-unit cells—our white blood cells.

Care and Support of the Blood

Juice fasting has been used to cleanse the blood, as well as all the other channels of elimination. Indeed, it is a powerful means for healing the entire body. (See Chapter Six.)

Chlorophyll, the phytonutrient that gives plants their green color, is known as a blood purifier. That's one of the reasons why green juices, such as wheatgrass juice, are so beneficial. Chlorophyll is known to fight bacterial growth as well as yeasts and fungi and to help in removing drug deposits. It is also helpful in deactivation of many carcinogens. Wheatgrass, nettles, and hijiki are thought to keep the hair from falling out, and they may help if you are taking chemotherapy drugs.

Avoid salt. According to Chinese medicine, too much salt damages the blood, just as too much meat, dairy, and sugar can damage the kidneys and contribute to acidic blood. The only salt I recommend is Celtic Sea Salt.

In addition to cleansing and supporting all the body's organs and channels of elimination, it is important to avoid toxicity in every way possible. Eat a diet that consists of fresh, organically grown, whole foods and avoid eating animal products, refined foods, sugars, and foods that contain additives and preservatives. You can clean out your home and work environment of all toxic materials such as stored or leaking chemicals and all household agents that are toxic. (See Chapter Eight.)

It is impossible to completely avoid toxicity, but you can greatly reduce toxins in your environment and keep them off your body and out of your home. To support your efforts to make this happen, the next five chapters are devoted to practical steps you can take each day to cleanse your body and to cleanse your home and working environment.

4

WHOLE FOODS FOR CLEANSING

Let food be your medicine, and medicine be your food.

—Hippocrates

Having shown that Mom was right about eating vegetables to prevent colds and drinking cranberry juice to cure a bladder infection, scientists are now showing the importance of a "balanced diet" to prevent and heal cancer. *Balanced* certainly does not mean one vitamin pill from the white pile, one from the red pile, and one from the yellow pile, while scarfing down a chocolate doughnut with a chaser of orange juice. A balanced diet involves *whole foods*—especially fruits, vegetables, whole grains, and legumes—that pack the disease-preventing and healing wallop. That's because they contain a whole ratatouille of compounds that have never seen the inside of a vitamin bottle (and probably never will).

The National Cancer Institute estimates that one in three cancer deaths is diet related, and eight out of ten cancers have a nutrition/diet component.[1] Therefore, an essential part of our healing process is learning about whole foods and nutritious dietary choices. We cannot control many toxic aspects of our existence, but the food we eat is our own choice, and it is up to us to select foods that are cleansing and life supporting.

WHOLE FOODS FOR CLEANSING AND HEALING

Whole foods is a term for foods that have not had any of their elements removed by processing. This term also refers to foods that do not contain foreign ingredients such as additives, preservatives, or colorings. These whole foods are the same foods that were eaten by our ancestors before industry got hold of our food supply, turning it into products that fit neatly into colorful little packages on the supermarket shelf. These products, many of which did not even exist fifty years ago, have become staples of our Western diets, which many of us cannot imagine living without. They have replaced the wholesome grains and vegetables that sustained life for centuries. Although to some, whole foods may seem like a trend indulged in by health fanatics, aging hippies, and radical youths, there is really nothing new or exotic about them. These foods were consumed by our grandparents, great grandparents, and every generation before them.

WHY ARE WHOLE FOODS BETTER?

To help us silence our inner child who occasionally demands a bowl of double-chocolate almond ice cream or a bag of potato chips, let's look at some interesting facts as to why a change to a whole foods diet is necessary for regaining health. Many diets claim to assist in curing cancer, and although each has its followers who have had their health restored, these diets are based on widely divergent theories. One thing that all successful healing and cleansing diets have in common, however, is an insistence on whole, unprocessed foods of all or mostly vegetable kingdom origin. Whole foods are better than processed foods for two reasons: first, for what whole foods have that is missing in processed foods; and second, for what processed foods have that is missing in whole foods. Sound confusing? Think about it for a moment.

Ingredients Missing in Processed Foods

One of the most important components missing in refined or processed food is fiber. A diet that is high in meat and refined flour products, which is what most of us in the Western world eat, is very low in fiber. In fact, Americans eat about ten to twenty grams of fiber daily, which is a far cry from the thirty to forty grams recommended by the National Cancer Institute. Fiber is the indigestible part of the plant, which is present in all plant tissues but is totally missing in foods of animal origin. In refined grain products, most of the fiber is removed, along with the highly nutritious bran and germ as whole grain flour is transformed into white flour and brown rice is made pristine fair.

The fiber content of foods is not a glamorous subject, but the benefits of fiber are many. Because it does not digest, fiber goes through the intestines, cleansing the colon and making bowel movements easier and more copious, as I've mentioned before. This helps prevent colon cancer and cures bowel problems, and prevents such problems as constipation, polyps, diverticular disease, and hemorrhoids, but this is only part of why fiber is so important.

Fiber also binds with toxins that we may have absorbed through our lungs, skin, or ingestion. These toxins make their way into our intestines after they have been filtered through our liver and mixed with bile from the gallbladder. Without sufficient fiber, these toxins risk being reabsorbed back into our system, but when plenty of fiber is present, it can absorb them and carry them out of the body. Fiber also binds with cholesterol, removing it from the body, which is equally important. In estrogen-sensitive cancers such as breast cancer, fiber may be even more protective, because it *increases* the removal and *decreases* reabsorption of estrogen in the stool.[2]

Another advantage of fiber is that it aids in stabilizing blood sugar, which keeps our energy level on a more even keel. We sometimes hear that carbohydrates are bad because they quickly turn into sugar, but this is true only for *refined* carbohydrates, such as most breads, rolls, pasta, pastry, and pizza dough that have been stripped of their nutrients and fiber. When we consume complex carbohydrates in the form of whole grains, legumes, fruits, and vegetables, the fiber that is naturally in these foods ties up some of the sugars, releasing them slowly into the bloodstream. By eating a plant-based diet of whole foods, we are getting about six times as much fiber as a person on the Standard American Diet. This gives our body extra cleansing power with every meal and a more even energy level to get through the day.

Besides fiber, other important elements such as vitamins and minerals are removed from refined and processed foods. Take salt for an example. Common table salt, a highly refined product, is grossly overused in processed foods. On a whole foods diet, a moderate amount of unrefined Celtic Sea Salt (also known as gray salt) is allowed. This salt has been used by every culture on earth for as long as we have record. It was mentioned in the *Peng-Tzao-Kan-Mu,* which was written in China around 4,700 years ago and is more than likely the earliest known treatise on pharmacology. Whole sea salt has a mineral profile that is similar to our blood; in Chinese medicine whole sea salt is thought to have a grounding effect that leads to clarity of mind, when used in moderation. It is also used in Chinese medicine for its detoxifying properties.

When salt is processed, its minerals are removed and what remains is primarily sodium chloride. Anticaking chemicals, potassium iodide, and dextrose (sugar) are added to make table salt. Perhaps the reason that so many people tend to overeat salty foods is because their bodies are craving the minerals that have been refined out of the salt—a craving that will never be satisfied with this product.[3]

Likewise with grains, when the germ and bran are removed, not only will fiber be lacking, vitamins and minerals will be stripped away. Grains, including wheat—which is the grain most commonly used in Western culture—kamut, spelt, rice, corn, millet, barley, amaranth, quinoa, and oats are all made by nature in a similar fashion. They have a hard, inedible, protective husk, which covers the grain. Cornhusk, which everyone is familiar with, is an example of this. Under the husk lies the bran, which covers and protects the endosperm, the part of the grain that is left after refining. Hidden within the endosperm is the germ, which holds the life essence of the grain and gives it the power to sprout, creating a new plant. As long as the grain remains intact, it can last for many years.

Along with fiber, other important minerals such as chromium, zinc, and manganese are stripped away from grains in the refining process. Interestingly, these minerals are also factors that control blood sugar levels and may help fiber in blood sugar stabilization.[4] Other nutrients that are removed from grains in the refining process include the B vitamins, vitamin E, important essential fatty acids, and plant sterols.

Additions to Processed Foods Can Be Just as Harmful

What is added to processed and refined foods can be just as harmful as the refining process, if not more so. Additives and preservatives are used in food processing for a variety of reasons. They maintain product consistency, preventing the separation of oil and water in foods like peanut butter and salad dressings. They keep powders such as flours, baking powder, and various types of mixes flowing freely without caking. They also help maintain a desired acid-alkaline balance in products. Additives preserve the palatability of products by retarding the spoilage of foods, allowing them to be kept for long periods of time in warehouses and on supermarket shelves and still give the illusion of freshness.

Preservatives also inhibit the formation of microbes, which allows us to eat old food, long past its prime, without developing food poisoning. Additives can control leavening in baked goods, creating products that are lighter and fluffier than anything we could make at home. Some additives such as artificial colorings are thrown in purely as an attempt to make preserved foods appear appetizing. Last, but not least, some additives take a further shot at mimicking fresh, whole foods by "enriching" products with some of the vitamins and minerals that were refined out during processing.

The main problem with "enriching" is that these foods can never measure up to whole, natural foods that have a balance of nutrients, and although scientists have made great inroads in nutrition, whole food chemistry is very complex. We cannot simply add a vitamin or mineral and expect it to work the same as it would with all its cofactors that were removed.

New discoveries keep surfacing. Just a few years ago nutritionists did not know about phytonutrients, and many people believed that vitamins and minerals were the sole essential components of foods. Today, phytonutrients are known to be highly important for their synergistic effects with vitamins and minerals and for their protective and antioxidant properties. With an intricate configuration of elements, nature has designed whole foods to have exactly what we need for proper utilization of all the nutrients present in the food. An orange, for example, contains not only vitamin C but bioflavonoids and other nutrients that have a synergistic effect, making the vitamin C in an orange more efficient because of the bioflavonoids than an equal amount of a vitamin C supplement without bioflavonoids. Therefore, when industry adds vitamins and minerals, or even fiber, to foods that have been stripped of these elements, we must ask, "What are they forgetting?"

Some additives such as ascorbic acid (vitamin C) and alpha tocopherol (vitamin E) are helpful and safe. The seaweed-derived alginate is also likely safe, but many other additives are questionable, and some are harmful, even though the food industry assures us that additives on the market today are harmless and have been thoroughly tested.

Close to thirty different additives, which were once regarded safe, are now banned. Some of these were used for several years before it was discovered that they posed health risks. What kind of risks? Cancer is the number one risk studied; however, some additives have been shown to induce liver poisoning or to damage other internal organs.[5]

According to the Center for Science in the Public Interest, there are still numerous additives on the market that studies have shown to be unsafe in amounts that are commonly consumed. Others have been poorly tested and are not worth the risk. Some additives, although not proven to be carcinogenic, are unsafe for other reasons, such as simply promoting bad nutrition by making junk food more desirable, even addictive. These have all passed FDA regulation.[6] A good rule to observe when shopping for food is to avoid anything that has additives you don't recognize.

An important consumer-protection clause, called the Delaney Clause, is a part of the Federal Food, Drug, and Cosmetic Act. This clause prohibits the use of any additive that "is found to induce cancer when ingested by man or animal." Thanks to this clause many harmful substances have already been banned, but because the food industry is powerful and their primary motivation is their own profit and not our health, control of these substances is an uphill battle. The food and chemical industries (which are becoming more and more entwined) are seeking to repeal the Delaney Clause. (If you're so inclined, this protective clause is worth fighting for.)

The manufacturing and selling of processed foods is a far more lucrative business than selling whole foods in their natural state. There is a lot of competition in the processed food business, and the successful companies spend an unbelievable amount of money on advertising. In total, at the turn of this last century, the food industry was spending more than thirty-three billion dollars annually to advertise and promote their products.[7]

Never assume if something is on the market that it is safe, or even that the products in a health food store are safe. Read all labels. It is probably smarter to assume that if something contains an ingredient that you do not recognize or cannot pronounce it is potentially unsafe. I often say, "If you can't pronounce it, don't buy it!"

MAKING CHANGES IS AN EMOTIONAL ISSUE

I know that some people will have difficulty changing to whole foods because some refined foods have emotional attachments. Most of us have a list of "comfort foods" that we turn to when ill or emotionally distressed, foods that make us feel happy. And most of us prefer the foods our mothers served to us. In times past, this could, in most cases, assure people of eating a nutritious diet. Dietary problems were usually caused by lack of food, poor sanitation, absence of refrigeration, or limited variety, not by poor food choices like junk food, and processed stuff simply wasn't available.[8]

Today, however, many of us have grown up almost exclusively on brand-name products that have little in common with the whole, natural foods from which they were processed. Even for those of us who have eaten a whole foods diet for years, there are still, somewhere back in the subliminal recesses of our minds, fond memories of such things as steaming bowls of canned soup served with a sandwich made of soft, snowy, white bread grilled in margarine and stuffed with melted, orange-colored cheese. Mothers, who were either frazzled by overwork, or seduced by the concept of convenience, served processed foods to us with love, and although they may have been anything but wholesome, in our subconscious mind they are still desirable. Unfortunately, all of us who grew up on a diet of brand-name fare have some major rethinking and attitude adjustment to do if we wish to successfully adopt a whole foods diet.

It is never easy to make a major change, even if our better sense says that whole foods are essential to regain health. No matter how convinced or motivated we are, a little voice, somewhere in our inner depths, screams, "I want sugar-frosted breakfast flakes!"

One of the easiest ways to change our eating habits effectively is to associate the results of our actions with the outcome.

A CHOICE RESPONSE

In questioning individuals who have been successful in changing their eating habits, one characteristic stands out: these individuals were able to imagine the relationship between their present choices and the effect those choices would have on their future. A default response, as opposed to a choice response, is when an individual has only one automatic response in a situation and can't seem to get beyond that, even when the outcome is adverse. From time to time, many of us respond in this manner. But if we are rarely able to get beyond the default response, regardless of the outcome, it is time to assess our behavior and set new goals for change.

The Choice Response: Changing Your Eating Habits

John Calbom

I'd like to ask you a question: "Are you discouraged, angry, or depressed about all the things you can no longer eat or drink?" If you aren't now, you may be by the time you have finished Cherie's chapters on food. Frustration is normal. In the midst of frustration, however, change can happen; it's a matter of choosing the right responses.

When I was diagnosed with hypoglycemia, I was initially relieved to find out about the cause of my fatigue, irritability, and headaches. Then, as I heard about what I would have to give up to feel better, my enthusiasm quickly gave in to downright panic. I thought I'd never be able to let go of the food and drink that had become so much a part of my life. It's now funny to think about how matter-of-fact the doctor was as he read off the list of what I could and couldn't eat—never, ever again! My first thought was to chain myself up, but in actuality, I realized I had to figure out a way I could make the new diet work.

Setting Goals for Dietary Change

If you can relate to my story in any way, I suggest you go through the following process to keep yourself from sabotaging your efforts.

1. Get a plan clearly in mind about what you are going to do the next time you are tempted to eat foods you know aren't the best for you and will sabotage your healing process.
2. Associate your actions with the outcome of your choices. Be as graphic as you can and try to actually feel what you would

experience physically if you ate the things you shouldn't eat. Or, if you experience no adverse physical sensations, think about how this food might impact your recovery from disease.

3. Picture the foods that are detrimental to your health with a very negative symbol, such as the words *rat poison* written above them or any other negative association that is meaningful to you.
4. Associate the foods that are good for you with positive thoughts such as *Mineral water with a slice of lemon is a great party drink! It's better for me than alcohol and tastes just as good.*
5. Develop a list of healthy comfort foods that you can turn to when you're emotionally down. Make sure you have some of these foods on hand at all times so you aren't tempted to go out for ice cream or something else unhealthy when your emotions are screaming for comforting food.
6. The next time you go out to dinner or prepare a special meal at home, and you're tempted to throw caution to the wind and splurge a bit, remember that what you eat, even this one time, will impact the future state of your health. You've embarked on a special mission of recovery!
7. If you make a mistake, don't punish yourself. Start over with a positive plan to make wise choices in the future. And no matter what, never succumb to the temptation to throw the whole plan out because you've "blown it" a time or two. Just pick yourself up "and get back in the race."

IT'S EASIER THAN YOU THINK

After reading this, you must be thinking of the daunting chore that lies ahead if you are to forego processed foods and take control of your own food preparation. Yes, it will take an effort, especially in the beginning, because you are learning something new. However, it is not nearly as difficult as you might think once you get the hang of it.

Because advertising agencies emphasize the convenience and ease of using their products, and because we have grown so accustomed to using them, we have developed the belief that something as simple and natural as preparing our own food is a dreadfully difficult process that only a gourmet chef can do correctly. Believe me, it's not. When you learn how to prepare these foods, it will become as easy as any other part of your daily routine. And when you become accustomed to how much better fresh, whole foods taste, you will wonder how you ever settled for a diet of processed food products instead of real food.

LIVE FOODS FOR CLEANSING AND HEALING

Live food is whole food that has not been cooked or processed in any other way to destroy enzymes and other nutrients. The term *live foods* was coined by Ann Wigmore, a Lithuanian born in 1909. Ann learned about the healing powers of plants as she watched her grandmother treat wounded World War I soldiers with herbs that grew around her home. In 1925 Ann moved to the United States where she adopted the Standard American Diet (SAD) of refined and processed foods. Her health suffered, and she was eventually diagnosed with colon cancer. She was also the victim of a terrible automobile accident that shattered both her legs. Gangrene set into her legs and the doctors wanted to amputate. Ann refused the surgery and began to apply the knowledge of plants that she had acquired from her grandmother. She cured her cancer, the gangrene, and a myriad of other health problems. And then at the age of fifty, her white hair returned to its natural, rich brown color!

Because Ann's healing regime depended on having access to very fresh, organically grown plants, which were impossible to obtain year-round where she lived in Boston, she developed the technique of growing wheatgrass and sprouting seeds indoors. She founded the Hippocrates Health Institute in Boston in 1963, which later became the Ann Wigmore Center. Ann lived a vibrant life, traveling and teaching the live foods philosophy until her death in an accidental fire at the age of eighty-three.

Live foods are an integral part of this cleansing program. Usually, *live food* refers to any organically grown raw fruit, vegetable, nut, seed, or grain. The term developed because every whole seed, nut, or grain has the potential to sprout, creating new life. Root vegetables such as carrots, beets, parsnips, onions, turnips, Jerusalem artichokes, and sweet potatoes will also, if given the opportunity. These foods are literally *alive*. Other foods that can be considered live foods are all fruits and vegetables that contain seeds, such as tomatoes, apples, green beans, cucumber, and squash. Even a cabbage will begin to grow roots if it is kept in the right conditions long enough.

Some raw food proponents only consider foods alive after they have begun to sprout, but usually people are referring to uncooked plant foods as opposed to cooked foods and flesh food, which is dead and does not have the power to regenerate. Processed foods and foods that have been heated above 118 degrees Fahrenheit cannot regenerate. At temperatures usually above 118 degrees Fahrenheit, the enzymes, which are necessary to sustain the life of the plant, are killed, and the food is no longer considered live.

Most followers of raw food diets cite digestive enzymes as one of the major reasons for eating uncooked foods. We need enzymes to digest the food we eat, and enzymes are abundant in raw food to facilitate the process, unless it is heated above 118 degrees Fahrenheit or processed. When the enzymes are destroyed, the body must produce all the enzymes necessary to digest those foods.

Dr. Edward Howell, the father of the food enzyme concept, has argued that when the body is busy digesting food, it is not able to make enzymes that are necessary for other metabolic functions. This creates a tug-of-war between the digestive system's demands and other systems of the body that need enzymes for cleansing, healing, and rebuilding. Without a continual dietary supply of enzymes, our recovery can be hindered. Cooking also decreases vitamin and (sometimes) mineral content, as well as enzymes; therefore, it is much better to take the enzymes directly from the plant and spare our organs from overwork in making the lion's share of digestive enzymes.

Ann Wigmore believed that the key to health is detoxification and rejuvenation. Detoxification begins when the sources of toxins are removed and stored toxins in the body are eliminated. However, when an individual is seriously ill, simply removing toxins from the diet and environment is not enough; the process must be helped along. Rejuvenation can take place when vitamins and minerals are added to a diet that was lacking in these essential elements. The fastest and most effective way I know to detoxify is with an abundance of whole, live foods and the right nutritional supplements. Although everyone can benefit by adding live food to his or her diet for the purpose of detoxification and disease prevention, some individuals find that an exclusively live foods diet is necessary for a period of time to facilitate healing.

Individuals who benefit the most from an exclusively raw-foods diet are those who are overweight, tend to be easily overheated, and have a robust nature. These people suffer from diseases that stem from the excesses of a rich diet, and this describes the majority of Americans. An exclusively live foods diet, when done correctly and under proper supervision, can be tremendously healing for persons of this type of constitution who need rapid detoxification.[9]

RAW FOODS OR COOKED FOODS

Because of the success that many people have on a live foods diet, a fad has developed among health enthusiasts. This kind of diet is recommended by raw food proponents, not just for healing and for persons with conditions resulting from excess of rich food, but for everyone and every type of constitution. However, for persons who are frail and weak, who are cold natured, and who suffer more from deficiency rather than excess in food and drink, an exclusively raw foods diet is not recommended over the long term, though short term it may be helpful. Persons with this kind of constitution often need some cooked foods to keep up their strength. In traditional Chinese medicine, too much raw food is known to deplete the energy of the spleen, eventually causing a deficiency. Even individuals of a robust nature can become deficient by following a cleansing diet over a long time period.

The Sample-Day Raw Foods Menu Plan
Breakfast
Herbal tea
Freshly made organic juice (mainly vegetable juices)
Melon or papaya or fresh raw vegetables thirty minutes later

Mid-Morning Break
Herbal tea or fresh vegetable juice or wheatgrass juice
Lunch
Garden salad
Cold raw soup, such as Carrot Juice/Avocado Soup with Cumin or Gazpacho or Guacamole, and homemade dehydrated crackers (Dehydrated foods are allowed on a raw-foods diet.)
Mid-Afternoon Break
Herbal tea or wheatgrass juice
Dinner
Sprout salad
Homemade dehydrated crackers
Raw creamy corn chowder made in blender, or other raw soup
Vegetable sticks
Bedtime
Chamomile tea

As our physiology changes during the healing process, it is important not to be rigid about such issues as eating only raw or only cooked food. Following a healing diet is an ongoing practice, and our choices of foods should change as our physiology transforms with the healing process. Even the seasons and the climate we live in play an important role in deciding which foods are best for us. In winter, in a cold or damp climate, a weak, frail person will not do well on a diet of exclusively raw food. Adding simple cooked grains such as quinoa, millet, or wild rice with steamed vegetables and the easier to digest beans, such as mung or adzuki, will be much more beneficial than a diet of only raw food.[10] Therefore, it is important to work with a nutritionist or nutritional doctor throughout the healing process, if at all possible.

GOING VEGAN TO CLEANSE AND HEAL

If we examine the diets famous for healing cancer, such as the live foods diet and macrobiotic diets, the two elements they have in common are an insistence on whole, organic foods and the absence of animal products.

Research has shown that vegans, individuals who eat no animal products whatsoever, have a lower risk of cancer than vegetarians who eat eggs and dairy or than meat eaters.[11] According to the Food and Nutrition Science Alliance, the incidence of cancer could be cut by one-third by changing to a healthier diet, and by another third by quitting smoking. The Alliance recommends eating a wide variety of fruits, vegetables, whole grains, and beans and monitoring fat intake, reducing alcohol intake, and exercising regularly.[12] Because this diet is universally recommended for cancer prevention, it should also be the diet universally recommended as part of a comprehensive program for cancer healing.

Many studies confirm that vegan diets are both cancer preventative and healing.

- According to the American Medical Association, more than half of all cancers in women are related to diet.[13]
- When Japanese women begin to eat meat daily, they have an approximately six-times-higher risk of breast cancer than those who rarely or never eat meat.[14]
- An article in *Health Plus* from Vanderbilt University states that a diet rich in meat, cheese, and whole milk may increase the risk of developing cancer of the esophagus and the stomach.[15]
- In a report titled *Food, Nutrition and the Prevention of Cancer,* which was published by the World Cancer Research Fund in association with the American Institute for Cancer Research, it was estimated that dietary change alone could reduce global cancer incidence by 30 to 40 percent. When the cessation of smoking is added to dietary change, 60 to 70 percent of all cancers are considered preventable.[16]
- In a World Cancer Research Fund Report, it was stated that vegetable foods generally decrease the risk of cancer, whereas the foods that raise cancer risks are animal fats and meat.[17]
- Obesity is a significant and controllable cancer-risk factor, with animal products and processed foods being major contributing factors.[18]

- A study by Dean Ornish, M.D., showed that after three months on a low-fat vegan diet, men with prostate cancer saw a drop in their levels of prostate specific antigens.[19]
- Studies have found that vegan men have lower levels of a growth factor that is associated with prostate cancer than either meat-eaters or vegetarians.[20]
- An Italian study revealed that adult women who reduce their dietary intake of fat and animal protein substantially lower their risk of breast cancer; unhealthy fats stimulate the production of estrogens, which encourages the growth of breast cancer cells.[21]

A major reason for reduced rates of cancer in vegans is the fact that vegans consume much greater quantities of antioxidants and protective phytochemicals than omnivores. Antioxidants and phytochemicals are abundant in the fruits, vegetables, legumes, and whole grains that make up the vegan diet. Vegans also consume considerably more fiber, because virtually everything they eat is rich in fiber, which binds with toxins, allowing them to be eliminated. The goal of The Complete Cancer Cleanse Program is to eliminate toxins from our body, and a diet high in the natural fibers contained in whole vegan foods is an important step in our healing.

A vegan, whole foods diet is not only important for what it has but also for what it lacks. Animal foods are higher in heavy metals, environmental toxins, pesticide residues, and other carcinogens than plant foods because animals are higher on the food chain, so they absorb and store the toxins they take in through the plants or smaller animals they eat throughout their lifetimes. Because pesticides are directly sprayed on plants, it may at first glance seem that plants would contain more pesticides; however when an animal eats a plant with pesticides or industrial residues, the residues are absorbed into the animal's system and stored in its body fat, tissues, and bones. When we consume animal foods, we are eating the animal's lifetime accumulation of toxins!

In addition to the pesticides and environmental toxins in meat, dairy, and other animal products, growth hormones and antibiotics are profusely administered to livestock, poultry, dairy cattle, and farmed-raised fish on a regular basis. At least one in six farmers injects his cows with genetically engineered growth hormones, and around 90 percent of the twenty-nine billion pounds of beef consumed in the United States each year comes from cattle that have been fattened by hormone implants. The steroid hormone implants used in beef cattle are inserted under the skin to make the animals gain weight more quickly. At least one of these hormones is feared to cause cancer in humans.

A reason for avoiding dairy, apart from the animal fat, is the genetically engineered growth hormone given to cows called bovine somatotropin (BST). And although the manufacturer of this hormone insists that it is safe, it too has been linked to cancer. BST makes cows more susceptible to infection, which increases their need for antibiotics, the residues of which end up in the milk.[22] So it is with chickens and other farm animals—adverse raising conditions make it necessary to administer large amounts of antibiotics to control infections.

Carcinogenic byproducts resulting from cooking animal products is one more reason to eat vegan. Cooked meat contains carcinogens such as PhIP, which is shown to cause mammary carcinomas in female rats.[23] When chicken is cooked, it produces heterocyclic amines (HCAs), the same carcinogens found in tobacco smoke. HCAs are fifteen times more concentrated in grilled chicken than in beef. Undercooked meat (rare to medium rare) is not a solution because it can harbor dangerous bacteria and parasites. Additionally, one-third of the packaged chicken in supermarkets has live salmonella bacteria growing inside the plastic.[24]

Fish too are a source of environmental contaminants. Our lakes, rivers, and oceans are becoming increasingly polluted so the fish living in them ingest toxins that include pesticides and heavy metals like mercury. Chlorinated chemicals such as PCBs and dioxins and even human fecal waste are among the many poisons that are passed on to us when we eat them. Mercury contamination in fish is systemic throughout its tissues and cannot be removed by any cooking method.

Fish that are most likely to be contaminated are the large ones such as swordfish, marlin, tuna, and shark. These fish have long lives, and they eat at the top of the food chain, meaning they eat other fish. Fatty fish are more dangerous than leaner fish because toxins are stored in fat. Fish from more contaminated waters are, of course, a greater source of toxins than fish from cleaner waters. Healthy individuals should seek out the types of fish that are least likely to be contaminated if they wish to eat fish, but if you have cancer it is wisest to avoid fish altogether until you are well.

Apart from the man-made toxins that can contaminate fish, there are natural toxins such as *ciguatera,* which is not known to cause cancer, but can cause intense flu-like symptoms that can be especially weakening to anyone with a compromised immune system; cooking does not destroy ciguatera. Uncooked fish, as in sushi, may contain E. coli and salmonella and can also be a source of parasites. (Avoid eel; it can contain deadly parasites.) Shellfish are especially dangerous because they are filter (bottom) feeders, straining water and its pollutants through their bodies.[25]

In our daily life, we are faced with many environmental toxins that are impossible or difficult to avoid, such as those in the air we breathe. However, by avoiding animal products and eating organically grown, whole, unprocessed foods we can decrease most of the toxicity that we would otherwise absorb. To heal, it is best to eat the cleanest, most toxin-free food possible and give our body the greatest chance to cleanse.

If until now you have been consuming the typical American diet, this must seem overwhelming. First I tell you to eat whole, unprocessed, organic foods, and now I am asking you to cut out meat, poultry, fish, and dairy. I know this seems like an enormous undertaking, and to some, a dreadful deprivation, but it's not as bad as you may think. In fact, if you are open to it, going vegan and organic can become an exciting and scrumptious culinary adventure. It will give you the opportunity to discover wonderful new foods and tastes that are as deliciously life supporting as your old favorites were decadently unhealthy.

Going vegan and organic will require some time and effort. A vegan cooking class or at least a good vegan cookbook will be helpful to get you started. It is never easy to change old habits. There are new cooking methods to learn, new shopping places to find, and different foods to familiarize yourself with, but healthy vegan cooking is a skill that will be priceless to you and your loved ones because it will help to restore your health and that of everyone you cook for.

I'd also like to assure you that you don't have to think you can never eat a bite of animal product again in your life. Once you are well, you can have a little bit of animal product once in a while and not notice ill effects. But now, while you are trying to heal and create a new internal environment, it is very important to be strict with your choices. The one exception is if your doctor says you must have some animal protein; then choose from cold-water fish such as salmon, halibut, mackerel, or trout.

PROTEIN AND OTHER NUTRIENTS ON A VEGAN DIET

By now you may be wondering where your protein will come from if you don't eat meat, poultry, fish, or dairy products. The antioxidants, fiber, and phytochemicals contained in vegetable foods are all fine and dandy, but without meat and other animal products, many people feel they will be protein starved. In reality, this is far from the truth. Protein requirements are much easier to meet than most people think.

Protein Values of Popular Vegan Foods

Food	Protein Values (in grams)	Food	Protein Values (in grams)
2 cups cooked legumes	28 to 32	4 ounces tofu	9
1 cup brown rice	4 to 5	1 cup millet	6
1 cup oatmeal	52 tbsp.	1/2 cup almonds	2 to 5
2 tbsp. seeds	3 to 5	1 tbsp. nut butter	4
1 cup fresh peas	9	1/2 cup mung sprouts	2
1 medium stalk broccoli	6	1 cup leafy greens	3 to 7
1 cup brussels sprouts	7	1 avocado	4
1 cup carrot juice	2		

If you balance your day with at least 2 cups of legumes and 2 cups of whole grains, along with vegetables, sprouts, leafy greens, avocado, fresh vegetable juice, and seeds or nuts, you'll be close to or at your protein requirements. Add one protein shake or smoothie (with whey, soy, or rice protein), and you will have met your protein needs for the day.

As long as we consume a varied diet of whole foods and eat enough calories to maintain our weight, it is improbable that we will lack protein.[26] What we may have heard in the past about plants not adequately providing complete protein is simply a myth. When people speak of complete protein they are speaking of protein with the same ratio of amino acids as egg protein. Amino acids are the components of protein, and eggs, in the past, were considered to have the perfect balance of amino acids. Today, we know that it is not necessary to get all our amino acids from one "perfect" food, or even in one meal. Although plants do not have an amino acid balance that is identical to animal foods, by eating a variety of plant foods throughout the day, and balancing whole grains and legumes, we end up getting all the amino acids we need to have a "complete" protein.

Our Western diet is quite high in protein, ranging from 50 to 100 grams or more per day, but of this amount, healthy individuals can comfortably process 40 to 60 grams daily (8 ounces of fish contains 40 to 55 grams of protein). While our bodies need adequate protein for building and repairing tissue, excess protein must be broken down and excreted. Sulfuric acid and phosphoric acid are byproducts of this process. Excessive amounts of protein also negatively impact a person's acid/alkaline balance and accelerate a loss of alkalizing minerals such as calcium.[27]

However, protein needs often increase for many people who have cancer. There is evidence that tumors take up more amino acids from the blood than some of the normal tissues. If adequate protein is not supplied, the tumor will take protein from muscles and increase wasting. Also, conventional cancer therapy may increase the need for protein. It is estimated that during illness, treatment, and recovery, protein needs almost double and calorie needs increase somewhat. A general guideline when you have cancer is to consume about 90 grams of protein daily for men and 80 grams of protein for women.

Cherie's Energy Soup

Add more protein and essential fats to your diet with Energy Soup.

8 ounces carrot juice
1 peeled, seeded avocado
Dash of cumin

Combine all ingredients in a blender. You can top with grated veggies, such as zucchini, beet, chopped herbs, or chopped nuts.

The iron in plant foods is different from that in meat; it is more sensitive to factors that both inhibit and enhance iron absorption. Meats contain what is called *heme* iron and plant foods contain *nonheme* iron.

Nonheme iron is less absorbable than heme iron, but several nutritional factors greatly enhance its absorption. Ascorbic acid (vitamin C) is the most potent enhancer of iron known. It forms a soluble chelate with iron, significantly promoting absorption. This is easy to achieve because vitamin C is so abundant in the fresh raw vegetables that are plentiful when consuming the whole foods, vegan diet. Also, the presence of adequate calcium helps to remove phosphates, oxalates, and phytates that would otherwise combine with iron and inhibit its absorption.

Some conventional cancer therapies contribute to iron-deficiency anemia. In these instances iron needs increase. Good vegan sources of iron are legumes (beans, dried peas, and lentils); seeds such as pumpkin, sunflower, flax, and sesame; grains such as millet and brown rice; nuts including almonds, cashews, Brazil nuts, and pecans; vegetables such as sea vegetables and green peas; and leafy greens like spinach, parsley, and beet greens.

Zinc is another mineral that people with cancer need to increase in their diet. Ginger root is one of the best sources of zinc; pecans and Brazil nuts are good, as are split peas and lima beans. Whole grains are also a good source, and if the grains are soaked overnight before they are cooked, some of the elements that inhibit zinc absorption are reduced, and zinc absorption will be enhanced.

Calcium is an important nutrient in the Complete Cancer Cleanse Diet. However, with a vegan diet that is rich in dark-green leafy vegetables, beans, and seeds, such as sesame, there is no problem. In fact, vegans are less likely to be calcium deficient than those with diets rich in animal protein because meat contains a high level of phosphorus, which interferes with calcium absorption. Also, high consumption of animal products creates high acidity for most people, causing calcium to be leached from bones to help buffer the acidity. This is one reason why osteoporosis is quite prevalent in Western culture, despite our high consumption of dairy products, and is lower to nonexistent in other parts of the world where little dairy and smaller amounts of meat and fish are consumed.

The calcium from many plant foods is well absorbed; however, a few green leafy vegetables that appear to be good sources are not. These vegetables are high in oxalic acid, which, like high levels of phosphorus, interferes with calcium absorption. Such vegetables include spinach, Swiss chard, and beet tops. This does not mean that we should not eat these vegetables; it just means that we should make sure to eat plenty of other green vegetables without oxalic acid. Leafy vegetables that are a good source of calcium include collards, turnip greens, kale, broccoli, bok choy, and mustard greens. Collards and kale are the best calcium sources (one cup of cooked collards or kale contains more calcium than a cup of milk). Beans and tofu are also a good source of absorbable calcium. Sugar, colas, and coffee interfere with calcium absorption.

To enhance calcium absorption, make sure to get enough vitamin D. Food sources of vitamin D are difficult for vegetarians and nonvegetarians alike, but a few minutes of sunshine on our skin every day will give us the vitamin D we need. To absorb vitamin D from the sun, we do not need to sunbathe for hours in a bikini. Ten to fifteen minutes per day on our arms, hands, and face should be enough. Dark-skinned individuals need more sun exposure than those with pale skin, and those who live in a northern region with very little sun may want to occasionally take a supplement just to be sure they get enough vitamin D. Cod liver oil is especially good. A calcium-enhancing factor is the mineral boron, which boosts compounds that prevent bone loss. Although the standard Western diet is low in boron, the average vegan eats plenty of boron-rich foods such as leafy green vegetables, nuts, whole grains, and apples.

The only nutrients that vegans may wish to pay special attention to are vitamin B_{12} and the long-chain n-3 fatty acid docosahexanoic acid (DHA). Vitamin B_{12} is found mostly in animal foods. The requirements for this vitamin are small; however, as a safety measure, take a sublingual B_{12} supplement along with a B complex vitamin supplement.

The fatty acid DHA is used by the body for brain development and function and is especially important for children. Vision is also dependant on DHA. There is no DHA in the vegan diet, but this should not be a problem if the proper precautions are taken; our body is able to make DHA from another fatty acid, *alpha-linolenic acid.* However, if we eat trans fatty acids (such as in fried and processed foods, margarine, and refined vegetable oils) or if we eat too much *linoleic acid* (notice the spelling difference), our body has difficulty making DHA. Linoleic acid (the one that interferes with DHA production) is found in corn, sesame, and safflower oils. For this, and other reasons that we will discuss in Chapter Eight in the section "Cleansing Your Pantry" (see pp. 198–215), corn, soy, sesame, canola, peanut, sunflower, and safflower oils are not recommended. To help your body manufacture DHA, eat foods that are rich in alpha-linolenic acid, which include ground flaxseed and walnuts.

By becoming vegan, eliminating processed foods, and going organic it is possible to give your body an abundance of phytonutrients, antioxidants, vitamins, minerals, enzymes, essential fatty acids, and fiber, while decreasing your load of additives and toxins. Just be careful to eat a variety of grains, beans, seeds, nuts, and vegetables with a small amount of lower-acid or alkaline fruit. Supplement this with ground flaxseed, B_{12} and B complex supplements, and lots of fresh raw vegetable juice and wheatgrass juice, and you will be nurturing your body with the most wonderfully healing and cleansing foods this earth has to offer.

THE ACID-ALKALINE BALANCING FOODS

In the early 1960s, Dr. Maud Tresillian Fere, a New Zealand physician, reported curing herself of colon cancer by changing her diet to that of whole grains and excluding meat, fish, cheese, sugar, stimulants, spices, and salt. Her theory was that cancer and other degenerative diseases are a result of excess acidity or alkalinity. She said, "In good health our blood and lymph are slightly alkaline, as also are our bodies."[28]

Dr. Fere is among a growing number of health professionals who have observed that degenerative diseases result from systems that are too acidic. Dr. Myron Wentz, founder and director of Sanoviv Medical Institute, has noted that among the most frequent health issues at Sanoviv, tissue acidity is the foremost contributing factor to diseases—approximately 93 percent of the illnesses reported there at the time of this writing.

Because of our Standard American Diet and stressful lifestyle, many people are overacidic, which can contribute to diseases such as arthritis and cancer. Therefore acid-alkaline balancing is vitally important. A small percentage of individuals are high-alkaline producers and must balance their systems by increasing their acidity. (Below is information on tests to determine if you are overacidic, which is very common among individuals with cancer.)

Testing Your Acid-Alkaline Balance

A pH test of your saliva or urine can help to assess your acidity or alkalinity. Your local pharmacy should carry pH Hydrion test paper and a color-graph chart. A one-day measurement may not give you a true picture of your status, but measuring your bodily fluids over a seven-day period will give you a better indication of your pH balance and the effectiveness of your alkaline-balancing diet.

Saliva tests should be taken either one hour before or one hour after a meal. An average pH saliva measurement can be obtained by taking a sample twice a day at the same times for seven days. Add all numbers and divide by fourteen for your average. Repeat the test in four to six weeks. The normal pH of saliva is 6.0 to 7.5, which is necessary to digest starches in the mouth. Urine tests should be performed on the first urine voided in the morning. Normal urine pH is slightly acidic, but should range from 4.6 to 8.0. Diet has a direct effect on this pH measurement. Test your urine for seven days, add all the numbers together, and divide by seven. Try to maintain a pH of 6.5–7.0.

These tests should be looked at in conjunction with medical tests, because they do not always reflect your internal acid-alkaline status. The results may vary significantly in response to your diet (a highly acidic meal) or lifestyle (a stressful situation or strenuous exercise can impact results).

You can perform a simple test to give you an idea if you are an overacidic or a high-alkaline producer. At least two hours before or after a meal, take 1/8 to 1/4 teaspoon bicarbonate of soda (baking soda) in water. Overacidic people will usually not experience any adverse reaction; indeed they may feel better. High-alkaline producers may not respond well. They may notice a negative change in their energy level or feel a bit anxious or hyper. They may even experience a mild digestive upset. They will, however, be able to tolerate well highly acidic foods such as vinegar or lemon juice without any ill effects. People with healthy buffering systems (most often children and healthy adults in their twenties, thirties, and forties) can usually tolerate both tests (the baking soda and the vinegar or lemon juice) well.

Be aware that most people with cancer are acidic. Overacidic people tend to feel exhausted after strenuous exercise and often feel fatigue and lack of stamina, whereas high-alkaline producers tend to be high performers who are full of energy and need only a few hours sleep per night. They can work long hours without getting tired and rarely get a cold or the flu. High-alkaline producers do not fit the normal profile for cancer, but if you should be a high-alkaline producer with cancer, you will need to balance your diet with acidic foods such as citrus and other high-acid fruits, sauerkraut, and vinegar. (For more information on acid-alkaline balancing strategies, see *The Chemistry of Success* by Susan M. Lark, M.D., and James A. Richards.[29])

Some studies have suggested that an acidic environment appears to be predisposing to certain cancers. In 1952 Dr. Otto Warburg was the first to discover that a deficiency of oxygen (a highly alkaline element) at the cellular level causes changes in cells that can lead to the development of cancer. Additionally, many other factors such as free radicals, food allergies, a high acid-forming diet, electromagnetic fields, chemicals, and other toxins produce overacidity in the body. Overacidity causes a host of health problems, and the body's inability to neutralize acids eventually contributes to chronic, long-term health problems such as autoimmune diseases and cancer.[30]

Not only is cell function dependent on alkaline balance, but the blood also must maintain a very narrow range of slightly alkaline pH between 7.35 and 7.45. This is difficult for the body to do because the typical American diet is composed of foods that are either very acidic in their chemical makeup or cause an acidic reaction within the body once they are eaten. These foods include meat, poultry, dairy products, many fruits, nuts, refined sugar, corn sweeteners, chocolate, refined flour products, soda pop, beer, wine, liquor, coffee, and black tea.

The whole foods, vegan diet consists of predominantly alkaline foods, with the exception of certain fruits and nuts, and is the very best food for cancer prevention and healing. I recommend that you balance your diet with about 75 percent alkaline foods and no more than 25 percent acid foods. (See Chapter 5 for a list of the high-alkaline foods and dietary recommendations.)

ORGANICALLY GROWN: A CLEANSING IMPERATIVE

Organic is a word that is often used in conjunction with whole foods and live foods. In order to have the right to label products organic, a farmer must adhere to strict standards. Certified organic food is grown and/or processed without the use of toxic insecticides, chemical fertilizers, sewage sludge, herbicides, additives, growth regulators, genetic modification, irradiation, or fungicides. Organic growers use natural fertilizers or compost, rather than chemical fertilizers.

I urge you to purchase organic foods as often as possible in planning your whole foods cleansing program. Yes, I know that organic foods often cost a bit more than conventionally grown foods, and I also know that many people have to go out of their way to attain them, but it's worth it!

Sometimes organic produce is not even as nice looking as conventionally grown produce, but as we become informed organic shoppers, we will learn how to get the best value for our dollar. And we may be surprised to find that when we leave the expensive meats and processed foods out of our diet, we are spending less on groceries than we did before, even when we purchase organic foods.

WHY BUY ORGANIC PRODUCE?

It is easy to say, "Go organic," but we need to know why in order to be motivated. This will show us why the extra effort and money are worth it.

Organic Produce Has Far Lower Pesticide Levels

Pesticides are substances formulated for one reason and one reason only: to be toxic to living organisms. Most of the pesticides used today are classified as either organophosphates or n-methyl carbamates, developed during World War II as chemical warfare agents.

The book *Five Past Midnight in Bhopal,* by humanitarian authors Dominique LaPierre and Javier Moro, tells the story of that December night in 1984, when the Union Carbide plant manufacturing the n-methyl carbamate pesticide *Sevin* exploded. More than five thousand people died immediately from inhaling the poisonous gas that swept through the poorest areas of the city. Everyone did not die immediately, however. Some died slowly. Today, the death toll has risen to more than 16,000 people. And it is estimated that 500,000 people are now chronically ill from chemical exposure that night and from pesticide-contaminated groundwater.[31]

Both acute and chronic poisoning of humans has been reported from pesticides. Symptoms of acute poisoning include blurred vision, salivation, diarrhea, nausea, vomiting, wheezing, and sometimes seizures, coma, and death. When acute poisoning is less severe, the symptoms are similar to gastroenteritis, bronchitis, or intrinsic asthma. These symptoms are so common that in many cases doctors do not even relate them to pesticides.[32]

Chronic health effects from pesticide exposure include neurological problems such as shortened attention span and early onset Parkinson's disease. Endocrine disruption is another serious disorder that can result from pesticide exposure, because chemicals interfere with hormones by mimicking estrogen in the body, disrupting normal growth and development. Mammals, birds, reptiles, and human beings are all susceptible to endocrine disruption. Reproductive problems and interference with infant development, as well as breast and prostate cancer, have been traced to chemically induced hormone disruption.[33]

Dr. Lynn Goldman of the United States Environmental Protection Agency states that at least 101 pesticides in current use are probable or possible carcinogens. Couple that information with that of the National Academy of Sciences—namely, that our diets are a significant source of exposure to pesticides—and we have a major reason for purchasing organic food.

In 1995 the United States Department of Agriculture (USDA) tested nearly seven thousand fruit and vegetable samples and detected residues of sixty-five different pesticides, with two out of three samples containing pesticide residues. Crop spraying and treating is not where it ends; nonorganic produce may be treated with pesticide after it is harvested, *without informing the consumer.* Making matters worse, the U.S. General Accounting Office reports that only 1 percent of the fruits and vegetables that are imported to the United States are tested by the FDA for illegal pesticide residues; imported produce can be treated with pesticides banned in this country![34] In fact, foreign markets offer a good outlet to sell pesticides that are no longer salable in America.

Pesticide exposure from conventionally produced foods is an even more serious problem for children than for adults. Young children seem to prefer many of the foods that are the most heavily sprayed, such as apples and pears, and on a body-weight basis they consume these foods at levels from three to twenty-one times greater than the average American adult. A test commissioned by the Environmental Working Group, and conducted in an independent laboratory, indicated that two in every twenty-five apples have pesticide levels so hazardous that a two-year-old eating one half an apple per day would exceed the government's daily safe exposure level.[35]

On a pro-organic note, a study of children who consumed organic foods revealed that the level of pesticides in their urine was significantly lower than that of children eating a conventional diet. Organic produce appears to provide a relatively simple means for parents to reduce their children's (indeed the whole family's) exposure to organophosphorus pesticide.[36] (It is true that organic produce has been found with some pesticide contamination, probably due to air- and water-borne contamination, but the level is significantly lower than the conventional counterpart.[37])

Washing Produce

Because of the challenges that are sometimes involved with buying organic produce, I am frequently asked if there is a way to wash or soak produce to remove the pesticides. If you must choose between conventional produce and no produce at all, it is far better to choose conventional vegetables and fruits than not to eat them. The most effective way to deal with conventionally grown produce is first to wash, then peel. To wash, pour 1/4 cup of ordinary 3 percent hydrogen peroxide into a sink full of water. Soak the produce for twenty minutes and then rinse with clean water; this will also kill parasites. Although some pesticides can be at least partially washed off, there may still be some residue left. There is, however, a category of pesticides known as systemic pesticides that are actually taken into the plant tissues; neither washing nor peeling can remove them.

Organic Produce Has a Higher Nutritional Value

Apart from having much lower levels of pesticide contamination, another important reason for us to buy organically grown produce is its superior nutritional value. Plants absorb nutrients from the soil, and healthy soil is rich in minerals and alive with microorganisms.

Since the advent of agriculture, farmers regularly nourished and replenished their soil in order to have abundant and vigorous crops that were resistant to pests. They understood that healthy soil is essential to growing healthy plants. With the green revolution and the arrival of industrial farming, it was no longer necessary to nourish the soil because chemicals could replace proper stewardship of the land. Again, convenience has had a price, and the result of industrial farming is produce that is inferior in every way.

In a 2001 study published in the *Journal of Complimentary and Alternative Medicine*, on average, organic produce contained 27 percent more vitamin C, 21 percent more iron, and 29 percent more magnesium than conventional produce, and all twenty-one minerals compared in the study were higher in the organic produce.[38]

Tips for Buying Organic

To get the most value for your dollar, try to go directly to the farmer whenever possible. In late spring, summer, and early fall, all over this country, in cities as well as small towns, weekly farmers' markets sell fresh produce; in warm climates they may be open year-round. Almost every farmers' market has at least one organic grower. Get to know your local growers and get to know what is in season at different times of the year.

Purchase what is in season and make that an abundant part of your diet when it is plentiful. By the time you are tired of a certain food, nature will have provided something new. Local, seasonal produce tastes better and costs less than fruits and vegetables transported across the country. Doesn't it stand to reason that foods grown in your region, at any given season, are the best foods for you? God has a way of providing what we need, when we need it.

In springtime, we should emphasize tender greens such as dandelion leaves, all the varieties of lettuce, spinach, and peas. These foods are light and cleansing after a winter of heavier, more building fare. In summer we have luscious vegetables: summer squash, zucchini, tomatoes, corn, and green beans. In fall, hearty cabbages, kale, winter squash, and root vegetables will not only be the best value, they will provide the dense, nutrient-rich qualities needed to sustain us through the winter.

It may be a bit of an ordeal to get to an organic farm or farmers' market, but there is always a festive quality about these local markets; this can become a fun weekly ritual to enjoy with family or friends. Even if you buy from the health food store or co-op, look for produce that is in season, because there, too, the price will be better and the produce will be fresher.

Impact on the Environment: A Moral Responsibility

One last reason that buying organic food is important for our healing process is the correlation between our personal health and the health of all creatures on the planet. With an illness as serious as cancer, we begin to examine the essence of life, and it is almost impossible not to become aware of our interconnectedness with all of nature. The food we eat, the water we drink, the air we breathe, and our own body are all a part of the same creation, fashioned by the same Creator. Today's industrial agricultural practices are poisoning creation.

Many of the pesticides currently used are classified as persistent chemicals, which will continue to stay in the environment for many years after they have done their work on the plants and insects. This, in turn, is poisoning us. It is estimated that every person alive today—even babies and young children, and those in the most remote parts of the world—carries at least 250 different chemicals within his or her body. These chemicals, which did not exist before 1945, are mainly from agriculture.[39] We can manage to wash and peel a good deal of the pesticides away from our food, but we can't wash or peel them away from our environment. By buying conventionally grown produce we are buying into the economic system that is poisoning us and threatening our very existence.

We Have a Voice

Individuals often heal themselves by detoxifying their bodies, but if industry continues to destroy our environment, the cycle will continue and the cancer epidemic will continue to grow. Industrial agriculture exists because people buy into it, purchasing its products because they are cheaper, more convenient, and sometimes more attractive. According to spokespersons promoting industrial pesticide use in agriculture, this is the only way for crops to produce a sufficiently high yield to feed the world's population.

However, Dr. David Suzuki in *Science Matters* gives a different picture. Studies have shown that the average reduction in productivity for organic crops is just 20 percent. Without wasteful distribution practices, this is enough food to feed the world. Also, with organic agriculture, the study showed a 56 percent reduction in energy required per unit of yield. Of the organic farms studied, there was a 40 percent greater colonization by fungi that help plants absorb nutrients, three times as many earthworms, and twice as many pest-eating spiders.[40] Also, when we calculate the cost of industrial agricultural practices, we forget to add in the cost of groundwater pollution, soil depletion, and the health risks faced by farm workers and consumers.

Each of us has a voice. In the United States, we vote with our dollar, and if we refuse to buy foods that contribute to the poisoning of our earth and ourselves, food producers will look for alternatives.

Dean Ornish, M.D., author of numerous books on reversing heart disease, said that the difference between illness and wellness is that in *i*llness one focuses on the *I,* and in *we*llness, the *we* is emphasized. For our health, I recommend not buying into the "I" mind-set that ignores the rapid destruction of our planet. By buying, or growing, organic food, we are voting with our forks and with our dollars. We are saying no to the devastation that is taking place all over the world in the name of greed, helping not only to heal ourselves but to heal our earth by stepping on the little *i* and embracing the *we.*

THE EASY CLEANSE PROGRAM

As you read through the next four chapters, you will embark on a fascinating, healing journey with The Complete Cancer Cleanse Program. If you are overwhelmed because you are working full-time and tired, or too sick or weak to follow the complete program, look for the Easy Cleanse Programs, which start at the end of the next chapter. These will help you do some basic cleansing steps. When you feel better, are not so overwhelmed, or can take a vacation and have some time to focus on more aspects of your healing process, you can work through some of the other steps in The Complete Cancer Cleanse Program.

5

HEALING, CLEANSING FOODS

Truly the vegetable kingdom contains our best medicine.

—Henry G. Bieler, M.D.,
Food Is Your Best Medicine

From the days of Hippocrates until now it has been known that certain foods have disease-preventing and disease-fighting benefits. Just as chemists are beginning to understand how substances in whole foods can prevent cancers from forming, they are also coming to understand how certain nutrients in foods assist in cancer treatment.

There is not only health insurance in our outdoor gardens, there's healing. Much of the current nutritional research focuses on compounds called phytochemicals (*phyto* is derived from the Greek word for plant; these are the natural chemicals in plants) as well as the vitamins and minerals in whole foods. Every bite of broccoli or slice of tomato contains thousands of little verbal tongue twisters, like the tomato's lycopene, p-coumaric acid, and chlorogenic acid, and broccoli's isothiocyanates and sulforaphane. These compounds protect plants from sunlight and disease, and they also protect and heal us.

Although phytochemicals have been known to exist for a long time, study of their protective role in our health is relatively new. At present, tens of thousands of phytochemicals have been identified as food components, which give plants their colors, odors, and flavors. Studies suggest that many of these compounds may help prevent disease; these include pigments such as carotenes, flavonoids, and chlorophyll. One serving of vegetables can have up to ten thousand different phytochemicals—such as coumarins, allyllic sulfide, monoterpenes, and lutein—helpful in the prevention and treatment of cancer, as well as diabetes, cardiovascular disease, hypertension, and numerous other conditions.[1]

Phytochemicals are thought to work for us in several ways, one of which is through their antioxidant action. Antioxidants are substances that inhibit the destructive effects of oxidation in the body, and they are found mostly in fruits and vegetables. These substances protect cells from the toxic molecules called free radicals, those unstable molecules that attack healthy cells in an attempt to stabilize themselves by picking up another electron. Although free radicals are a result of the normal metabolic processes, their production increases with any kind of exposure to environmental toxins, infection, intense exercise, many processed foods, or excessive sunlight. Antioxidants "cut 'em off at the pass," before they make an attack.

Another way that phytochemicals are thought to protect us is by controlling certain substances and carcinogens that promote disease. Phytochemicals, like sulphoraphane (broccoli and cauliflower), work their magic by boosting the activity of Phase II enzymes—the enzymes that detoxify carcinogens by hooking them up to molecules that act like furniture movers' dollies. Within hours of broccoli's arrival in the stomach, carcinogens are wheeled out of cells.[2] Another phytochemical, indole (cabbage, brussels sprouts, kale) helps to induce protective enzymes that deactivate excess estrogen.

Although the foods we are about to discuss have been studied for their healing properties, do not think that any one food will be a "magic cure." All the fruits, vegetables, legumes, grains, nuts, and seeds that are commonly used as food contain phytochemicals, as well as vitamins, minerals, and enzymes; many are rich in fiber, and some have essential fatty acids. All are beneficial. Carrots, sweet potatoes, yams, and winter squash are especially good because of their high beta-carotene content, and certain mushrooms, such as shitake and reishi, show promise as potent cancer fighters.

Who knows which fruits and vegetables will be considered helpful for cancer prevention and treatment in the future? Therefore, it is important to eat a variety of whole, natural foods in order to have the widest scope of cancer-fighting nutrients, and not to focus solely on any one food or food group for our healing. That said, let's take a look at some of the foods that have been shown to be helpful in cancer treatment and prevention and discuss how we can harness their powers to work for us.

FOODS TO CLEANSE AND HEAL

Over the past few years, we have been reading in newspapers and magazines about certain foods that have been touted as "super foods" with exceptional powers to heal and to prevent disease. These are sometimes called "functional foods." According to the International Food Information Council Foundation, functional foods are foods that may provide a health benefit beyond basic nutrition. Some of these foods, such as garlic, have become quite famous for their purported health benefits and have almost developed a cult following. Other foods that have been praised by the media in recent years as functional foods include citrus fruits, cruciferous vegetables, flaxseeds, oats, and tomatoes.

You may be wondering what makes these foods so special. It may be simply that they have been studied. As we said earlier, when we were speaking of the importance of using whole, unprocessed foods, all natural foods are made up of extraordinarily complex groupings of chemical compounds. Some of these compounds are nutrients or substances that provide nourishment. Protein, carbohydrates, lipids (fats), vitamins, and minerals are nutrients. *Foods that are considered functional foods are rich in both nutrients and phytochemicals.*

VEGETABLES AND FRUITS

Eat your veggies! From Mom to the media, this admonition reaches us nearly every day—and for good reason. Vegetables are high in fiber, and they also contain many cancer-fighting substances. Over two hundred epidemiological studies regarding vegetables and fruits found that a variety of plant foods (not just one or two varieties) reduced the risk of nearly every type of cancer.

DNA damage has to occur several times before a cell becomes fully cancerous. At almost every stage of the cancer-development process, phytochemicals found in vegetables and fruits can alter the likelihood of cancer.[3] Our bodies are built primarily to process plant foods. Some experts believe that cancer is a "maladaptation" over time, due to reduced intake of nutrient-rich vegetables and fruits.[4] To our detriment, we have shifted to eat more animal products and processed foods and less and less whole, plant foods.

In 1992 the National Cancer Institute launched the "Five-a-Day for Better Health" campaign to get people to eat more of these cancer-preventing foods. I recommend that you go far beyond that goal and get eight to ten servings a day of vegetables and a small amount of the recommended lower-acid and alkaline fruits (see p. 118). Though that may sound like a lot, it's actually easy when you count in fresh juices, which are an integral part of this program (1 cup of vegetable juice equals one serving). Additional servings can be obtained easily. Each of the following equals one serving: 1 cup raw leafy vegetables, 1/2 cup nonleafy raw or cooked vegetables, one medium fruit, or 1/2 cup cut-up fruit. It is important to eat at least half of the servings raw, because many of the anticancer compounds are found in highest concentration in raw foods.

If vegetables and fruits reduce the risk of cancer, then they are even more important to the healing of cancer, for preventing metastases (spreading of tumors to other parts of the body) and for cleansing. Many fruits and vegetables are rich sources of glutathione, a powerful antioxidant and a key agent in converting fat-soluble toxins to less harmful water-soluble forms that can easily be excreted, making it one of the most important anticarcinogens in our cells. They are rich in other nutrients as well, such as vitamin C, beta-carotene, zinc, and selenium that help detoxify and eliminate toxins such as heavy metals, pesticides, and solvents.[5] Raw fruits and vegetables provide high levels of glutathione, whereas cooked vegetables and fruits offer much less. It's worth noting that the body absorbs glutathione when taken from food, but it absorbs very little when taken in supplemental form. So listen to your nutritionist—*eat your vegetables*!

Several vegetables and fruits are considered "superheroes" for cleansing the body and fighting cancer. Though citrus fruits have been studied for their cancer-preventative properties, they are not an integral part of The Complete Cancer Cleanse Program because they are highly acidic and a little higher in sugar than many other fruits. (See the Acid-Alkaline

Balancing Diet on pp. 128–29.) Take special note of the foods highlighted in this chapter and include them often in your daily meal planning.

Cruciferous Vegetables

It was first reported in the 1970s that cruciferous vegetables are associated with lower cancer risks. The complete family of cruciferous vegetables include bok choy, broccoli, brussels sprouts, cabbage, cauliflower, collard greens, kale, kohlrabi, rutabagas, mustard greens, horseradish, radish, watercress, and turnips and their greens.

Cruciferous vegetables are rich in phytochemicals known to fight cancer, which include sulforaphanes, indoles, indol-3-carbinols, and isothiocynates. Isothiocyanates fight cancer by stopping carcinogens before they have a chance to be activated. Like Pac-Man, they "latch onto the enemy," speeding up their removal from the body. This phytochemical is especially helpful in cases of lung and esophageal cancers. Consuming isothiocyanate-rich, cruciferous vegetables may also prevent cancers of the gastrointestinal tract and the respiratory system.[6]

Indole-3-carbinol has been associated with lower rates of breast and prostate cancer. A form of estrogen appears to promote cell division that can lead to cancerous breast tumors. It has been reported that a diet rich in vegetables, especially the crucifers, decreases the formation of this dangerous form of estrogen.[7] Indole-3-carbinol stimulates both Phase I and II detoxification enzymes in the liver and is a very active stimulant of detoxifying enzymes in the gut as well.[8]

Make cruciferous vegetables a daily part of your diet. They can be steamed, stir-fried with coconut oil, added to your fresh raw vegetable juices, and eaten raw in salads.

Tomatoes

Several epidemiological studies have shown that eating tomatoes and tomato products is related to a lower risk of a variety of cancers. Tomatoes, like all foods, are a complex mixture of chemical compounds, but the one in tomatoes that is getting the most attention is a phyto-chemical called *lycopene*. Lycopene is a carotenoid that is responsible for the red color in tomatoes, and it is a powerful antioxidant that fights cancer.[9]

Scientists at Cornell University reported that two other tomato phytochemicals (of tomatoes' multitude of phytochemicals), known as *p-coumaric acid* and *chlorogenic acid*, snuff out the formation of cancer-causing substances. During digestion, the body routinely makes compounds called nitrosomines out of nitric acid and amines (components of proteins). P-coumaric acid and chlorogenic acid "act like Dustin Hoffman in *The Graduate*; they grab hold of the nitric acid and whisk it out of the church—er, cell—before it can marry amine."[10]

Tomato juice lovers take note. Cornell's Joseph Hotchkiss gave volunteers tomato juice and discovered that their bodies made fewer nitrosomines.[11] And lovers of Italian food will be happy to learn that the most available form of lycopene is in tomato sauce, not in raw tomatoes.[12] All forms of tomatoes are beneficial, however. Because pasta and pizza are not a part of The Complete Cancer Cleanse Diet, the best way to enjoy tomato sauce is over brown rice, millet, or quinoa, which can be quite delicious. Throw in some garlic and lightly steamed broccoli, kale, or other vegetables, and you have a tasty meal with loads of protective phytonutrients. And bake or steam spaghetti squash (rich in beta carotene) and top it with marinara sauce. Tomatoes are also delicious raw in salads and homemade juice.

Garlic

Since antiquity, garlic has been revered for its strengthening, protective, and stimulating properties. In recent years, many of the folk claims surrounding garlic have been studied by modern science. A number of promising assays show garlic as a cancer-suppressing agent.

Among garlic's scientific proponents, one of the most esteemed is Dr. Benjamin Lau, M.D., Ph.D., a professor of microbiology, immunology, and surgery at Loma Linda University School of Medicine in California. According to Dr. Lau, garlic's role in preventing cancer may be due to its ability to detoxify heavy metals in the body. Heavy metals, such as lead, cadmium, cobalt, and mercury, can be absorbed into our systems through exposure to polluted air, paints, drinking water, contaminated fish, and dental amalgams. Dr. Lau cites numerous studies that confirm garlic's ability to detoxify toxic substances. One in particular reported that four of the sulfur compounds isolated from garlic protected liver cells against damage caused by the toxic chemical carbon tetrachloride. Dr. Lau also claims that garlic nullifies the effects of radiation.[13] Additionally, garlic is said to help kill parasites and other pathogens.

In a 1991 study, garlic was shown to stimulate the production of an enzyme that occurs naturally in the body and protects against cancer by detoxifying potent carcinogens. A research team based in New Zealand concluded that one of garlic's compounds produces enzymes in the gut that can clear it of cancer.[14]

Garlic's ability to kill mold, viruses, and bacteria has been well documented over the years. Aflatoxin, a carcinogenic mold that contaminates peanuts, grains, beans, and sweet potatoes, is inhibited by garlic. Garlic works against aflatoxin, both outside the body, when mixed with foods that contain the mold, as well as inside the body. Maybe an intuitive sense of garlic's antimicrobial powers is why Indonesians, who eat lots of peanuts, traditionally combine garlic with their peanut dishes.

Several epidemiological studies also link garlic intake with lower rates of cancer across populations. In northern China where people commonly eat five to ten cloves of garlic per day, there is a lower incidence of stomach cancer. Other studies from Sweden, Italy, and the Netherlands have also shown lowered risk of stomach cancer in people who eat garlic. The Iowa Women's Health Study determined that the women who ate significant quantities of garlic were approximately 30 percent less likely to develop cancer of the colon.[15]

Although cooking destroys garlic's antimicrobial properties, its anticancer agents are not affected as long as garlic's sulfur compound allicin has the chance to develop. Allicin, thought by many to be the most active ingredient in garlic, develops from an enzyme that is freed only after a garlic clove is cut or damaged. Although allicin is destroyed by heat, if garlic is chopped and allowed to sit for ten to fifteen minutes before cooking, the allicin transforms into other compounds that have anticancer qualities, which are not destroyed by heat. When garlic is cooked whole, as in oven-roasted garlic, it does not have anticancer qualities. Therefore, to get the most of garlic's anticancer properties, it is best to chop it and then wait for ten to fifteen minutes before cooking or eating it raw.[16]

In epidemiological studies concerning garlic consumption, there is a good possibility that the populations that consumed the most garlic also consumed the most vegetables and ate less animal fat and refined vegetable oils. Any way you look at it, though, garlic is a healthy and protective dietary addition. Not only does it have therapeutic benefits, it is a natural way to make almost anything taste better. Therefore, if you love garlic, eat all you wish. If it's not your favorite, find ways to incorporate it into dishes you like. The only people who need to limit their garlic intake are those who tend to become easily overheated, because garlic can aggravate this imbalance.

Onions

Onions are one of the richest sources of the flavonoid quercitin. In fact, the onion is the highest quercitin source in the Western diet. Quercitin has been shown to inhibit proliferation (rapid spread or increase) of human breast cancer cells in test tubes and to delay mammary tumor growth in the body.[17]

Onions are one of the earliest known food medicines that have been used to drive impurities from the body. Because they contain a large amount of sulfur, they are excellent for liver detoxification. So don't worry about your breath! Eat onions. Get everyone around you to eat them, too. Include them in stir-fries, steamed vegetables, soups, and salads.

Sea Vegetables

Sea vegetables, or seaweeds, if you must, have been used by sea-dwelling cultures for thousands of years. Although most Americans are not too familiar with these foods, the Japanese have brought the use of sea vegetables to a level of *haute cuisine.* In traditional Oriental medicine, sea vegetables are used to soften hardened areas and masses in the body, detoxify, moisten dryness, remove residues of radiation in the body, alkalize the blood, and alleviate liver stagnancy. They are also seen as beneficial to the thyroid and are used to improve water metabolism and cleanse the lymphatic system.

Sea vegetables contain lignans, although they are not as rich a source as flaxseeds. Sea vegetables are a gold mine of minerals, however, and if for no other reason than this, they should be a regular part of everyone's diet.[18]

In Western trials, the wisdom of the East has been confirmed. An experiment on rats at the Harvard School of Public Health showed that sea vegetables have a consistent antitumor activity. Scientists at the National Cancer Institute in Bethesda, Maryland, have studied the chemical components of a particular algae (a sea vegetable) that appears to be more potent in cancer treatment than the drug taxol, which is a drug that has been used to treat breast and prostate cancer. Research at McGill University in Montreal has shown that sodium alginate, a derivative of the sea vegetable wakame, binds with radioactive strontium 90 in the body, allowing it to be excreted. Agar agar, a sea vegetable that is used in making vegetarian gelatin, has also been shown to bind with heavy metals and radiation, carrying them out of the body.[19]

To benefit from sea vegetables, only a small percentage of our diet needs to consist of them. One Harvard study showed that rats benefited when just 5 percent of their diet consisted of sea vegetables. In our diet this could mean eating a daily bowl of miso soup with sea vegetables, adding some dulse to a salad, cooking beans or rice with a strip of kombu, preparing vegan nori rolls, or making an unsweetened jelled dish with agar agar.

ESSENTIAL FATTY ACIDS

After several years of hearing about the perils of fats, we are now being bombarded with information about *good* fats. Good fats are essential for optimal health; indeed they are part of our healing and cleansing program. They are the omega-3 fatty acids, which are an important component of The Complete Cancer Cleanse Diet. These oils are abundant in certain fish and in flaxseeds. In The Complete Cancer Cleanse Program I emphasize ground flaxseeds and cod liver oil.

Studies have shown that omega-3s (high in alpha-linolenic acid) have pro-oxidant activity in tumor cells. They help make cell membranes more permeable, potentially increasing a cancer cell's sensitivity to therapies.[20] In one study, oils rich in omega-3s or vegetable oils (rich in omega-6) were given to twenty-five women at high risk for breast cancer. The biomarker for breast cancer was measured, and the marker in the omega-3 group significantly decreased, whereas in the omega-6 group, markers did not change.[21]

In the 1950s two independent researchers, biochemist Johanna Budwig and cancer researcher and physician Max Gerson, working independently, discovered the benefits of omega-3 oils in cancer treatment. Gerson found that his regime of live foods and juices was much more effective in dissolving tumors when cold-pressed flax oil was added.

In a study presented at the Twenty-Third Annual San Antonio Breast Cancer Symposium in 2000, Dr. Paul Goss, from the University of Toronto and director of the breast cancer prevention program at the Princess Margaret Hospital and the Toronto Hospital, presented a study that he had conducted with fifty women who had newly diagnosed breast cancer tumors. While waiting for surgery, each woman ate a muffin containing 25 grams (slightly less than 2 tablespoons) of ground flaxseeds every day. At the end of the study, the tumor growth rate in the women who had eaten the flaxseed muffins was significantly reduced compared to those in a control group who ate muffins without the flaxseeds.[22] Another study showed that the higher the level of alpha-linolenic acid (an omega-3 fatty acid), "the less likely the cancer was to spread into the lymph nodes of the armpit or be invasive."[23]

The component of flax that is getting the most attention is lignan, a fiber-related substance with estrogen-like qualities that can bind to estrogen receptors and interfere with the cancer-promoting effects of estrogen on breast tissue—kind of like Meg Ryan's character in *Sleepless in Seattle,* who won the heart of Tom Hanks's character and beat out the "competition." Lignans also increase production of SHGB (sex hormone binding globulin), which regulates estrogen by ushering the excess out of the body.[24]

Lignans also have been shown in animal studies to reduce colon cancer tumors by slowing down cell division and inhibiting the formation of blood vessels around cancer cells.[25]

Although flax oil is an excellent source of omega-3 fatty acids, you have to eat the seeds to get sufficient amounts of the lignans. To get the most benefit from the seeds, they must first be ground because they are very difficult to chew otherwise, and if they aren't broken down, they tend to go through the system unused. To grind flax seeds, just place about 1/3 cup of seeds at a time in a blender or coffee grinder. You can grind enough seeds for a week or two at a time and keep them in an airtight container in the refrigerator. Add a pinch of ascorbic acid powder to the jar of ground flaxseeds to help keep them fresh. The oil in flaxseeds goes rancid very quickly after they are ground, so it is best to grind your own seeds—and don't keep them around too long. I recommend eating two tablespoons of ground flaxseeds per day, which you can add to your breakfast cereal, smoothies, protein shakes, salads, or muffins.

Flaxseed oil is excellent to use in salad dressings or dips. Or you can swig down a tablespoon and chase it with juice. Flaxseed oil goes rancid very quickly; buy it in opaque bottles and keep it in the refrigerator at all times. Date it at purchase and throw it out after three months. Never use this or any oil that has a rancid or bitter taste. And *never cook with flax oil.* It has high amounts of polyunsaturates, which are easily damaged by heat, and oxidized oils are very unhealthy. I recommend virgin organic coconut oil for cooking. Coconut oil, which is high in medium-chain triglycerides, is the most heat stable of the cooking oils, meaning less damage is done to the oil when it is heated.

WHOLE GRAINS AND LEGUMES

Whole grains and legumes (beans, lentils, and split peas) are an important part of The Complete Cancer Cleanse Diet. They are rich in fiber, which helps the body eliminate harmful wastes and expel estrogens. In 1970, British physician Dennis Burkitt observed that a high-fiber diet of whole grains, legumes, vegetables, and fruits reduces diseases of the digestive tract. He reported that in countries where diets are high in fiber, there were fewer cases of colon cancer. Animal products and refined foods contain no fiber, so countries such as the United States and other Western nations that base their diets upon these foods have the highest rates of colon cancer.[26]

Under normal conditions, as the liver filters the blood, it removes excess estrogens and sends them through the bile duct into the intestinal tract. There, fiber soaks them up like a sponge, carrying them out of the body with the other wastes.[27] When there is not sufficient fiber from plant-based foods like whole grains, vegetables, and legumes, estrogens and other toxic substances can pass back into the bloodstream. Also, bile acids are secreted into the intestinal tract to help digest fat; bacteria in the gut can change the acids into chemicals that promote colon cancer. Fiber binds with these bile acids and evicts them, like a bad tenant, before they can damage their dwelling.[28]

Whole grains and legumes are hearty, strengthening foods that will go a long way toward providing us with the calories, protein, fiber, and other important nutrients like vitamin E and selenium (rich in whole grains) that we need to cleanse and heal. Please do not let yourself be duped by the dangerous hoopla being spread by high-protein faddists who say that all carbohydrates are bad and that we should eat a high-protein, animal-based diet.

As we have said before, refined carbohydrates, such as sugar, white flour, refined flour products, and white rice, need to be completely avoided because of their additives, lack of fiber, loss of nutrients, and because these carbohydrates are rapidly converted to glucose (sugar) when digested. Whole grains and legumes cannot be thought of in the same category as refined carbohydrates. They are excellent foods that sustain the body and have a low glycemic effect (lentils are the lowest), which means they have a low insulin response and promote a slow and very low rise in blood glucose. Legumes and whole grains are the most neglected foods in the modern, Western diet, but historically, they have been the primary staple foods for most of humankind.

When adding grains to your diet, always make sure to buy them in the whole form. By this I mean do not buy grains that have been ground into flour, cracked, or transformed in any way. The reason is that whole grains contain natural oils that can easily go rancid, which contributes to toxicity in the body. When grains are intact, the oil they contain is protected from exposure to oxygen (which causes these oils to go rancid). Grind your own grains and use them shortly after they have been ground. Ground, cracked, or flaked grains that sit for a long time period run the risk of containing rancid oils, which can be carcinogenic. When you buy whole grain flours, cereals, or flour products, you do not know how long they have been on the shelf; therefore, it is best to avoid them.

The grains I recommend include whole millet, brown rice in all its varieties, quinoa, buckwheat, amaranth, spelt, barley, and oats. Millet should be emphasized because it has alkalizing properties. This grain is good for people with *Candida albicans* because it has mild antifungal action; candida is very common in cancer patients. Millet's cooling properties make it a good grain for summertime, especially for people who tend to become overheated. Barley also has cooling properties, but it contains gluten, as do oats, and these grains should be limited if you are gluten sensitive. (In the West, we tend to overeat grains high in gluten such as wheat, rye, barley, and oats, and many people become sensitive to gluten as a result. Sensitivity reactions stress the body, create more toxic byproducts, and can cause inflammation of the intestinal tract.)

Oats, quinoa, and buckwheat have warming qualities and are especially good to help warm you up in wintertime. When you are traveling, oatmeal may be the best choice for breakfast in most restaurants. Quinoa is particularly high in protein; it is great as a bed for steamed vegetables or as a breakfast cereal. Brown rice is a good grain to eat year-round because it has a neutral thermal nature; cream of brown rice cereal makes a great breakfast, and you can grind brown rice for delicious cereal. Wheat should be avoided as much as possible because many people have allergies, intolerance, or sensitivities to it. We have completely overeaten wheat in this country, causing high sensitivity to it in many individuals.

All grains can be cooked whole and served as a bed for vegetables, beans, tofu, and tempeh. They can also be ground in small quantities, using a blender, and made into creamy porridges for breakfast.

Legumes: Beans, Lentils, and Split Peas

Once the center of a meal in times past, beans have been nearly forgotten in American cuisine; however, they are an important part of our Cancer Cleanse Program. One study has found a lower rate of breast cancer in Hispanic women, who eat twice as many beans as white women. An estrogen-blocking phytoestrogen in beans may account for the difference.[29]

The best beans to cook are mung and adzuki beans because they are easy to digest. Mung beans, in both traditional Chinese and Ayurvedic medicine, are thought to have detoxifying properties. Chickpeas (garbanzos) are a good source of iron—a mineral that many cancer patients can become deficient in. Lentils—very stabilizing for blood sugar level—are practical because they cook in less than an hour. All legumes are good, so give beans, lentils, and split peas some prominence in your meal planning. Get Beano (available at most pharmacies and supermarkets) if beans cause gas.

The nutritional benefits of both grains and legumes are enormous;

therefore, add them to your diet daily, except when following a specific cleansing regime. Legumes can be sprouted, making them a good alkalizing food that is highly nutritious. All legumes are high in amino acids, but when sprouted and eaten raw or juiced, they have some of the highest protein available in vegan foods.

Preparing Legumes and Grains

Both legumes and grains benefit from being soaked in filtered water for eight hours, or overnight, before cooking them. Before you soak them, sort through the beans, peas, lentils, or grains to remove any dirt, small stones, or broken or discolored legumes or grains. Rinse them, and then place them in a bowl. Cover them with filtered water and add a pinch (about 1/4 teaspoon) of ascorbic acid powder (vitamin C), which is available in most natural food stores. The pinch of ascorbic acid will help to neutralize any harmful molds (such as the carcinogenic aflatoxin) that may be present in the grains or legumes. It is not necessary to measure how much water you use to soak the grains or beans, just cover them by about two inches of water.

After soaking, pour the beans or grains through a strainer to drain off the water. Then place them in a pan with fresh, filtered water. (A pinch of Celtic sea salt may be added to grains, but not beans. It will make them tough. Add salt after they are cooked.) Always rinse quinoa before cooking or it could have a bitter taste. It is best to measure the cooking water when you cook grains. Except for millet and barley, use 2 cups of water for each cup of grain. Millet is best cooked with 2 1/2 to 3 cups of water per cup of grain; to cook barley, use 3 cups of water to each cup of barley. Barley, oats, and rice take about forty-five minutes to cook; millet and quinoa take about twenty minutes; buckwheat takes about fifteen minutes.

For beans, lentils, or split peas, it is not necessary to measure the cooking water. After pouring off the soaking water, place the legumes in a pan with fresh water and cover them by about two inches. Bring them to a boil, then turn down the heat, cover, and let them cook over low heat, stirring occasionally until they are very tender. Add salt, vegetables, and seasoning near the end of cooking. Cooking time will depend on the type of bean; add more water if necessary. A strip of kombu (a sea vegetable that can be purchased at health food stores and Asian markets) can be added to the pot along with beans or rice at the start of cooking; this sea vegetable adds minerals and makes beans easier to digest.

Cooking beans and grains is really quite easy. Still, a good whole foods vegan cookbook or a cooking class can be invaluable. Just remember to presoak the beans or grains with a little ascorbic acid in the water to help eliminate molds. Most cookbooks do not use this method, but grains and beans prepared this way are healthier; you will also find that they taste cleaner.

SPICE UP YOUR LIFE!

Spices are also an important part of The Complete Cancer Cleanse. The American Institute for Cancer Research has noted several herbs and spices that are cancer-preventative as well as cleansing and healing. The Institute will send you a free set of markers for your herb garden if you call them at 1-800-843-8114, extension 10, and request "Herb Markers." The following is a list of cancer-fighting herbs and spices:

Turmeric

A ground spice that is an essential part of curry dishes, turmeric contains the yellow compound known as *curcumin.* Curcumin is known to inhibit Phase I detoxification while stimulating Phase II and can be very beneficial in the cleansing programs, especially The Liver Cleanse. This spice is very helpful in cancer prevention as well, since it has been found to inhibit carcinogens such as benzopyrene (found in charbroiled meat).[30] This spice has also been shown to directly inhibit the growth of cancer cells.[31] Curcumin tends to stay in the gastrointestinal tract, where it appears to block the release of damaging substances that can turn on cell proliferation, resulting in colon polyps or colon cancer. In cell culture studies, it has been shown to slow prostate cancer cell proliferation.[32] I recommend that you make lots of curry dishes and add turmeric to rice and bean dishes.

Rosemary

A pine-scented herb with needle-like leaves, rosemary contains carnasol, a phytochemical with strong antioxidant action. Carnasol may help detoxify substances that initiate the cancer process and help prevent skin and lung cancers. It can be added to soups, bean and rice dishes, and vegetables.[33]

Oregano

An herb associated with Italian food, oregano contains quercitin, a powerful antioxidant also in onions (see p. 98), and farnesol, a phytochemical that has blocked the growth of a fast-growing skin cancer in mice. Oregano is delicious in Italian dishes (especially marinara sauce), vegetarian chili, and Mexican dishes.[34]

Ginger Root

The National Cancer Institute lists this spice as one of the foods with the strongest anticancer activity. Ginger's pungent flavor comes from the phytochemical gingerol, which is believed to induce cancer-cell death. This is one reason I include ginger in nearly all of my fresh juice recipes. This spice is also delicious in Asian dishes, stir-fry, and with beans and rice.[35]

Mint

A good source of the phytochemical limonene, mint can be added to herbal tea, juiced with cucumber for a refreshing beverage, or added to melons or salads. Limonene has been found to be a powerful anticancer agent that can block the development of breast tumors and shrink them.[36]

Parsley

Not just a garnish on our restaurant plate anymore, parsley is an herb of prominence studied by The National Cancer Institute. These green sprigs have a subtle flavor, but they are a not-so-subtle inhibitor of cancer. Parsley packs a wallop of protection against carcinogens. This herb is rich in polyacetylenes, phytochemicals that offer protection against a certain carcinogen in tobacco smoke. Parsley may also help regulate the body's production of prostaglandin, a substance that is a powerful tumor promoter. Add a handful of parsley to your juice recipes. It is also good in salads, tomato sauces, soups, salad dressings, and with most vegetables.[37]

THE POWER OF FRESH RAW JUICE

Raw juices do most of the excellent things that solid raw foods do, but they put minimum strain on the digestive system because they are broken down into an easily absorbable form. And you can juice more of them for a glass than you would probably eat in a day. It is believed that the nutrients from fresh juices are at work in the bloodstream within about thirty minutes of drinking them. The alkalinity of raw vegetable juices, in particular, is a powerful ally in our fight against cancer, because cancer cells thrive more easily in an acidic environment. Raw juices are "alive" and packed with an abundance of nutrients—from the phytochemicals discussed earlier to a cornucopia of cancer-fighting vitamins and minerals. Juices are also replete with enzymes, which greatly benefit the digestive system.

Juicing is the best way I know for us to get a high concentration of all the beneficial elements found in fruits and vegetables that will help us fight cancer. Fresh raw juices made from organic vegetables and fruits give us a concentration of these beneficial nutrients far superior to any supplement we can buy. Our Creator has designed fruits and vegetables with the perfect proportions of elements that act synergistically to give our body what it needs. No matter how sophisticated a pill or man-made formula may be, it cannot come close to the balanced perfection of these whole foods. Juicing unlocks this power and gives it to us in a concentrated, easily assimilated form. It would be difficult, if not impossible, to eat the amount of vegetables in one meal that we can drink in a glass of juice.

Can freshly made juices become powerful healing tools in our fight against cancer? Just ask a close family member of mine. She discovered an unfriendly looking mole, made a trip to her dermatologist, waited a long, long time for results from a test, and finally got an answer—from one of the top labs in the nation that had eventually received the specimen from another lab.

Her dermatologist said she stupefied the experts! They said it looked like a melanoma that had regressed to a precancerous state. Pondering the whole matter, the only thing she saw that could possibly have made the difference, the only real health change she'd made in her lifestyle, was to faithfully start juicing vegetables and fruits every morning.

Add one to three or more glasses of fresh juice to your daily diet of fresh, whole, unprocessed, organic foods, and you will be providing your body with a "bushel basket" of healing, cleansing, and protective agents. (For delicious juice recipes, see my book *The Juice Lady's Guide to Juicing for Health*.)

The fresh juice program is a major part of the one that worked for my own cleansing and healing. This is the reason I'm known today as the Juice Lady.

Numerous alternative cancer treatments are available that successfully rely on fresh raw juices as an integral part of their treatment, such as those at Sanoviv Medical Institute and the Gerson Institute. Pioneers in juice therapy include Max Gerson, M.D., Rudolph Breuss, Alec Forbes, M.D., and Norman Walker. These researchers of the mid-twentieth century all used fresh raw juices to treat cancer patients with great success, often cases that the medical establishment deemed hopeless. (For stories of cancer cures that used juice therapy, read *A Cancer Therapy: Results of Fifty Cases,* by Max Gerson, M.D.) Although there have been no published studies to scientifically affirm the life work of these great healers, a wealth of current research illustrates the protective powers of fruits and vegetables, and with all that we know about them, juicing makes a lot of sense.

A number of years ago juicing got a "bad rap" in the sense that many individuals in the media began telling people that eating the vegetables and fruits is better than juicing because juice has no fiber. That statement simply is not true. Juice is replete with soluble fiber, such as the pectins, which are very good for the colon. But most importantly, juice offers the opportunity to consume produce, and parts of produce such as leaves, stems, seeds, and peels, which we would probably never eat otherwise, along with amounts of produce we'd probably never be able to consume in a day. It has *never* been recommended that people give up eating vegetables and fruits in trade for juice, but rather that people do both. Juice is a marvelous supplement to a high-fiber, whole foods diet that includes the insoluble fiber, and a great way to cleanse and heal the body. I do not recommend that you drink very much fruit juice, however, because of the sugar content and acid. Through juice fasting and other cleansing programs that incorporate fresh juice, we can greatly facilitate the elimination of toxins and restore balance to our body. If you want to make juicing a way of life, you will need a good juicer—one that is easy to clean and use. It should have a strong motor—1/2 horse power (hp) is best. Avoid those that don't eject the pulp, need a tool to loosen the blade, and are time-consuming to clean. I recommend the Juiceman® juicer by Salton. I tried nearly every juicer on the market and chose this one as the easiest to use (see Products and Information).

"Superhero" Juices

I have found the following juice ingredients to be very helpful in fighting cancer. The recommendations are adapted from *The Juice Lady's Guide to Juicing for Health.*[38]

- *Beet* juice has been used traditionally to cleanse and support the liver. It has been used to reverse and prevent radiation-induced cancers.
- *Cabbage* juice contains a high concentration of two phytochemicals: indole-3-carbinol and oltipaz, which help increase the enzymes that protect us from cancer.
- *Carrot* juice is one of nature's richest sources of beta-carotene. It is also believed by some to have powerful cancer-fighting properties. Virginia Livingston, M.D., had her patients drink 2 pints of fresh carrot juice every day. Max Gerson, M.D., prescribed ten 8-ounce glasses of juice daily, alternating carrot-apple and green juices throughout the day.
- *Garlic* juice has been found to inhibit tumor growth.
- *Green* juices such as parsley, spinach, kale, chard, mustard greens, and wheatgrass are rich in chlorophyll. Research at the University of Texas Systems Cancer Center found that chlorophyll might block the genetic changes that carcinogenic substances produce in cells.
- *Tomato* juice is rich in lycopene, which has been widely studied for prostate cancer prevention. Tomatoes are also rich in p-coumaric and chlorogenic acid, two phytochemicals that block formation of highly carcinogenic nitrosomine compounds within the body.

Carrots and beets are considered high glycemic vegetables, compared with other healthy vegetables. But if you compare carrots and beets with other foods, they are moderate to low, and their health benefits are many. Beets are a moderate glycemic index food at a value of 64 and carrots are in the low glycemic index food range (that's anything below 55) at a value of 49.[39]

WHEATGRASS JUICE

Apart from raw juices, the other foods that we have reviewed thus far have been the object of numerous scientific studies that support their use in cancer prevention and, in some cases, treatment. Wheatgrass, however, has had very few studies to back up the antidotal claims by hundreds, if not thousands, of cancer survivors who swear that wheatgrass juice saved their lives.

Yoshihide Hagiwara, M.D., and other Japanese scientists found that wheatgrass juice helps to deactivate the carcinogenic and mutagenic effects of benzopyrene, a substance found in smoked fish and charbroiled meat. The enzymes in wheatgrass have also been found to neutralize and detoxify toxins from automobile exhaust and other pollutants. Dr. Chin-Nan Lai at the University of Texas showed that wheatgrass has a powerful antimutagenic effect and antineoplastic ability (the ability to fight tumors).[40]

Wheatgrass juice has never been found to have any toxic properties or negative side effects. Its proponents claim that it increases hemoglobin production, rebuilds the bloodstream, purifies the blood, improves the body's ability to heal wounds, creates an unfavorable environment for candida growth, eliminates drug deposits from the body, and neutralizes toxins and carcinogens in the body. It is also said to help purify the liver, lower blood pressure, and improve blood sugar metabolism.

A double-blind scientific study published in the *Scandinavian Journal of Gastroenterology* showed wheatgrass juice to significantly improve symptoms for persons suffering from ulcerative colitis. It also significantly reduced the severity of the rectal bleeding and abdominal pain associated with the condition.[41]

Wheatgrass is grown by first soaking wheat berries overnight, then planting them, usually in a tray with about two inches of soil, and letting them grow until the shoots are about seven inches high. The freshly harvested wheatgrass is then cut, rinsed, and forced through a special juice extractor to press out the rich, green juice from the tender shoots. The chlorophyll-rich cocktail is drunk, one or two ounces at a time, two times a day, for the most benefit. Wheatgrass is easy to grow at home, and a high-quality, manual wheatgrass juicer can be purchased for less than two hundred dollars. A good electric juicer, however, can cost as much as six hundred dollars.

Many health food stores, juice bars, and natural foods restaurants offer wheatgrass juice by the one- or two-ounce shot. It is best always to drink wheatgrass juice immediately after it is made to get the most benefit. Some people like the taste of wheatgrass juice, but most do not. If you don't like it, it is comforting to know that you only have to take it in small doses and swig it down quickly. John and I say, "Forget savoring this juice! Just get it down." But then, you may love the flavor of green grass and do better than we do.

WATER

In his book *Your Body's Many Cries for Water: You Are Not Sick, You Are Thirsty,* F. Batmanghelidj, M.D., says, "The simple truth is that dehydration can cause disease."[42] Neither Dr. Batmanghelidj, nor anyone else I'm aware of, has ever alluded to the fact that failing to drink enough water can cause cancer, but it's well recognized that dehydration can contribute to the overall diseased state of the body.

The body is composed of approximately 75 percent water. We need to replenish our water daily for efficient functioning of all our organs and systems. In addition, water is a key part of cleansing because it flushes toxins from the body. The "water rule" is eight-to-ten 8-ounce glasses (64 to 80 ounces) of purified water per day for a person weighing 120 to 160 pounds. If you are over that weight, divide your weight in half to determine the suggested number of ounces of water per day to drink. For example, if you weigh 200 pounds, you should drink close to 12 glasses or 100 ounces of water. Herbal teas and mineral waters count for your water quota. Black tea, coffee, alcohol, and commercial beverages do not. Though they contain water, they are also dehydrating.

If you have never been a water drinker, you may be quite dehydrated. Start adding water slowly, with one or two extra glasses of water per day, and judge how you're doing. If your feet and ankles swell, drink more diuretic juices, such as cucumber and parsley mixed with carrot, and eat more asparagus; add no more than the one or two extra glasses of water daily until your system balances out. Then add a third extra glass of water, and so forth, until you work up to the recommended number of ounces of water per day. Make sure that the water you drink is purified. (See Chapter Eight for water purification recommendations.)

GREEN TEA

Epidemiological data show that green tea has a potentially preventative effect against cancer in humans. Green tea contains polyphenols, which may protect against certain cancers by inhibiting chemical carcinogens. One cup of green tea contains about 100 to 200 milligrams of tannins; the main constituent being EGCG. EGCG has been shown to reduce the number of tumor promoters in tissue.[43] Even though green tea does have some caffeine, its benefits may outweigh its liabilities. You may benefit by drinking a cup of organic green tea each day.

HARMFUL FOODS

Logic says that if certain foods are known or thought to contribute to cancer, then once a person has that disease, he or she should avoid those foods and substances even more. Diet is more important once someone is diagnosed with cancer, because not only do we want to get rid of the cancer present in the body, we want to prevent metastases (spreading of cancer to other parts of the body) and the return of cancer in the future.

The Complete Cancer Cleanse Program is about getting rid of all harmful substances in our diet, our body, and our personal environment so we can completely cleanse our system, give it every opportunity to heal, and supply superior nutrition to assist in the healing process.

SWEETEN NO MORE

I have placed sweeteners in the harmful foods section because they are among *the most* detrimental foods available, along with alcohol, meats, animal fats, refined foods, and junk food. Otto Warburg, whom I mentioned earlier, stated, "The prime cause of cancer is the replacement of the respiration of oxygen in normal body cells by a fermentation of sugar." Sugars have been shown to feed cancer cells, and possibly to contribute to the formation of the protective coating that envelopes cancer cells, preventing the white bloods cells of the immune system from detecting and destroying them.

High-sugar diets are associated with an increased risk of breast, biliary (bile duct or other systems of ducts within the liver), pancreatic, and colorectal (colon/rectal) cancers. Refined sugars cause a rapid rise in blood sugar levels, because they are quickly absorbed into the bloodstream. The pancreas, in response, releases insulin. And too much insulin can cause a host of physical problems, among them the promotion of certain kinds of cancer cell growth, including breast, colon, stomach, ovarian, endometrial (the lining of the uterus), lung, and prostate cancer.[46] High insulin levels may also be a predictor of whether breast cancer returns after treatment, because high insulin levels increase the risk of recurrence and death at least eightfold.[47]

The wisdom of the East also recommends *no sweets* for anyone with cancer. Oriental medicine states that foods having a "sweet flavor" may contribute to cancer because "they are moistening and promote dampness and mucous." (Mucous is a primary substance we are working toward detoxifying on The Complete Cancer Cleanse Program.) Additionally, Tibetan medicine warns against sweet, white foods during cancer.[48] Avoid the following: white and brown sugar, dried sugarcane, turbinado sugar, sugar alcohols such as manitol and sorbitol, honey, maple syrup, malt barley syrup, brown rice syrup, fructose, and all other sugars and sweeteners. Although some sugars that are not refined are billed as healthier fare, all sugars have a similar effect in the end. If you want a bit of sweetener in something, use stevia, an herbal sweetener, which can be found at most health food stores. Stevia actually helps regulate blood sugar levels.[49]

Artificial sweeteners are even worse than sugars. In 1991 an article appeared in the *Journal of Advancement of Medicine,* reviewing the potential detrimental effects of aspartame (popularly known as NutraSweet) as the cause of brain tumors. According to the National Cancer Institute

Whole Foods Glycemic Index[44]

The *Glycemic Index* was developed by David Jenkins in 1981 to measure the rise of blood glucose after consumption of a particular food.[45] This index shows the rate at which carbohydrates break down to glucose (sugar) in the bloodstream. The best way to keep insulin levels low is to eat carbohydrates that rank low on the glycemic index. Foods with a high glycemic index release glucose into the bloodstream rapidly, causing a fast rise in blood sugar and a subsequent rise in insulin.

High Glycemic Index Foods—greater than 70

Food	Index
Dried dates	103
Baked potato	100
Red-skinned potatoes	93
Rye bread	76
Whole grain bread	72
Watermelon	72

Moderate Glycemic Index Foods—55 to 70

Food	Index
Cantaloupe	65
Raisins	64
Beets	64
New potatoes	62
Banana	62
Brown rice	55
Sweet corn	55
Popcorn	55

Low Glycemic Index Foods—below 55

Food	Index
Sweet potato	54
Kiwi	52

Carrots	31 to 51*
Oatmeal	49
Green peas	48
Orange juice	46
Grapes	46
Oranges	44
Apple juice	40
Plums	39
Pears	38
Apples	38
Chick peas	33
Beans	31
Lentils	29
Cherries	22

*NOTE: There's a 10 to 15 percent variation in these numbers, depending on the standards used to define the index. I have found greater than 15 percent glycemic value differences for carrots; however, both values place carrots in the low glycemic index. They are considered a high glycemic food compared to most other vegetables, but they are low glycemic compared to other foods.

there has been a significant increase in primary brain cancers and brain lymphomas since 1985; previously these conditions were rare. This sharp increase occurred within one to two years following licensing in July 1983 of the chemical aspartame for use in beverages. Prior to that, there was a high incidence of brain tumors in rats after experimental administration of aspartame. The Food and Drug Administration scientists and a public board of inquiry strongly recommended delaying this license pending further investigation, but that did not happen. There is a long list of central nervous system reactions to aspartame, which suggest brain aggravation by this chemical.[50] If aspartame is heated, it is even worse. When the temperature of aspartame exceeds 86 degrees Fahrenheit, it converts to formaldehyde.

In light of these findings, I recommend that you do not use *any* artificial sweeteners, for any reason—that means no packets of artificial sweetener and no artificially sweetened soda pop or other artificially sweetened beverages or desserts. Be wary of all new artificial sweeteners coming on the market such as sucralose (Splenda®), which has chlorine molecules substituted for some of the sugar molecules (see www.red-ice.net/specialreports/sucralose.html). Tampering with and changing natural foods has not produced good outcomes in the past, and there is no reason to believe that it will in the future.

MEAT AND OTHER ANIMAL PRODUCTS

Why are animal products a bad choice on The Complete Cancer Cleanse Program? Animals are at the top of the food chain, and the toxins they take into their bodies through toxic air, soil, feed, and water are stored in their flesh, just as they are stored in ours. Add to that the way factory farm animals are raised—overcrowding, unsanitary conditions, high-stress situations, poor feed that has completely deviated from animals' intended fare, antibiotics, and continual injections, such as growth hormones to make them grow faster or produce more milk. All this contributes to disease for the animals, and toxic flesh and fat for us to ingest.

Rather than give factory farm animals more humane conditions, such as fresh air, decent food, and freedom to move around, the majority of them are pumped full of antibiotics and fed food sprayed with pesticides and filled with additives that are sometimes unthinkable. When we eat the flesh of sick animals (growing numbers have been found to have cancerous tumors at the time of processing), we take this unhealthy flesh into our bodies. All this disease at factory farms leads to new and more lethal strains of bacteria, such as E-coli, that contaminate our food supply. The commercial answer to this problem is irradiation of animal products, which leads to more free radicals, generated when gamma rays break up the molecular structure of food; or the latest—spraying meat with a virus designed to kill E-coli. These are moral issues as well as valid health concerns that cannot be ignored.

Studies have found that up to 80 percent of breast, bowel, and prostate cancers are attributed to diet. International studies show a strong correlation between meat consumption and these cancers. When meat is cooked, substances known as heterocyclic amines form, which require acetylation by P450 enzymes. People with fast acetylation can have an increased risk of colon cancer.

Also compounds such as NH3 and N-nitroso compounds form from meat residues by action of bacteria in the colon. NH_3 is a promotor of colon tumors and is chemically induced by N-nitroso compounds.[51] Actually, more than twenty heterocyclic amines are produced in cooked meats that are highly mutagenic to bacteria in the colon.[52]

SMOKED, PICKLED, AND SALT-PRESERVED FOODS

In a study evaluating ten thousand people who developed colon cancer, high amounts of NDMA (nitrosodimethylamine) were found in their systems, which doubled their risk of developing colon cancer. NDMA compounds are found in smoked and pickled foods, those preserved with salt, and in beer.[53]

ALCOHOL

We constantly hear reports in the news that wine and beer are good for the heart and help to lower the risk of cardiovascular disease. We need to ask, "Who is funding these studies and how are they being conducted?" to see if they are really valid. And more importantly we need to ask ourselves, "What about the liver? And what about cancer?" Alcohol is hard for the liver to metabolize, interferes with the detoxification process, and is very acidic. Alcohol will actually stop the cleansing process.

The Iowa Women's Health Study evaluated over 41,000 women between the ages of fifty-five and sixty-nine, comparing 109 females with lung cancer to 1,900 females without lung cancer, and found that those with lung cancer consumed more alcohol. The difference was largely related to beer consumption, which was a significant predictor of lung cancer risk. Those who drank one beer per week had a higher risk of developing cancer, compared to those consuming less than one glass per week.[54]

In addition, there is indication that all alcoholic beverages—beer, wine, and hard liquor—are risk factors in cancer of the colon, liver, breast, oral cavity, pharynx, larynx, and esophagus.[55] Ethanol or its metabolites may be the culprit. Some of the possible cancer-contributing mechanisms are as follows:

- Alcohol contains contaminates and generates metabolites that may be carcinogenic.
- Alcohol acts as a solvent, increasing the penetration of other carcinogens into target tissue.
- Alcohol reduces the bio-availability of cancer-preventative nutrients.
- Alcohol inhibits detoxification of carcinogenic compounds.
- Alcohol increases the rate at which some compounds become carcinogenic.
- Alcohol can affect hormonal status, increasing the risk of hormone-related cancers.

- Alcohol may increase cellular exposure to oxidants (substances that oxidize other substances, creating more free radicals).
- Alcohol can suppress immune system function, which needs to be at its peak to destroy cancer cells.

On The Complete Cancer Cleanse Diet, no alcohol—beer, wine, or hard liquor—is allowed. And though beer and wine may have shown promise for preventing heart disease, it is not a good idea to drink every day. In that case the liver never gets a rest. There are other far more effective means of preventing heart disease, which have been shown by such distinguished doctors as Dean Ornish, M.D.

AVOID CARCINOGENIC FOODS

Peanuts and peanut products like peanut butter contain aflatoxins. Other foods that contain natural toxins are black pepper, button mushrooms (the common kind), carrot tops (don't juice them), and alfalfa sprouts. Limit these foods in your diet. Throw away celery that is wilted, yellow, or has brown spots; it can be carcinogenic. Completely avoid salted and smoked foods and pickled foods. Avoid all barbecued and blackened foods. Avoid all artificially colored, flavored, and preserved foods and *all* artificial sweeteners.

Food Substitutes

For foods not on The Complete Cancer Cleanse list, you can substitute the following:

Excellent Cleansing Food Choices

Wheat Products	**Substitutions**
Wheat bread	Breads made with rice, millet, amanranth, quinoa (look for labels that say "gluten free")
Wheat crackers	Rice, flaxseed, dehydrated veggie crackers
Wheat pasta	Rice, corn, quinoa, or buckwheat pasta
Breakfast cereal	Cream of brown rice, millet, quinoa, oat groats, oatmeal
Dairy Products	**Substitutions**
Cow's milk	Almond, rice, hazelnut, soymilk (homemade is best)

Cheese	Almond cheese
Eggs	Tofu scramble
Meat	Tofu or tempeh
Sweeteners	Stevia
Beverages	**Substitutes**
Coffee	Grain-based coffee substitutes
Black tea	Herbal tea
Soda pop	Mineral water; iced herbal tea
Condiments	**Substitutes**
Commercial mayonnaise	Healthy or homemade mayonnaise
Salt	Celtic sea salt (gray salt)

THE ACID-ALKALINE BALANCING DIET

As we reduce the acid load of our body and restore our mineral reserves and buffer systems (the blood and kidneys have a buffer system to balance pH), and reduce stress on our organs of elimination, we should see astounding results in our health. In Chapter Four, we looked at the reasons for choosing The Acid-Alkaline Balancing Diet. What follows are the diet and foods that are part of The Acid-Alkaline Balancing Plan.

SELECTING THE RIGHT FOODS

Among health educators, there is considerable misinformation and conflicting information concerning the relative alkalinity or acidity of foods. The following information is based on the work of Susan M. Lark, M.D., and the information from technical sources compiled at the University of California Davis, Department of Food Science and Technology, and Cornell University, Department of Food Science.[56]

The following is a summary of the acid-forming foods and the high-alkaline foods.

Acidic Foods

Though many other foods are considered highly acidic, I am only listing whole foods that could be considered part of The Complete Cancer

Cleanse Diet. Until one's system is pH balanced, these foods should be kept to a minimum, meaning only a few servings. Just how many servings depends on your system, but a good rule might be no more than 25 percent of your diet from the high-acid group. The rest should come from the high-alkaline foods.

Highly Acidic Foods (pH between 1 and 4.6)

Fruit Juice: Lemon, lime, cranberry, grapefruit, currant, orange, apple, pineapple, prune, and tomato juice

Fruit: Lime, lemon, cranberry, gooseberry, loquats, orange, plum, rhubarb, apple, raspberry, grapefruit, boysenberry, strawberry, blackberry, kumquat, quince, blueberry, pineapple, crab apple, kiwi, apricot, and raisins

Vegetables: Sauerkraut, cucumber, and tomatillo

Condiments: Vinegar, pickles, olives, and mayonnaise

Moderately Acidic Foods (pH between 3.1 and 5.6)

You can have the moderately acidic foods listed a bit more often, but they should still be limited.

Fruit: Peach, cherries, pear, mango, Asian pear, guava, and banana

Vegetables: Tomato, eggplant, and string beans

Low Acid to Alkaline Foods (pH between 4.6 and 9.5)

Choose from these low-acid to alkaline foods most often as part of the cleansing program.

Fruit and Fruit Juice: Figs, papaya, persimmon, avocado, cantaloupe, and melon other than watermelon, which is high on the glycemic index

Vegetables: Pumpkin, sweet peppers (green, red, yellow), spinach, carrot, squash, kale, asparagus, turnip, cabbage, broccoli, parsnip, sweet potato, onion, peas, turnips, red potatoes (high on the glycemic index), artichoke, cauliflower, parsley, celery, corn, lettuce, and brussels sprouts

Legumes: Beans, lentils, and dried peas. These legumes become very alkaline when sprouted and are highly nutritious.

Nuts and Seeds: Almonds, walnuts, flaxseeds, hazelnuts, pecans, macadamia nuts, poppy seeds, sesame seeds, pumpkin seeds, and sunflower seeds

Grains: Rice, millet, quinoa, amaranth, hominy, and spelt, which contains gluten

Chew, Chew, Chew Your Food!

Have you ever heard that you should chew your food at least twenty to thirty times before you swallow it? Now, studies reveal the real truth. A Japanese study evaluating 242 cases of gastric cancer (compared with 484 matched controls) found that insufficient chewing put stress on the digestive system, which promoted cancer. Those who ate meals rapidly, had intense stress, or had lost teeth were at the highest risk.[57] It is possible that the cancer that resulted from insufficient chewing was due to incompletely broken-down food particles and their toxic metabolites in the gastrointestinal tract or maldigestion of important nutrients, or immune suppression from stress, causing people to eat rapidly (or all of these).

Part of The Complete Cancer Cleanse Program is "complete chewing" of all food. As the saying goes, "We should liquefy our food and chew our juice." This means that whatever we are eating should remain in our mouth long enough for digestion to begin there, where it was intended to begin.

TRAVELING AND EATING IN RESTAURANTS

When dining out or on the run, there are nearly always choices that complement The Complete Cancer Cleanse Program. Look for the following selections at these differing restaurants:

- *Vegetarian restaurants:* select almost anything that is dairy free
- *American restaurants:* select salads, salad bars, and vegetable, bean, lentil, or vegetarian split pea soup
- *Italian restaurants:* select polenta, eggplant dishes, salads, escarole soup, white bean soup
- *French restaurants:* select vegetable dishes, dairy-free soups, bean dishes

- *Thai and Vietnamese restaurants:* select tofu dishes, vegetarian spring rolls, vegetable dishes, rice dishes
- *Indian restaurants:* select vegetarian curries, lentils, rice dishes, cucumber salad
- *Chinese restaurants:* select sizzling rice soup, tofu or bean curd dishes, vegetable dishes
- *Mexican restaurants:* select beans and rice, tostado with corn tortilla and no cheese, vegetarian taco with corn tortilla
- *Japanese restaurants:* select miso soup, vegetarian sushi, tofu and vegetable dishes
- *Coffee bars:* select herbal tea
- *Fast-food restaurants:* select salads

WHERE ARE THE EMPEROR'S CLOTHES?

Some individuals in the medical and scientific community would tell us there is nothing about food that can heal or cleanse our bodies. These are the people who recommend chocolate milkshakes for cancer patients who have lost their appetites, or Jell-O when nauseated "just to keep something down," even though such fare is known to be very unhealthy, even contributing to cancer due to the sugar and other unhealthy ingredients. I've always wondered how anyone could heal on such unhealthy food.

Why some individuals in the health-care community have adopted the idea that once a person has cancer it really doesn't matter what someone eats—as long as the patient gets ample calories and protein and is able to "keep something down"—is a mystery to me. In looking over popular books from government agencies and various organizations, published as guidelines for cancer patients, I have read about recommendations of ice cream, ginger ale, milkshakes, or eggnog to inspire the taste buds of cancer patients who aren't hungry. When food just doesn't taste right, they're encouraged to cook on a barbecue or add bacon bits or ham strips to vegetables. Wine, beer, or mayonnaise makes soups taste better, we're told. To get rid of a strange taste in the mouth—eat hard candy. Nauseous? Try flavored gelatin, Popsicles, or carbonated beverages.

These recommended foods and cooking practices are the very ones people who don't have cancer are cautioned not to eat or do in order to prevent cancer. They have prompted me to ask, "Where are the emperor's clothes?"

HOW STRICT SHOULD WE BE?

When I was taking organic chemistry as a prerequisite for my master's degree in nutrition, I learned about the importance of not letting a drop of anything foreign get into my test tube when I was attempting a reaction. Once the reaction was achieved, those extra drops of stuff weren't so important—up to a point, that is. When it came to test time, I was religious about guarding what went into my test tube.

The same thing was true for me when I was trying to get well. I instinctively knew I had to be absolutely strict with everything I ate and drank, and it paid off quickly. I was bounding out of bed in just three months.

How strict should you be? Very strict—as strict as I was with my chemistry test tubes during a test. You're attempting to create new biochemistry in your body and that takes diligence, especially in the beginning. Take heart if the endeavor seems daunting. Thousands have succeeded in the past. *And you can, too!*

The Easy Cleanse Food List

I've rated foods from Excellent to Good/Fair to Poor Choices for quick referral in menu planning and shopping. All these foods should be purchased as organically grown whenever the choice is possible.

Excellent Cleansing Food Choices

Vegetables	Fruits	Grains	Legumes	Herbs/spices
Artichoke	Avocado*	Amaranth	Beans	Anise
Asparagus	Cherry	Brown rice	Lentils	Basil
Beetroot and greens	Guava	Millet	Split peas	Bay leaf

Bok choy	Mango*	Quinoa`	Hummus	Cardamon
Broccoli	Melons	Wild rice		Cilantro
brussels sprouts	Papaya*			Cumin
Cabbage	Pear			Dill
Carrot	Peach			Dry mustard
Cauliflower				Fennel
Celery				Ginger root
Chicory				Marjoram
Chinese lettuce				Oregano
Chives				Parsley
Dandelion greens				Rosemary
Endive				Saffron
Escarole				Tarragon
Green/yellow beans				Thyme
Green peas				Turmeric
Kale				
Kohlrabi				
Leeks				
Lettuce (green leaf, Romaine, Bibb, spring greens)				
Okra				
Onions				
Radish				
Seaweed				
Snow peas				
Spinach				
Summer squash				
Sweet potato				
Swiss chard				
Watercress				
Winter squash (all varieties)				
Yam				
Zucchini squash				

*The starred fruits are the best choice because of their low acidic rating, except watermelon, which is poor because of its high glycemic index.

Nuts/Seeds	Milk Substitutes	Condiments	Oils	Beverages
Almonds	Almond milk	Celtic sea salt	Flax	Herbal tea
Hazelnuts	Rice milk	Stevia	Olive	Green tea
Flaxseeds	Hazelnut milk	Kelp powder	Coconut	Fresh juice
Pumpkin seeds	Coconut milk	Soy sauce		Wheatgrass juice
Sesame seeds		Tamari		Coconut water
Sunflower seeds		Spike/Mrs. Dash		
Nut/seed butters, such as almond and tahini		**Other Foods** Homemade healthy dressings and sauces		

NOTE: Though tomatoes are quite acidic, I rated them excellent because of their lycopene content and the fact that studies have proven their cancer-fighting properties. Tomatoes and their products such as tomato sauce and juice should still be included in the acid category of no more than 25 percent of the daily diet.

Good to Fair Cleansing Food Choices

Fruits*	Vegetables	Other Foods	Animal Products**
Apple	Cucumber	Corn tortillas	Salmon
Apricot	New potato	Italian dressing	Halibut
Blackberry	Sauerkraut	Sun-dried olives	Trout
Blueberry	Tomatillo	Carob	Mackerel
Boysenberry			Healthy commercial dressings
Cranberry			
Kiwi			
Kumquat			
Lemon			
Lime			
Loquat			
Pineapple			
Plum			
Raspberry			

*I have rated these fruits and vegetables in the fair category because they are rated high to moderate in acidity (new potatoes are ranked here because of their higher glycemic index). This does not mean you shouldn't eat them, but that they should be limited to no more than 25 percent of your diet. Also, frozen vegetables and fruits are better than canned, but they are only a fair choice when compared to fresh produce. However, when fresh is not available, frozen is the best choice.

**If your doctor or nutritionist advises you that you need some animal protein, these fish are the best choices.

Poor Cleansing Food Choices

Fruits	Vegetables	Cereals/Grains	Other
Banana	Red-skinned potato	Boxed/commercial cereals	Mayonnaise
Grapes	Russet potato	Packaged flours	Pickles
Grapefruit	Sweet corn	Packaged crackers	Olives
Orange	White rice		Animal products other than fish: butter, cheese, milk, molasses, honey
Watermelon			Maple syrup, fructose
Dried fruits of all kinds (because of potential molds and higher sugar content)			Coffee Refined oils Most commercial salad dressings

Harmful Food Choices

Animal Products	Prepared Foods	Desserts
Bacon	Pizza	Cakes
Barbecued foods	Anything with hydrogenated oil	Chocolate
Bologna	Peanuts and peanut butter	Cookies
Hot dogs	Waffles	Doughnuts
Fried fish/chicken/steak	Pancakes	Ice cream
Salami	Frozen dinners	Pie
Smoked ham	Jell-O	Popsicles
Smoked fish	Sweetened yogurt	All other desserts

Beverages	Misc.
Beer	Aspartame
Hard Liquor	Hydrogenated or refined vegetable oils
Wine	MSG
Soda pop/diet soda	Shortening/lard
	Syrups, both sugar and sugar free

6

THE CLEANSING PROGRAMS

The doctor of the future will give no medicine but will interest his patients in the care of the human frame, in diet, and in the cause and prevention of disease . . . The physician of tomorrow will be the nutritionist of today.

—THOMAS EDISON

Whatever treatments or cancer-care programs we choose, there's one aspect of cancer treatment and prevention that we can't ignore, and that is *cleansing our body.* Although many treatment protocols are available, toxins in the body prevent most methods from being completely successful. To get the maximum benefit from any and all cancer-care treatments, it is imperative to rid the body of the buildup of waste, overacidity, toxins, drugs, heavy metals, parasites, fungi, other pathogens, and dead cells.

As we clear our organs and systems of unwanted substances, we speed our healing and help to prevent incidence of cancer in the future. The eleven programs in this chapter have worked for me and for countless numbers of people I have advised through the years. I will begin with The Acid-Alkaline Balancing Cleanse, because many people with cancer are acidic. Then I will suggest eight cleanses—The Intestinal Cleanse, The 7-Day, Kick-Start Liver Cleanse, The Gallbladder Cleanse, The 3-Day Kidney-Bladder Cleanse, The Lung Cleanse, The Skin Cleanse, The Lymphatic System Cleanse, and The Blood Purifying Cleanse—to get rid of the toxins in these organs of elimination. Then I will present two specialized cleanses: The Parasite Cleanse, in case you have parasites in your body, and The 30-Day Heavy Metal Detoxification Program to assist in ridding your system of heavy metals. If you are weak or experiencing cachexia (wasting caused by cancer), you may not be able to do many of these programs until you are stronger. However, four of these cleanses are appropriate for everyone: The Acid-Alkaline Balancing Cleanse, The Lymphatic System Cleanse, The Lung Cleanse, and The Skin Cleanse. Each of the cleanses is presented so that it can be followed individually; therefore some of the directions will be repeated. If you are working full time, are especially weak, or are overwhelmed with treatment schedules, follow the Easy Cleanse Programs at this time.

I encourage you to take full advantage of these cleansing programs and to stick with the detoxification process until you have cleansed your body and are enjoying a high level of wellness.

THE ACID-ALKALINE BALANCING CLEANSE

Many people with cancer tend to be overacidic and can greatly benefit from an alkalizing program. Restoring proper acid/alkaline balance is one of *the most* important steps we can take in prevention and recovery from cancer. This is a program everyone can follow, no matter how weak or debilitated one may be. (See Chapter Four for information on acid/alkaline testing to determine your body's pH.)

The mainstay of this cleanse is The Acid-Alkaline Balancing-Cleansing Diet. A sample menu plan follows:

Easy Acid-Alkaline Balancing Cleanse

Everyone can follow the guideline of this sample menu and choose foods from the Easy Cleanse Food List at the end of Chapter Five.

Sample Menu Plan for The Acid-Alkaline Balancing-Cleansing Diet

Breakfast

Fresh vegetable juice
Herbal tea or green tea
For your main breakfast course, choose from:
Papaya Smoothie (See box on p. 130.)

Cream of brown rice cereal, millet, amaranth, or quinoa with almond or rice milk
Toasted rice bread with melted soy cheese or almond butter
Tofu scramble with onions, mushrooms, and green pepper and melted almond cheese on top

Mid-Morning Break

Fresh vegetable juice, wheatgrass juice, or herbal tea

Lunch

For your main lunch course, choose from:
Vegan split pea soup and green salad
Hummus sandwich with broccoli sprouts and grated zucchini on rice bread
Garden burger on spelt or rice flour "hamburger buns" or rice bread (avoid spelt if you are gluten sensitive) or garden burger lettuce wrap
Vegan chef salad with beans and cooked or sprouted grains such as quinoa and spelt berries

Mid-Afternoon Break

Fresh vegetable juice, homemade lemonade (sweetened with stevia), homemade cranberry juice, or herbal tea

Dinner

First course:
Vegetable or lentil soup
Garden salad or spinach salad
For your main dinner course, choose from:
Vegan stir-fry with tofu over a bed of quinoa or wild and brown rice
Tostado: black beans, brown rice, grilled onions, shredded greens, cilantro, avocado on a corn tortilla with salsa dressing
Rice tabbouleh
Steamed vegetables over a bed of wild and brown rice with melted almond cheese on top
Vegan Caesar salad topped with avocado and sunflower seeds

Bedtime

Herbal tea: chamomile, peppermint, or rose hips are good

A diet composed of menu plans like the sample Acid-Alkaline Balancing Diet Plan will restore the body's buffering capabilities when used along with alkalinizing supplements and alkaline-enhancing habits.

Papaya Smoothie*

Nutrition tip: Papaya contains the enzyme papain, which helps with digestion and helps alleviate inflammation.

3/4 cup almond, rice, or coconut milk
1 papaya, peeled, seeded, and cut into chunks
2 tablespoons protein powder**
1 1/2 teaspoons freshly grated organic lemon peel
1 teaspoon pure vanilla extract
4 ice cubes (optional)

Pour the milk into a blender and add the papaya, protein powder, lemon peel, vanilla, and ice cubes, as desired. Blend on high speed until smooth and serve immediately. If you want it cool without ice, make sure the milk and papaya have been chilled before blending. It's best not to add too much ice, however, because ice-cold drinks cause the colon to contract, which is not good for digestion.

*From *The Ultimate Smoothie Book* by Cherie Calbom

**Whey protein is recommended for those with cancer because it is the protein with the highest concentration of glutamine, an amino acid, and branched chain amino acids. It's good fuel for white blood cells, and it has been found to help prevent mouth ulcers and suppression of the immune system in those receiving chemotherapy.[1] If you are sensitive to dairy whey, try goat whey. If you are sensitive to both of these, then choose rice protein. (For product recommendations, see Products and Information, p. 326.)

ELECTROLYTES

Calcium, magnesium, potassium, and sodium are the electrolytes that help the body achieve a normal pH balance. Restoring the alkaline mineral reserves, especially the electrolytes, is necessary for promoting and maintaining proper pH balance and for detoxification of toxins. Consume lots of vegetables and vegetable juices. You may also wish to take a mineral supplement.

BUFFERED VITAMIN C

Buffered vitamin C can be used daily as part of an alkalinity restoration program. Human beings do not make vitamin C, so we need to constantly replenish our supplies. It is estimated that if we were to produce vitamin C, our body would produce as much as 10 grams (10,000 milligrams) per day.[2] Vitamin C in its natural form as ascorbic acid is mildly acidic. In addition, most vitamin-C products on the market are acid-based. Therefore, if you are acidic it is best to take a buffered vitamin C, which is combined with alkaline minerals. Vitamin C is most effective when taken with bioflavonoids (a naturally occurring compound in plants) in half to equal amounts.

ALKALINE WATER

Alkaline water can be used daily as part of an alkalinity restoration program. Several devices use an innovative technology to convert ordinary tap water, through filtration and electrolysis, into alkaline water that can greatly benefit health and restore and maintain proper pH balance. Some individuals have attributed their recovery from cancer directly to restoring their acid-alkaline balance and credit drinking alkaline water as a significant contributing factor.[3] (See Products and Information.)

ALKALINE-ENHANCING HABITS

Moderate Aerobic Exercise
Stress Management Techniques

Follow this acid-alkaline balancing program for the first four weeks and continue to follow it as recommended throughout the cleansing cycles. Include the supplements as needed to restore alkalinity.

Now that you have achieved an acid-alkaline balance, you are ready to begin the eight organ-cleansing programs.

THE INTESTINAL CLEANSE

A toxic, underactive bowel promotes disease in several ways:

- It creates a disease-friendly environment where parasites and yeasts such as *Candida albicans* can grow.

- It contributes to slower transit of feces; therefore, more toxins penetrate the bowel wall and move into the bloodstream and lymph. From there they are carried throughout the body, causing increased vulnerability to disease in weakened tissues and organs.

- The immune system becomes depressed when it is overwhelmed with toxic substances because it takes a host of white blood cells to get rid of toxic debris. Cancer and other degenerative diseases develop more readily when the immune system is depressed. It contributes to inflammation in the intestinal tract, which depresses the immune system.

If these reasons aren't enough for cleansing the intestinal tract, toxic drugs (such as chemotherapy drugs), effects of radiation, or drugs associated with surgery must be detoxified and eliminated, and dead cancer cells discarded. Therefore, it is imperative that the intestinal tract be cleansed so that it is as clear and clean as possible and able to move waste efficiently from the body.[4]

BOWEL CARE

Throughout our life, our bowel has probably not been fed or cleansed properly, and there's no doubt it has been sluggish due to standard American dietary choices, our stressful lifestyles, and our failure to always heed nature's call. Cleansing the intestinal tract doesn't happen in a week; it may take several months to years for the intestinal cleansing and healing process to be completed. I advise starting with The Easy Intestinal Cleanse Program, and as your body gets stronger and healthier, you can move on to experience more intense cleanses, as desired. These intense cleanses release toxins very quickly, and only a body that has reached a significant level of strength and health can handle this type of cleansing. When you are weak and fighting cancer, the cleansing process should be slow.

If at any time you start feeling considerably worse for more than a few days, you can slow the cleanse by drinking one less cleansing cocktail. In this way you can reduce cleansing reactions.

I have started with this system of elimination because the intestinal tract is the primary channel to carry waste from the body as the other organs of elimination are cleansed and toxins are released; throughout the cleansing process it will need special attention. The easy, outlined Intestinal Cleanse schedule is followed by The Complete 7-Day Intestinal Cleanse and an explanation of each part of the program.

The 7-Day Easy Intestinal Cleanse

Various aspects of this program are explained on pages 134–38.

Phase I:

7:00 AM Cleansing Cocktail Fiber Shake: psyllium and bentonite with 8 ounces of water or flax fiber and bentonite. (NOTE: Psyllium can be drying and somewhat irritating to the colon.)

8:00 AM 3 ounces beet juice; see the Beet Juice Express on page 136

Take supplements:

- Calcium-magnesium supplement
- Vitamin C (buffered is best if you are acidic) or an antioxidant supplement
- Digestive enzymes (see p. 137) and/or herbal colon cleanse supplements

8:30 AM Breakfast: Cooked whole grain cereal such as millet or amaranth with rice or almond milk

10:30 AM Cleansing Cocktail Fiber Shake

11:30 AM Take herbal colon cleanse supplements and/or between-meal digestive enzymes with 1 cup flaxseed; chamomile or peppermint tea

12:30 PM Lunch: garden salad with lemon juice and olive oil dressing and vegetarian soup (preferably homemade) or other vegetarian foods chosen from the cleansing foods list in Chapter Five (pp. 122–24)

- Digestive enzymes

2:00 PM	Cleansing Cocktail Fiber Shake
3:00 PM	Green juice: wheatgrass juice or any fresh greens juiced, such as kale, parsley, and spinach, juiced with cucumber, celery, carrot, and lemon for flavor
3:30 PM	Herbal colon cleanse supplements and/or between-meal digestive enzymes
5:30 PM	Dinner: garden salad with vegetarian chili or steamed vegetables or stir-fry vegetables over a bed of wild and brown rice or quinoa; choose from the cleansing foods on page 122–24 of Chapter Five ➤ Digestive enzymes
6:30 PM	Herbal tea
7:30 PM	Colon flush: colonic or enema
9:00 PM	Herbal tea such as chamomile or peppermint; one calcium-magnesium supplement before retiring*

*It is best to retire early, between 9:00 PM and 10:00 PM, because you need extra rest when your body is working hard at cleansing.

During the day, consume a minimum of 64 ounces (eight 8-ounce glasses) of purified water in addition to the other liquids.

NOTE: Though this cleanse is titled The 7-Day Easy Intestinal Cleanse, it often takes six months or more to completely cleanse and heal the colon. This seven-day program should be repeated for as many weeks as it takes to free the colon of all encrusted, putrefactive buildup. See the cycle of cleanse programs schedule at the end of this chapter.

THE COMPONENTS OF THE 7-DAY COMPLETE INTESTINAL CLEANSE

Now let's look at the individual components that are part of The 7-Day Complete Intestinal Cleanse.

THE CLEANSING COCKTAIL FIBER SHAKE

The Cleansing Cocktail consists of 8 ounces purified water to which we add 1 tablespoon bentonite (clay water), 1 teaspoon psyllium husk powder (flax fiber may be substituted), and 1 to 2 teaspoons organic black cherry juice concentrate or cranberry concentrate or 2 ounces papaya or apple juice as desired. Place in a container with a lid screwed on tightly and shake well. Drink immediately because the fiber thickens very quickly to a gel-like consistency.

Drink three shakes per day. I recommend hydrated bentonite and psyllium husk powder or flax fiber. Make sure the psyllium husk powder you use has been heat-sterilized rather than treated with ETO or irradiation treatments; hydrated bentonite is better than powdered bentonite. Black cherry juice concentrate, cranberry concentrate, and organic papaya juice can be found at most health food stores and at some grocery stores.

This cleansing cocktail is designed to remove unwanted substances from the alimentary canal. Derived from the colloidal mineral montmorillonite, bentonite is an absorptive substance that has been used by Native Americans for centuries for internal purification. It is a drawing and binding element that facilitates the binding effects of psyllium husk powder or flax fiber. Apple juice is also good for the colon because it is rich in pectins—soluble fiber. Black cherry juice has been used traditionally to improve the blood. Cranberry juice is beneficial for the kidneys. And papaya juice is good for digestion.

BEET JUICE

Beet juice has a laxative effect and is excellent for the liver. Because of its strong taste, it's best combined with other milder-tasting juices such as carrot, celery, and cucumber (cucumber is acidic, but acceptable when balanced with high-alkaline vegetables). Try the Beet Cleansing Express Cocktail, listed as follows.

NOTE: When you consume this much beet juice, it will often affect the color of your stool; don't be alarmed if it is a color similar to beet juice. Also, if you are sugar sensitive (hypoglycemic or diabetic), you may not be able to tolerate beet and carrot juices. (I am very sugar sensitive but have no problem with these vegetable juices; however, if you are not able to tolerate them, substitute green juices in their place, as desired.)

Beet Juice Express

5 medium carrots, scrubbed well, green tops removed, ends trimmed
1 small or 1/2 large beet, with green top, scrubbed well
1 cucumber, scrubbed well, or peeled if not organic
2 stalks celery with leaves, scrubbed well, ends trimmed
1 handful parsley, rinsed well
2-inch piece ginger root, peeled

Bunch up the parsley and push it through the juicer feed tube with the carrots, beet and beet greens, cucumber, celery, and ginger. Stir the juice and pour into a glass. Drink as soon as possible to maximize the nutritional benefits.

CALCIUM-MAGNESIUM SUPPLEMENT

The minerals calcium and magnesium are important for muscle contraction and relaxation and, therefore, good for bowel movement and tone. They also promote restful sleep, which is very important in the cleansing and healing process.

VITAMIN C AND BIOFLAVONOIDS OR ANTIOXIDANT SUPPLEMENT

A good vitamin C and bioflavonoid supplement or antioxidant formula will help to eliminate free radicals and is needed for deep tissue cleansing. Use buffered vitamin C if acidic.

HERBAL COLON CLEANSE SUPPLEMENTS

The herbs that are the best to help rid the colon of putrefactive debris are listed below. They help to soften and break up the putrefactive material in the colon. Look for products that contain barberry bark, cascara sagrada bark, fennel seed, ginger root, golden seal root, lobelia leaf, myrrh gum, peppermint leaf, plantain leaf, red raspberry leaf, turkey rhubarb root, and sheep sorrel leaf. The herbs I use for strengthening the body are in Herbal Nutrition; they include: alfalfa leaf, dandelion root, Atlantic kelp, rose hips, shavegrass, yellow dock root, chickweed leaf, hawthorne berry, Irish moss, licorice root, and marshmallow root.

NOTE: It is never recommended that you prepare your own herbal cleansing formula, as the ingredients mentioned are not combined in equal parts. And always seek medical advice before taking herbal supplements because they may have adverse reactions with drugs you are taking.

DIGESTIVE ENZYMES

A mixture of digestive enzymes can help digestion and facilitate the cleasning process. There are enzymes formulated to take with meals and enzymes formulated to assist digestion in between meals. (See Products and Information.)

THE CLEANSING FOODS

Follow The Acid-Alkaline Balancing Diet and choose foods mainly from the list of alkaline-forming foods (Chapter Five, pp. 118–20).

Beside these cleansing foods, I recommend flushing the colon during The 7-Day Complete Intestinal Cleanse.

COLON FLUSH

Flushing the colon with colon hydrotherapy (popularly known as colonics) or enemas is an important part of the cleansing process. While not commonplace today, or too popular I might add, enemas have a long history and were recorded as early as 1500 B.C. in an Egyptian medical document called the *Eber Papyrus.* In the early 1900s, John H. Kellogg, M.D., used colon therapy on some forty thousand patients in Battle Creek, Michigan. He reported his findings in the *Journal of the American Medical Association,* noting that in all but twenty cases, surgery was not necessary for the treatment of gastrointestinal diseases in his patients. Enemas fell out of vogue in the 1950s.[5]

You don't need a gastrointestinal disease, however, to benefit from daily enemas while you are cleansing. Everyone benefits from flushing the colon during a cleanse. When you are detoxifying, more toxins can build up in the intestinal tract than your body can eliminate quickly and efficiently, and that can lead to headaches, flu-type symptoms, and a host of other reactions. Flushing the colon can offer quick relief from such symptoms, and it also offers protection from toxins being reabsorbed back into the system. There is a school of thought that one can become dependent on enemas and therefore should not perform them. For the many people who have benefited from enemas during cleansing, this hypothesis is completely unfounded. When the colon is cleansed, the intestinal tract should perform *better* than in the past.

Enemas are something you can do at home each day. Most independently owned drug stores have enema bags for sale. I also recommend a professional colonic or two each week of the colon and liver cleanses for a more thorough cleansing. Or, if you wish to perform colonics at home, several companies sell colema boards and other specialized equipment.

NOTE: You can make your cleanse more intense and speed the process by eating just one or two meals a day and adding another freshly made vegetable juice in place of the omitted meal. The most intense cleanse, The 7-Day Intense Cleanse (not outlined in this book), involves no solid food, just fresh juices in place of meals along with three Cleansing Cocktail Fiber Shakes. I don't recommend this intense cleansing unless you are well on your road to recovery or have been determined by your health-care professional to be healthy and strong enough for this process.

THE 7-DAY, KICK-START LIVER CLEANSE

In her book *The Chemistry of Success,* Susan Lark, M.D., says, "When a person is undergoing chemotherapy or any cancer treatment that results in the killing of tumor cells at an accelerated rate, it is imperative that both the toxic by-products of this tumor cell destruction and the drugs themselves be quickly eliminated from the body. If these toxic chemical residues remain in the system, they can overburden the liver's detoxification capabilities and greatly increase the risk of death."[6] Dr. Lark and many other doctors practicing complementary alternative medicine (CAM) recommend that cancer patients do everything possible to detoxify harmful substances and dead cancer cells as efficiently as possible.

It is very beneficial for every person with cancer to embark on a liver cleanse. Also, everyone who wants to prevent cancer from returning needs to periodically cleanse the liver in order to remain healthy. Though this program is a seven-day plan, the process needs to continue over a period of time, alternating various cleanses within this chapter with the liver cleanse and focusing attention continually on this hard-working organ of detoxification.

The 7-Day, Kick-Start Easy Liver Cleanse Menu

For seven days, follow this easy menu plan for liver cleansing.

Breakfast:

7:30 AM 1 cup lemon juice (1/4–1/2 lemon) and hot water with a dash of cayenne pepper

7:45 AM Fresh juice: Beet Juice Express

8:00 AM Whole grain cereal such as millet, amaranth, or cream of brown rice cereal with almond or rice milk

Supplement: Milk thistle or liver cleansing herbs

9:00 AM 1 to 2 teaspoons Beet Salad

10:30 AM Dandelion herbal tea

11:00 AM 1 to 2 teaspoons Beet Salad

Lunch:

12:00 PM Vegan soup such as split pea, bean, or lentil and green salad; or vegan tostada and rice and beans; or hummus sandwich on rice bread with grated veggies and sprouts with a cup of vegan soup; or veggie-stuffed avocado on bed of lettuce with gazpacho soup

Supplement: Milk thistle or liver cleansing herbs

1:15 PM 1 to 2 teaspoons Beet Salad

3:00 PM Green Drink: Juice any fresh greens you wish; cucumber, celery, and lemon make a nice base for other greens such as kale, parsley, spinach, and sprouts

3:15 PM	1 to 2 teaspoons Beet Salad
4:00 PM	Protein shake or smoothie (as a pick-me-up)
5:15 PM	1 to 2 teaspoons Beet Salad
Dinner:	
5:30 PM	Carrot Salad with lemon-olive oil dressing
	Potassium broth
	Vegan Entrée
	Supplement: Milk Thistle or Liver Cleansing Herbs*
7:15 PM	1 to 2 teaspoons Beet Salad
8:30 PM	Chamomile or peppermint herbal tea

*Avoid eating after 6 PM if possible (except for the beet salad) to give your liver a chance to do its cleansing work as you sleep.

Recipes and explanations of the various parts of the liver cleanse follow.

COMPONENTS OF THE 7-DAY COMPLETE LIVER CLEANSE

EAT A VEGAN DIET

Eat only a vegan diet, which means you'll exclude all animal products (meat, poultry, fish, eggs, and dairy). Completely avoid all sweets, gluten-containing grains (wheat, barley, rye, and oats), soft drinks, alcohol, junk food, caffeine, and tobacco. Make at least 50 percent or more of your vegan diet raw food—salads, sprouts, fresh fruits, veggie sticks, and freshly made vegetable juices; choose from the list of alkaline-forming foods as much as possible. (See Chapter Five.) You may eat three vegan meals a day; breakfast and dinner should be the lightest meals with your largest meal at noon. Drink at least 64 ounces (eight 8-ounce glasses) of purified water daily. If you miss a day, you will need to start the cleanse over again. You can follow the preceding Easy Liver Cleanse Menu and add the addtional supplements and procedures for the Complete Liver Cleanse.The following foods and supplements will be part of this program.

FRESH BEET JUICE

Beets are used traditionally to cleanse and support the liver. Drink from 3 to 8 ounces of fresh beet juice each day; it is also best to start the day with this juice. Because of its strong taste, mix beet juice with milder tasting juices such as carrot, cucumber, celery, and lemon. To this mixture, add freshly juiced ginger root for a spicy burst of flavor and a big helping of zinc. For the Beet Juice Express cleansing cocktail, see page 136.

NOTE: If you are extremely sugar sensitive (hypoglycemic or diabetic), you may not be able to tolerate the beet juice, the beet salad, or the carrot salad. Omit as needed. Your cleanse will still be effective without these. Add one more green drink for the morning in place of the beet juice and substitute 1 tablespoon of extra virgin olive oil and 1 tablespoon lemon juice on a green salad to replace the carrot salad. I am quite sugar sensitive, and I have no problem with these foods.

MILK THISTLE (SILYMARIN)

Take one capsule of the herb milk thistle with each meal. Milk thistle contains some of the most potent liver-cleansing compounds known. Silymarin, the most active ingredient in milk thistle, enhances liver function. It has excellent antioxidant properties that help prevent damage to the liver from environmental pollutants. It is also a powerful antioxidant and inhibits the depletion of glutathione, an important liver enzyme. Or you can take a liver-cleansing herbal formula that includes milk thistle.

LIVER CLEANSE HERBS (OPTIONAL)

You may wish to add a liver cleanse formula that contains the following: milk thistle, curcumin, dandelion root, bupleurum root, barbery root bark, stillingia, burdock root, turmeric root, and mandrake root. If you use this formula, you do not need to take additional milk thistle with each meal. (I do not recommend that you formulate your own combination of these herbs, since they are not combined in equal amounts.)

Traditionally, these herbs have been used to "kick start" the liver into normal function, to improve bile flow, and to help the liver remove toxic drugs, including chemotherapy. This formula is also known to help bring to the surface old, stored-up anger, grief, depression, and other toxic emotions that have been stuck in organs and tissues.

TAKE HERBAL SUPPLEMENTS

Once you have completed The 7-Day Liver Cleanse Program, continue with the vegan, alkaline-forming dietary suggestions and continue to take the herbs until you've used all the capsules. Follow label directions accordingly. If you are following the cleansing program cycles at the end of this chapter, continue with the Liver Cleanse as recommended or as desired.

Be Aware

Some herbs have powerful liver-cleansing properties. Individuals who are quite sensitive may not be able to process these herbs, and their detoxification pathways can become overwhelmed. There may be reactions such as abdominal bloating, congestion, nausea, and pain or discomfort in the abdominal area. If this occurs, discontinue the use of herbs until the detoxification pathways are strengthened.

The liver is a doorway into our emotional library. Unexpressed or denied emotions have the ability to shut down important liver functions. Always watch for emotions [that surface] when working on the liver. More than any other organ, the liver is affected by negative thoughts and feelings. Feelings such as anger, hate, fear, jealousy, resentment, depression, self-pity, and hopelessness have a powerfully detrimental impact [on the liver].[7]

—Richard Anderson, N.D.

MINERAL SUPPORT

Minerals, and especially the electrolytes (sodium, calcium, potassium, and magnesium), are very important in the detoxification process and the healing of the liver; they should be added to the daily regimen.

LECITHIN

An important nutrient for the liver, lecithin helps speed up regeneration of damaged liver tissue and helps prevent accumulation of fat in the liver. Dissolve 2 tablespoons lecithin granules in water or juice daily.

VITAMIN C AND BIOFLAVONOIDS OR ANTIOXIDANT SUPPLEMENT

Vitamin C and bioflavonoid supplement or antioxidant formula will help to eliminate free radicals and is needed for deep tissue cleansing. Choose buffered vitamin C if you test acidic.

LIVER-FRIENDLY FOODS

Eat an abundance of liver-friendly foods for the seven days of cleansing, which include: beets, artichokes, peas, parsnips, pumpkin, sweet potatoes, squash, yams, green beans, broccoli, brussels sprouts, cabbage, carrots, cauliflower, celery, chives, cucumber, eggplant, garlic, kale, kohlrabi, mustard greens, okra, onion, and parsley. Choose organically grown produce as often as possible to avoid pesticides and thereby lighten your body's toxic load.

Finally, below are recipes for The 7-Day, Kick-Start Liver Cleanse.

Recipes for The 7-Day, Kick-Start Liver Cleanse

Beet Salad

1 cup raw beets, finely grated or chopped
2 tablespoons extra virgin, cold-pressed olive oil
Juice of 1/2 lemon, organic is preferable

Whisk the olive oil and lemon juice together and mix with the grated beets. Eat 1 or 2 teaspoons of this salad every two hours during an eight-hour period for seven days.

Carrot Salad

Place one cup of finely shredded carrots, or carrot pulp left over from juicing, in a bowl. If shredding the carrots, they should be a mushy consistency; use a food processor or fine grater. (Believe me, it's easiest to use the carrot pulp.) For the dressing, combine 1 tablespoon extra virgin, cold-pressed olive oil with 1 tablespoon fresh lemon juice. Whisk together. You may add more dressing, but not less. (I like to add a dash of cinnamon to the dressing.) Pour the dressing over the shredded carrots (or carrot pulp) and mix well.

Green Drink

Preferably in the afternoon, drink 10 ounces freshly juiced green drink: cucumber, parsley, spinach, kale, celery, or any other green herb or vegetable. You can add fresh lemon juice and/or freshly juiced ginger root to improve flavor. Fresh mint also makes a nice addition with cucumber and other milder-tasting greens.

Potassium-Rich Vegetable Broth

This vegetable broth provides important nutrients, especially minerals, that your body needs during the cleansing process. Eat 1 to 2 cups of the broth daily.

2 to 3 cups chopped fresh string beans (green beans) (frozen is acceptable when fresh is not available)
2 to 3 cups chopped zucchini
2 to 3 stalks celery
1 cup coarsely chopped onion
1 to 3 tablespoons chopped parsley
1 tablespoon chopped garlic

Steam the string beans, zucchini, celery, and onion over purified water until soft, but still green and not mushy. Place the cooked vegetables, plus the raw parsley and garlic, in a blender and puree until smooth. Add a bit of the steaming water, as needed, but keep the broth fairly thick. Season to taste with minced ginger, cayenne, vegetable seasoning, or herbs of your choice.

During The 7-Day Easy Liver Cleanse, your body can benefit from colon cleansing in the form of colonics and enemas.

THE COLON FLUSH

Flushing the colon can greatly facilitate the elimination of toxins and speed your liver cleansing process. (For more information, see the Colon Flush in this chapter under The Intestinal Cleanse.)

HERBAL WRAPS

Herbal wraps use sheets of cloth that have been soaked in a hot herbal solution and wrapped around the body to encourage perspiration. They are very helpful to cleanse toxins from the body and also for relaxation. I recommend them especially during The Liver Cleanse; they may also be used with any of the other cleanses.

Having completed The Intestinal Cleanse and The Liver Cleanse, you are now ready for The Gallbadder Cleanse.

THE GALLBLADDER CLEANSE

The Gallbladder Cleansing Programs can help purge the gallbladder of stones, including the "silent stones"—those that don't cause symptoms—and what is known as gallbladder *sand* or *mud*. If you know that you have gallstones, suspect that you might, or if you are over forty and have eaten a typical Western diet most of your life and have not done much cleansing, it is advisable to start with The Easy Gallbladder Cleanse. You should complete two to three weeks of the gentle phase of gallbladder cleansing before you proceed to The 7-Day Complete Gallbladder Flush.

If you try The Complete Gallbladder Flush prematurely, the gallbladder could release a large stone that could block the bile duct, which would require immediate surgery. Before embarking on The Gallbladder Flush, you may wish to consult your health-care professional.

The 7-Day Easy Gallbladder Cleanse Menu

The 7-Day Easy Gallbladder Cleanse is designed to soften stones and increase bile solubility. For seven days follow this easy menu plan for gallbladder cleansing.

Breakfast:

7:30 AM Liver/Gallbladder Flush Cocktail (see p. 147)

7:30 AM 1 cup peppermint or chamomile herbal tea

8:00 AM Fresh juice: Carrot, beet, and cucumber juice or Beet Juice Express (see p. 136)

8:30 AM Cooked cereal such as cream of brown rice, millet, or

	amaranth with a tablespoon ground flaxseeds and rice or almond milk
	Supplement: Lipotropic formula
9:00 AM	1 to 2 teaspoons Beet Salad
10:30 AM	Fresh juice: Carrot, beet, and cucumber juice or Beet Juice Express
11:00 AM	1 to 2 teaspoons Beet Salad (see p. 147)
Lunch:	
12:00 PM	Vegetable soup and green salad or vegan entrée
1:00 PM	1 to 2 teaspoons Beet Salad
2:00 PM	Fresh juice: Carrot, celery, kale, or endive
3:00 PM	1 to 2 teaspoons Beet Salad
3:30 PM	Fresh juice: Beet Juice Express (optional) or herbal tea
5:00 PM	1 to 2 teaspoons Beet Salad
Dinner:	
5:30 PM	Soup or green salad
	Vegan entrée
	Supplement: Lipotropic formula*
7:00 PM	1 to 2 teaspoons Beet Salad
8:00 PM	Herbal tea

*It is best not to eat after 6 PM (with the exception of the Beet Salad) to give your body a chance to cleanse.

COMPONENTS OF THE 7-DAY EASY GALLBLADDER CLEANSE

The 7-Day Easy Gallbladder Cleanse is composed of the following elements:

A VEGAN DIET

Vegan means no animal products; therefore, you will be avoiding all meat, poultry, fish, eggs, and dairy products. Avoid all fried foods.

Use only extra virgin, cold-pressed olive oil for dressing, and only organic, virgin coconut oil for cooking. Make a large portion of your diet vegetables and choose most of these from the list of alkaline-forming foods. In addition, avoid all sweets, alcohol, caffeine, gluten-containing grains (wheat, rye, barley, oats), soft drinks, junk food, caffeine, and tobacco.

BEET SALAD

1 cup raw beets, finely grated or chopped
2 tablespoons extra virgin, cold-pressed olive oil
Juice of 1/2 lemon, organic is preferable

Whisk the olive oil and lemon juice together and mix with the beets. Eat 1 or 2 teaspoons of this salad every two hours during an eight-hour period for seven days.

THE LIVER/GALLBLADDER FLUSH COCKTAIL

Combine 6 ounces of freshly made apple juice (preferably Pippin or Granny Smith) with 2 ounces of fresh lemon juice and 1/2 teaspoon ginger juice (or grated ginger). Pour the juices into a blender and add one or two cloves of peeled garlic; blend until liquefied. Add 1 tablespoon extra virgin olive oil and 2 to 4 ounces purified water; blend until thoroughly mixed. Sip slowly on an empty stomach. Follow with peppermint or chamomile herbal tea. This is best taken early in the morning, but if that does not work for you, take it just before bedtime. (NOTE: if you are sensitive to fruit sugar, omit the apple juice and combine juice of 1/2 lemon and 1/2 lime with 1 cup water, a few ice cubes, a clove of garlic, a chunk of ginger, and 1 Tbsp. of extra virgen olive oil.)

THREE TO FOUR GLASSES OF FRESH VEGETABLE JUICE DAILY

Drink two to three 8-ounce glasses of a mixture of carrots, beets, and cucumbers; or the Beet Juice Express (recipe on p. 136); also, drink one 8-ounce glass of a mixture of carrot, celery, and endive or kale juice.

NOTE: If you are extremely sugar sensitive (hypoyglycemic or diabetic) and react to carrots or beets, add cucumber and more greens and flavor with lemon juice and/or ginger.

LIPOTROPIC FORMULA

A lipotropic formula includes choline, methionine, lecithin, betaine, folic acid, and vitamin B_6. This combination of nutrients helps remove fat from the liver and increases bile solubility. Take as directed. (See Products and Information.)

THE 7-DAY COMPLETE GALLBLADDER FLUSH

This is the program I completed when I was thirty years old. It was very effective, and I have tried different versions of this flush at various times since then. Each time, I've observed different results, from stones to sand and mud being eliminated. The bottom line—the program works. (See comments on recent medical observation on p. 55.)

EAT ONLY A VEGAN DIET

Vegan means no animal products; therefore, you will be avoiding all meat, poultry, fish, eggs, and dairy products. Avoid all fried foods and nuts. Use only extra virgin olive oil or flaxseed oil in cold-food preparation; and virgin organic coconut oil for sautéing. Make a large portion of your diet vegetables. Choose most of your foods from the list of alkaline-forming foods (see pp. 122–24). In addition, avoid all sweets, alcohol, caffeine, gluten-containing grains (wheat, rye, barley oats), soft drinks, junk food, caffeine, and tobacco.

DRINK THE INTESTINAL CLEANSING COCKTAILS

Follow instructions under Intestinal Cleanse for the Cleansing Cocktail Fiber Shake (psyllium husk fiber and bentonite). (See p. 135.)

BEGIN THE PROGRAM WITH AN ENEMA OR COLONIC

It's important to flush the colon at the start of The 7-Day Advanced Gallbladder Cleanse. (For more information on enemas and colonics, see pp. 137–38.)

And use the following foods to facilitate the cleansing process:

CLEANSING FOODS

Apple Juice

For the first five days, preferably Monday through Friday if you work outside the home, drink two 8-ounce glasses of freshly made apple juice. Choose any kind of apples you wish—Golden or Red Delicious, Granny Smith, or Pippin. Choose organic whenever possible. If you have a sugar metabolism disorder (hypoglycemia or diabetes), choose the lowest-sugar green apples such as Granny Smith or Pippin. Dilute the apple juice with at least 4 ounces of purified water. Or you can substitute fresh lemon juice and water; mix the juice of 1/2 lemon in 10–12 ounces of purified water.

Carrot/Beet/Cucumber Juice

Each day drink a glass of freshly made carrot, beet, and cucumber juice, combined in nearly equal parts, or the Beet Juice Express (recipe on p. 136). Choose organic vegetables whenever possible.

Beet Salad

For three days, eat Beet Salad (see p. 143). Eat one teaspoon of this salad every two hours during an eight-hour period for three days.

Olive Oil and Lemon Juice

Upon rising on day three (Wednesday if you began on Monday), mix 2 tablespoons extra virgin olive oil and 1 tablespoon fresh lemon juice in 4 to 6 ounces of purified water. Mix vigorously; down quickly! Drink this mixture for three days—Wednesday through Friday.

Chamomile Tea

Drink 3 to 4 cups of chamomile tea each day—mid-morning, mid-afternoon, evening, and before bed, or as desired.

Drink Eight 8-Ounce Glasses of Purified Water

Each day of The Complete Gallbladder Flush drink a minimum of eight 8-ounce glasses of purified water in addition to the other liquids.

DAY 6—THE INTENSIVE FLUSH

- Choose a day like Saturday when you can rest most of the day.
- Take no nutritional supplements on this day.
- Drink only fresh vegetable juices for breakfast and lunch; eat no solid food.
- After 2:00 PM do not drink juices, only water.
- Prepare Epsom Salts by mixing 4 tablespoons of Epsom Salts in 3 cups cool purified water; this makes four servings. Store the mixture in a jar in the refrigerator.
- 6:00 PM Drink 3/4 cup of cold Epsom Salts water. This does not taste good. You may want to have a mouth rinse ready. It's okay to yell, sigh, and carry on a bit! But don't neglect this part of the flush, because the Epsom Salts water helps to open up the bile duct so stones can pass easily.
- 8:00 PM Drink another 3/4 cup of the Epsom Salts water.
- 9:45 PM Pour 1 cup of extra virgin olive oil into a saucepan and add 1 cup apple juice; gently warm. Pour the mixture in a jar and shake or mix in the blender. Mix thoroughly and drink it all down within five minutes. You may want to rinse your mouth after this as well; it's not much better tasting than the Epsom Salts water.
- 10:00 PM Lie down in bed on your right side, the sooner after drinking this mixture, the better. Try to lie still for at least twenty minutes; hopefully, you can go to sleep.
- The next morning, upon awakening, take your third dose of Epsom Salts water. (Yes, this is your breakfast.) Two hours later, take your final 3/4 cup Epsom Salts water.
- In one hour, you may have fresh vegetable juice.
- You may have a fresh garden salad for lunch.

WHAT TO EXPECT?

Though this program is an insult to one's taste buds, this regime is worth it because it works. Here's what you can expect.

You may experience diarrhea after taking the Epsom Salts drinks. Sometime during the morning of the seventh day, you should pass gallstones, sand, or mud. Gallstones are usually about pea-size and green, but can range in size from that of lemon seeds to dimes, and they float. Sand or mud looks about like it sounds. Colors can range from tan, black, light-to-dark green, and turquoise. I only mention this so you won't be too alarmed by what you see. The upside of what to expect is greatly improved digestion. I can attest to this firsthand.

THE COMPLETE KIDNEY CLEANSE

The fourth cleanse, The Kidney Cleanse, is an important part of the elimination process. The bladder and kidneys are important elimination sites for toxins in the bloodstream. Their job is to maintain a healthy internal environment and control the acid-alkaline balance of the body. They must get rid of proteins, salts, and chemicals, but if they are congested, we can experience mild symptoms such as water retention or more severe symptoms such as inflammation of kidney tissue. Concentrated protein wastes can cause inflammation of kidney filtering tissues (nephritis), causing the bloodstream to become overloaded with toxins. Therefore, it is important to cleanse and support the kidneys as we cleanse the entire body.[8]

It is best to start a kidney cleanse by using gentle diuretic remedies, which strengthen the kidneys and promote excretion of metabolic waste via the urine. The Easy Kidney Cleanse Program incorporates the following:

3-DAY JUICE FAST

For three days drink primarily fresh vegetable juices and vegetable broths for breakfast, lunch, dinner, and snacks. (Limit fruit juice in order to limit sugars and acid in your diet.) Drink at least four 10-ounce glasses of vegetable juice each day.

Choose from the following combinations:

- Carrot, beet, celery
- Watermelon (quite good for the kidneys)
- Asparagus, carrot, cucumber (asparagus is a tonic for the kidneys)
- Carrot, beet, and coconut milk
- Cucumber and fresh mint
- Cucumber, celery, parsley, and ginger
- Sprouts, carrot, celery, jicama
- Papaya shake

NOTE: Cucumber, watermelon, cantaloupe with seeds, asparagus, lemon, kiwi, and parsley are all considered natural diuretics.

MORNING START

Herbal tea upon rising: agrimony, marshmallow, juniper, nettles, and buchu are diuretic herbs that also benefit the urinary system.

Morning drink: Make a fresh 8- to 10-ounce glass of vegetable juice such as carrot, celery, cucumber, beet with leaves, parsley, and ginger or Papaya Smoothie.

DRINK A MINIMUM OF EIGHT 8-OUNCE GLASSES OF PURIFIED WATER

The kidneys will be able to cleanse efficiently only if the volume of water is adequate to carry off wastes. It is helpful to drink about 1 pint of purified water before going to bed to insure the "flushing out" continues through the night. Sixty-four ounces is the recommended minimum amount of water to drink daily. Eight glasses of water are for a person weighing up to about 130 pounds. If you weigh more or live in a very dry climate, drink ten to twelve glasses per day. (NOTE: If you have not been a water drinker, start slowly, with one or two additional glasses of water per day and see how you do. If you retain water—e.g.

your feet and ankles swell—don't add any more water until your system adjusts.)

NETTLES TEA

The herb nettles is used traditionally for kidney cleansing and support; it helps eliminate uric acid. Drink a cup of this tea the night before starting the cleanse and drink 1 cup each day of the cleanse.

HERBAL TEAS

For mid-morning and mid-afternoon tea breaks, watermelon seed, oatstraw, or cornsilk are good.

HERBAL SUPPLEMENTS

You may wish to take an herbal formula that is helpful in cleansing the kidneys, bladder, and the entire urinary tract system. Look for herbal supplements that combine gravel root, juniper berries, uva ursi, burdock root, hydrangea root, parsley leaf, marshmallow root, ginger root, and lobelia leaf.

NOTE: It is not recommended that you attempt mixing individual herbs yourself, as these herbs are not combined in equal amounts in various products; and always seek professional advice about combining herbs with your current medications.

KIDNEY STONES AND GRAVEL

Being confined to bed for a long period of time or not exercising for a while can encourage mobilization of calcium from bones into the blood and increase calcium in the urine, which can contribute to kidney stones or gravel. These stones can range in size from that of a grain of sand to a large stone the kidneys cannot pass. An acid-rich diet can cause stones to form, especially if a lot of meat, dairy, coffee, sweets, and soda pop are consumed. Once you've completed the kidney cleanse, an alkaline-forming diet is very helpful in preventing stones and gravel.

A traditional remedy for clearing out deposits in the urinary tract calls for daily drinking 1/4 cup parsnip juice with 3/4 cup liquid chlorophyll (green juices are rich in chlorophyll) until cleansed.[9]

The Easy Kidney Cleanse

For seven days, drink the following along with eating the recommended vegan diet (see p. 73).

1. Mix 1 tablespoon unsweetened cranberry concentrate* in 24 ounces of purified water with a pinch (or a few drops) of stevia to sweeten. Drink this cranberry cocktail throughout the morning.

2. Drink 1 to 2 cups of nettles tea.

*Cranberry concentrate can be purchased at most health food stores.

THE LUNG CLEANSE

The fifth cleanse is The Lung Cleanse. The lungs are a major organ of elimination. You can perform this lung cleanse process throughout your cleansing program.

DEEP CLEANSING BREATHS

Use your diaphragm to fill up the belly and the upper chest; hold for a count of two and then expel the air. Take deep cleansing breaths throughout the day. And remember not to hold your breath, especially when tense or anxious.

Exercise That Promotes Deep Breathing

Many exercises promote deep breathing—walking, biking, hiking, stretch classes, aerobic exercise, and swimming. Find something you enjoy and have the energy to perform, and remember to breathe during your activity. The more you can exercise outside, the better, because indoor air is usually more polluted than outdoor air. (Chapter Eight discusses the problems with indoor air.)

Air Purifier

Breathing deeply is good, but the quality of the air we breathe should also be good. A quality air purifier is an excellent investment to facilitate your overall cleansing process.

Release Emotions That May Impede Lung Health

Grief is the toxic emotion most often associated with the lungs. Repressed grief can contribute to long-term contraction in the lungs, which can interfere with nutrient delivery and life force. (See Chapter Nine for more information on emotional cleansing.)

THE SKIN CLEANSE

During the cleansing processes in this chapter, the skin will eliminate wastes through perspiration. It is important that the pores not get clogged and thus hinder your elimination process. The sixth cleanse is The Skin Cleanse.

The skin is a supporting organ of elimination. You can do several things to facilitate your overall cleansing process and support the skin's role in detoxification of the body.

DRY SKIN BRUSHING

Brushing the skin with a natural bristle, vegetable fiber brush is very helpful in removing toxins and opening pores through eliminating dead skin cells and other wastes. This process also stimulates the lymphatic system. Each day before you shower, brush your skin as follows:[10]

- Use a natural vegetable-fiber brush (synthetic is not good; it scratches the skin); use no water.
- Start with the bottoms of your feet, and using circular motions, move upward toward the heart.
- Use circular, counterclockwise strokes on the abdomen.
- Always move outward to inward, starting with the hands and moving up the arms.
- Brush lightly around the breasts; do not brush the nipples.
- Brush the entire body for best results.

- Placing sea salt on the brush will cause the pores to open more.
- Wash your brush every few weeks and let it dry.

This type of brushing is best done in the morning; before bedtime can be too stimulating and can interrupt sleep.

NOTE: If you have psoriasis, eczema, or any other skin condition, you will want to omit this step.

SAUNAS AND STEAM BATHS

Heat will cause the body to release toxins through sweat. Dry or moist saunas and steam baths create intentional perspiration for therapeutic purposes. Intentional sweating not only facilitates the release of toxins through the skin but also helps to lighten the toxic load from the kidneys and liver.

If you have trouble staying in a conventional sauna, you may want to try an infrared sauna (lower temperatures—110 to 130 degrees Fahrenheit.). Infrared heat is radiant heat that heats objects directly without excessively heating the air in between—only 20 percent heats the air; 80 percent is converted to heat within the body. Infrared heat penetrates more deeply without the discomfort and draining effect of conventional saunas and produces more sweat volume. Saunas, especially infrared saunas, accelerate the removal of toxic metals as well as organic toxins like PCBs and pesticide residues, which are stored in fatty tissues and are not easily displaced. Sweating caused by deep heat also helps remove dead skin cells, thus opening the pores for better elimination of toxins. The infrared sauna has an energizing effect on its users, making them feel good as it rids the body of unwanted toxins.[11] Conventional saunas are usually found in gymnasiums and health clubs, and infrared saunas are more apt to be found in holistic clinics and spas.

THERAPEUTIC BATHS

Creating your own therapeutic bath at home can be quite helpful in releasing toxins through the skin.

1. Fill a tub with comfortably hot water.
2. Add therapeutic ingredients:

    - Epsom Salts contains magnesium, which helps muscles relax, and sulfur that aids in detoxification; 1 cup is a good start, but you can increase it to 2 cups.
    - Ginger is a favorite of mine. You can juice or grate fresh ginger root and pour 1/4 to 1/2 cup ginger into the water. Ginger helps the body sweat and draws out toxins.
    - Baking soda and sea salt make a good alkalinizing bath; add 1 cup baking soda and 1 cup Celtic Sea Salt to hot water.

Thalassotherapy, which is bathing in seawater, is very therapeutic as well as detoxifying. (Sanoviv Medical Institute has several heated seawater pools at their facility.)

Hot mineral springs are excellent for detoxification and relaxation. There are many natural hot springs throughout the United States, Canada, and Europe. See the publication *The Spa Finder* for locations.

EXERCISE

Aerobic exercise such as fast walking can enhance circulation and increase perspiration, thus promoting excretion of toxins more efficiently through the skin. For in-home exercise, I recommend a video series called "Walk Away the Pounds." It comes with hand weights and is an excellent way to get started if you haven't been exercising for a while, whether you want to lose weight or not. You can choose the lightest program to begin and work up to more intense movements as your energy increases. I do recommend that whenever possible you get outside, even if it is only for a short walk, because fresh air and oxygen are so important for your recovery.

WATER

It is very important to get enough water when cleansing in order to flush toxins from your body, especially when you are perspiring and losing fluids. Drink eight to ten 8-ounce glasses of purified water per day; or make part of your water intake the alkalizing water (see p. 131). Drink water at room temperature; iced water is hard on the digestive system, causing the colon to contract. Fluids are best taken between meals, but a small amount of water (4 to 6 ounces) can be drunk with a meal.

THE LYMPHATIC SYSTEM CLEANSE

You can use the The Lymphatic System Cleanse at any time during your cleansing program. The lymphatic system has no pump; it depends on exercise and breathing to move the lymph through the system. Known as the "garbage arteries," the lymphatics are responsible for picking up intracellular waste and discarding it in the bloodstream to be carried to the organs of elimination. Therefore moving lymph through the vessels is another key aspect in the cleansing and healing process. During this cleanse you will want to continue The Skin Cleanse Program. Dry brushing, sauna and steam baths, therapeutic baths, exercise, and drinking plenty of water are all pertinent to cleansing the lympathic system. In addition, add the follow cleansing steps.

DIAPHRAGMATIC BREATHING

Deep breathing is very beneficial in helping move the lymph through the vessels. Use your diaphragm to fill up the belly and upper chest with air, hold for a count of two, then expel the air. Do this several times a day. Remember to breathe deeply throughout the day and be sure not to hold your breath when you're tense.

MINI TRAMPOLINE (THE REBOUNDER)

This form of exercise is particularly beneficial for the lymphatic system and helps to clear clogged lymph nodes.

LYMPHASIZER (AEROBIC OXYGENATOR—ALSO KNOWN AS THE SWING MACHINE)

After noticing how well toned and healthy fish are, Dr. Shizuo Inoue developed a machine with rhythmic side-to-side movement that creates a wavelike motion up the body and spine—like a fish swimming. This type of machine provides gentle massage as it oxygenates muscles, tissues, and organs. It also helps move lymph along so it does not stagnate. If you are not able to do much exercise because of weakness or time constraints, this machine is a must. However, this machine is beneficial for everyone. John and I have a swing machine that we use regularly.

Lie on the floor with your feet in the grooves so the machine can do the work. It is believed that fifteen minutes on the Aerobic Oxygenator provides oxygen to the body equal to about a ninety-minute walk. This is very important in the cancer cleanse process because cancer cells are anaerobic (living in a lack of oxygen). Oxygen is known to weaken or kill cancer cells.

LYMPHATIC DRAINAGE MASSAGE

This particular type of light touch massage works on the lymphatic system to move the lymph through its vessels. It can be very helpful in assisting lymphatic cleansing. You need to see a professional massage therapist who is trained in this type of massage.

WATCH YOUR CIRCULATION

Decreasing circulation can hinder our body's natural ability to remove carcinogenic fluids, which can become trapped in the saclike glands known as the lymph nodes. These glands make up the largest mass of lymph nodes in the upper part of our body's lymphatic system. Wearing a bra fourteen hours or more a day tends to increase the hormone prolactin, which causes decreased circulation in breast tissue.

In 1997, medical anthropologist Sidney Singer compared the incidence of breast cancer in two groups of women on the Fiji Islands whose diet, environment, and lifestyle were the same. Half the women wore bras; the other half did not. Singer discovered that those who wore bras had the same rate of breast cancer as American women, whereas those who did not wear bras experienced almost no breast cancer.

It is recommended that women should always remove their bras during sleep, and as much as possible at home. Also, women should purchase bras without underwires and remove wires from their old bras; underwires are the most constricting. It is also suggested that women perform a light, gentle breast massage at night before bed to enhance lymphatic drainage.[12]

Finally, do not use antiperspirants; the chemicals are absorbed through the skin and can cause the underlying lymph nodes to constrict and block lymph flow. Antiperspirants contain aluminum, which adds to the heavy metal toxicity of the body. Use only the natural deodorants that can be found at most health food stores.

THE BLOOD PURIFYING CLEANSE

The eighth cleanse, The Blood Purifying Cleanse, is not part of the schedule recommendations for the cleansing programs at the end of this chapter; this cleanse can be done at any time during the program.

Any serious immune-deficient disease, of which cancer is one, indicates a need to cleanse the bloodstream. A blood-purifying cleanse can be followed for months, until the toxins are cleared. When there are large amounts of toxins in the bloodstream, a prolonged, all-liquid diet can cause more toxins to be released into the bloodstream than the body can handle. Therefore, it is not recommended that one do a prolonged juice fast because it is too harsh for an already weakened system. If you are relatively strong, then one or two days of vegetable juice fasting per week will be beneficial.

VEGAN DIET

Your diet should be as pure as possible. Eat only a vegan diet; avoid all animal products (meat, poultry, fish, eggs, and dairy). Select fresh organic produce as much as possible and choose most of your food from the list of alkaline-forming foods (see pp. 122–24). Make frozen foods your second choice after fresh foods, but avoid canned and packaged foods. Avoid all foods with preservatives, additives, and flavorings. Completely eliminate sweets, artificial sweeteners, caffeine, soda pop, and fried foods. Drink only purified water, alkalinizing water, non-carbonated mineral water, herbal teas, vegetable juices, and a small amount of low-acid fruit juice.

FRESHLY MADE JUICES

Vegetable juices and a small amount of low-acid fruit juice, such as melon or papaya, promote detoxification. Include two or three glasses of primarily fresh organic vegetable juices each day. For juice recipe ideas, see my book *The Juice Lady's Guide to Juicing for Health*.

BUFFERED VITAMIN C AND BIOFLAVONOIDS

Taking buffered vitamin C and equal amounts of bioflavonoids will help keep the body alkaline and encourage oxygen transport and uptake.

ELECTROYLYTES

Electrolytes (calcium, sodium, magnesium, potassium) are important for maintaining healthy blood and a proper alkaline-acid balance in the blood.

HERBAL TEA

Drink several cups of blood-cleansing herbal teas daily. Choose from the following: Pau d'Arco, dandelion, Oregon grape, burdock, red clover, yellow dock, and goldenseal.

DIGESTIVE AND SYSTEMIC ENZYMES

Digestive enzymes such as protease, amylase, and lipase assist in the digestive process. Systemic enzymes, taken on an empty stomach about two hours after eating, help clean up undigested proteins and help maintain healthy blood and tissue functions. Enzymes can also help relieve the body of some of its digestive burden.

SHORT JUICE FASTS

One- or two-day juice fasts once a month to once a week can be quite beneficial in purifying the blood. Start your day with a 10-ounce glass of vegetable juice; have an herbal tea for mid-morning break; make another 10-ounce glass of vegetable juice for lunch; mid-afternoon have a juice break; make a 10-ounce glass of vegetable juice or warm vegetable broth for dinner; mid-evening drink another cup of herbal tea. Throughout the day consume eight to ten 8-ounce glasses of purified water between juices. Mineral water can be substituted for some of the water. Make one or two of your juices a green drink—cucumber, parsley, celery, spinach, kale, mustard greens, beet greens, or any other greens you like; add mint, ginger, or lemon for flavor. Greens are rich in cholorphyll and chlorophyll is known to be a blood purifier.

THE PARASITE CLEANSE

The Parasite Cleanse is a specialized cleanse that is appropriate for those who have parasites, which is many Americans. Parasitic infestation is growing at an alarming rate in North America; many believe it has reached epidemic proportion. A growing number of health-care professionals believe parasites are the cause or a contributing factor to many cancers. Often the problem goes undiagnosed or misdiagnosed because these pathogens are difficult to detect and many times hide in the lining of the intestinal tract or in other organs. Parasites can cause damage to the body and the waste they discharge is toxic and harmful. These microscopic pathogens disrupt the digestive process, and good digestion is critical to good health, because whatever disrupts digestion also negatively impacts the immune system.

Parasites produce a mucous overlay that protects them and interferes with their destruction and with nutrient absorption; they thrive, while the host (that's us) experiences nutritional deficiencies. Tests for parasites are often inconclusive, and stool tests are completely ineffective if the parasites are localized in areas other than the colon, such as the brain or lungs.[13]

We can do many things to rid our body of these destructive pathogens. The program that follows has been highly effective for many, and sometimes life saving.

EAT A CLEANSING DIET

The Standard American Diet contributes to parasitic infection by causing a buildup of wastes and toxins—food for the parasites. The purer the diet, the easier it will be to get rid of them. Start by following The Acid-Alkaline Balancing Diet. Include an abundance of beta-carotene-rich foods, which are converted to vitamin A as needed in the body. It appears that vitamin A increases resistance to tissue penetration by parasitic larvae. Beta-carotene-rich foods include: carrots, sweet potatoes, yams, squash, broccoli, parsley, kale, spinach, dandelion greens, and other dark leafy greens. A good rule is to choose foods that are brightly colored—red, orange, yellow, and green.

Avoid foods that cause flatulence and irritate the gastrointestinal tract, as this interferes with nutrient absorption. Many of the protein-rich vegan foods such as beans, lentils, split peas, nuts, and seeds can cause irritation or flatulence; they need to be limited or avoided during The Parasite Cleanse. (Sprouted nuts, legumes, and seeds should not cause a problem.) You may need to eat fish for protein at this time. Avoid all gluten-containing grains such as wheat, rye, oats, spelt, and barley, which can cause irritation to the intestinal tract. During this cleanse, you may need to supplement your diet with natural free-form amino-acid protein such as whey protein to meet your protein needs.[14] As you change your internal environment, the parasites die off.

OZONATED WATER

A study at the Tenth World Ozone Conference in 1991 reviewed eighty patients with *G. lamblia.* Half the patients were treated with ozonated water four times a day for twelve days, while the remaining patients were given ozonated oil for five to ten days. The treatments were highly successful, with a cure rate of 97.5 percent for each group.[15]

GARLIC

Garlic has been used since ancient times for deworming, effective against roundworm, pinworm, and hookworm. Take two raw garlic cloves per day; mince fine, place on a teaspoon, and swallow with water; don't chew it, and you won't taste it. (Avoid if you are allergic or sensitive to garlic). Other foods that have antiparasitic properties are onions, radish, kelp, raw cabbage, ground almonds, blackberries, pumpkin, and sauerkraut.[16] Include these foods often in your diet.

HERBS

A variety of herbs are available to help us kill and expel parasites and worms. Green/black walnut hulls tincture is used for parasites in the blood as well as other parts of the body. However, many black walnut tinctures and capsules are not effective because of preparation methods or because they are weak. (See Products and Information for specific recommendations.) For roundworms, the following combination of herbs is effective: green/black walnut hulls, wormwood, ground cloves, gentian root, ginger, and mandrake root. Pink root, also known as Indian Pink, was used by Native Americans to kill intestinal worms, especially roundworms. For removing flatworms such as tapes and flukes, the following combination of herbs is effective: male fern, pumpkin seeds, pink root, wood betony, chamomile, and senna.[17]

The combination of green/black walnut hulls, wormwood, and ground cloves is recommended and used by Dr. Hulda R. Clark, who writes about the connection between parasites and cancer in her book *The Cure for All Cancers*.[18] She notes that this herbal combination kills both the egg and adult stages of one hundred different parasites, including amoebas, giardia, worms, and liver flukes, which she attributes to serious illnesses in those who are infected.

Dr. Clark has observed that flukes are a cancer-causing parasite. The adult fluke stays tightly stuck to the intestinal wall. Most of us get small lesions in our intestines from time to time, allowing fluke eggs, which are microscopic in size, to be pulled into the bloodstream; this is the way other parasite eggs get into the bloodstream as well. Some of the eggs hatch in the bloodstream as well as the intestines. It is the liver's job to kill them, but when it is sluggish, toxic, and not functioning efficiently, it too can become infested.[19]

Many people have experienced excellent results in eliminating parasites by using grapefruit seed extract and enzymes such as bromelain, papain, and protease. These enzymes can break through the mucus barrier that overlays most parasitic cysts. Grapefruit seed extract has been shown to eliminate protozoa and fungi on contact.[20]

NO SUGAR, NO SWEETS, NO ARTIFICIAL SWEETENERS, NO FRUIT

Parasites flourish on sugars; therefore, it is very important *not to eat any sweets.* They are on the "completely avoid" list. Sugars are detrimental to the cleansing of parasites.

CLEANSE THE INTESTINAL TRACT

Until the mucous-encrusted layer in the intestinal tract is removed, parasite cleansing will not be completely effective, because parasites become embedded in this matter and treatments cannot reach them until the plaque is removed. Follow The Complete Intestinal Cleanse Program for several weeks before beginning The Parasite Cleanse. Avoid all iced drinks as they can cause the intestines to contract, thus holding in toxins that should be released.

DIGESTIVE AND SYSTEMIC ENZYMES

Digestive enzymes assist in the digestive process. Systemic enzymes, taken on an empty stomach about two hours after eating, help clean up undigested proteins and also help maintain healthy blood and tissue functions. Additionally, enzymes can help relieve the body of some of its digestive burden. The supplements bromelain and papain can be taken with meals, and enzymes such as protease, amylase, and lipase can be taken between meals.

THE 30-DAY HEAVY METAL DETOX PROGRAM

Another specialized cleanse is The 30-Day Heavy Metal Detox Program. Metal intoxicants pour into our environment from numerous sources all around us; no one is immune to heavy metal contamination. Lead reaches us from solder used to seal food cans; leaded dust from ceramic glazes; vegetables and fruits grown in lead-contaminated soil; atmospheric lead from glass manufacturers, printers, smelters, and various other sources of industrial lead; and—for those of us who were living in the '50s, '60s, and '70s—leaded gas and paint.

Mercury toxicity comes from fish, shellfish, chicken (fish meal is often fed to chickens—which they were never meant to eat), and dental amalgams (silver fillings).[21] Cadmium exposure comes from residues or runoff from phosphate fertilizers, sewage, fossil fuels, gasses released from zinc, lead and copper smelters, and tobacco smoke. Arsenic, tin, copper, aluminum, and a host of other heavy metals may contribute to heavy metal toxicity. These metals tend to accumulate in the brain, kidneys, and immune system, where they can severely disrupt normal metabolic function.[22] It is suspected that heavy metals play a role in the development of some cancers.

It is a conservative estimate that up to 25 percent of the U.S. population suffers from heavy metal poisoning.[23] Dr. Myron Wentz, director of Sanoviv Medical Institute, has found that about 85 percent (at the time of this writing) of the individuals coming to Sanoviv for medical treatment have heavy metal/chemical toxicity.

When any type of detoxification program is undertaken there is usually a redistribution of heavy metals within the body. Therefore, it is very important to follow the guidelines in this section for heavy metal detoxification.

FOLLOW THE ACID-ALKALINE BALANCING DIET

When cleansing heavy metals from the body, it is very important to eat alkaline-forming foods and include plenty of the cruciferous vegetables such as cauliflower, broccoli, brussels sprouts, kale, and cabbage along with dark leafy greens for extra minerals and calcium. Get adequate amounts of protein as well; choose from vegan protein foods such as beans, lentils, split peas, whole grains (exclude wheat), raw nuts, and seeds. Nuts and seeds can be sprouted. Never fast while you are detoxifying heavy metals. Specific amino acids could be carrying around heavy metals, and fasting can break down the protective protein layers, exposing metals and causing damage. You may benefit from one or two protein shakes per day. (See information on whey protein on pp. 190–92.)

CARROT JUICE

Drink two glasses of carrot juice each day; you may add celery, cucumber, parsley, sprouts, jicama, any greens such as kale, spinach, or beet leaves; and flavor with ginger, one-half green apple (Pippin or Granny Smith), lemon, or herbs such as cilantro.

CILANTRO AND GARLIC

Thought to help in removing mercury from the body, cilantro can be added to salads, soups, juices, and salsas. Sulfur-containing foods such as garlic and onions help to combat heavy metal toxicity.[24]

WATER

Drink eight to ten 8-ounce glasses of purified water each day; alkalinizing water is very beneficial.

COLON CLEANSING FIBER SHAKES

Drink one to two of the Colon Cleansing Fiber Shakes each day. It is also advisable to take the herbal formulas recommended in The 7-Day Intestinal Cleanse once or twice daily. The fiber and bentonite will help to absorb the metals, preventing them from being reabsorbed into the system.

DO NOT TAKE ENZYMES DURING THIS CLEANSE

Enzymes can remove the protein that carries heavy metals out of the body, exposing the metals and causing damage.

SUPPLEMENTS WITH MEALS

- Calcium and vitamin C are nutrients that are necessary to protect tissues from heavy metal damage. Electrolytes (calcium, sodium, magnesium, potassium) and glutamine are necessary for proper pH balance and elimination of toxins.
- Alkalizing minerals are also important in the metal detox program.

SUPPLEMENTS AFTER MEALS

- Probiotic formula: two after each meal. (Probiotic formula is a friendly bacteria formula that helps restore good intestinal bacteria that may have been compromised by antibiotics and heavy metals.

SUPPLEMENTS BETWEEN MEALS

- Antioxidant formula: take as directed. (Antioxidants destroy free radicals and assist in liver cleansing.)
- L-Methionine: 500 mg, twice a day. L-methionine is an amino acid that binds to heavy metals and carries them out of the body.
- L-Cysteine: 500 mg, twice a day. L-Cysteine is an amino acid that binds to heavy metals and carries them from the body.
- Zinc: 50 to 100 mg daily. Zinc helps bind toxic metals to amino acids.

REMOVE ALL MERCURY AMALGAM FILLINGS

Research indicates that amalgam (silver fillings) surfaces release mercury vapor into the mouth, and this release rate is increased when you brush your teeth or chew your food. Once a surface is stimulated by such activities, mercury vapor from amalgams is released into your system. The authors of *Biological Monitoring of Toxic Metals* say that "the estimated release rates from amalgam appear to be consistent with levels of mercury found in autopsy tissue in the general population and with increases in brain and urinary levels due to amalgam fillings."[25] They also state that mercury from dental fillings is the predominate contribution to human exposure to inorganic mercury. The World Health Organization (WHO) has confirmed these conclusions, which are published in WHO *Environmental Health Criteria 118* titled "Inorganic Mercury."[26]

It is important to your Complete Cancer Cleanse Program that your amalgam fillings be removed by a dentist trained to prevent further mercury intoxication during the removal process. Also, the materials that replace amalgam fillings should be tested to determine that they are compatible with your body chemistry. (See *Dental Mercury Detox* by Sam Ziff, Michael Ziff, and Mats Hanson for further information.)

NOTE: Root canals can cause severe problems for some people that can contribute to cancer. If you have a root canal(s), see a holistic dentist who can advise you on your options of treatment.

IMMUNIZATIONS AND MERCURY

Thimerosol is a preservative that is found in many infant vaccines; it contains 49 percent ethyl mercury by weight and generally contributes as much as 25 micrograms of ethyl mercury per dose. Vaccines during the first eighteen months of an infant's life may put the infant at risk for neurobehavioral alterations, may contribute to autism, and will contribute to mercury toxicity. Hair analysis of mercury concentrations in infants exposed to vaccines containing thimerosol were in excess of the Environmental Protection Agency safety guidelines. To prevent mercury toxicity in children, avoid immunizations with thimerosol or any other vaccine that contains any form of mercury.[27]

CLEANSING REACTIONS

The Heavy Metal Detox Program can activate cold symptoms or numerous other cleansing symptoms that preceded or contributed to your current physical problems. Don't be alarmed if this happens; it simply means the process is working. Old symptoms can manifest for a short time as heavy metals are being released. This is part of the cleansing reaction, known as the Herxheimer Reaction.

BUILDING, REGENERATIVE FOODS

Thorough cleansing is never complete in our toxic world, and you will always need periodic detoxification. Once you've finished the cleansing programs appropriate for you, you are now ready to rebuild your body. Continue to choose building, regenerative foods that include whole grains, particularly millet, quinoa, brown and wild rice of all types, and amaranth; seaweeds; traditional soy foods only, such as organic, non-GMO tofu, tempeh, and soy sauce; beans such as black beans, mung beans, and aduki beans; sprouts; soups; salads; vegetables; nuts; seeds; fruits; and fresh juices, especially vegetable juices.

Make at least half of your food choices raw food unless you are very weak, frail, or anemic. In this case, you may need to eat more of your food gently warmed or cooked. If you decide to include some animal products, make sure they are organically grown and free-range raised; fish is the best choice (avoid farm-raised). And eat only small portions of animal products. Continue to make most of your meals vegan. Limit your choices of high-acid foods; no more than 25 percent of your diet. And continue to avoid all foods on the list that are harmful, such as refined foods, junk foods, alcohol, sugar, soda pop, and all products with artificial ingredients.

THE EASY CLEANSE SCHEDULE

For those who work full time and those who are particularly tired, weak, or overwhelmed, I have designed an Easy Cleanse Track, which is a modified cleansing process for you to begin your detoxification program. The schedule that follows is the best order in which to proceed with the cleansing programs.

Weeks One and Two:

The Acid-Alkaline Cleanse*; The Lymphatic Cleanse; The Skin Cleanse; The Lung Cleanse

Weeks Three and Four:
The 7-Day Easy Intestinal Cleanse

Week Five:
The 7-Day, Kick-Start Easy Liver Cleanse

Week Six:
The 7-Day Easy Gallbladder Cleanse

Week Seven:
The 7-Day Easy Kidney Cleanse

*This diet should be followed throughout your cleansing and healing process. The Lymphatic Cleanse, The Skin Cleanse, and The Lung Cleanse can also be carried out throughout the cleansing process and with any of the other cleanses.

THE COMPLETE CLEANSE SCHEDULE

Weeks One to Four:
The Acid-Alkaline Balancing Cleanse, The Lymphatic System Cleanse, The Skin Cleanse, and The Lung Cleanse

Weeks Five through Eight:
The Complete Intestinal Cleanse

Week Nine:
The 7-Day, Kick-Start Complete Liver Cleanse (This program can be continued for additional weeks, as needed.)

Week Ten:
The Complete Gallbladder Flush

Week Eleven:
The Kidney Cleanse

Weeks Twelve to Fourteen:
The Parasite Cleanse (If you do not need this cleanse, go on to Heavy Metal Detox.)

Week Fifteen:

The 30-Day Heavy Metal Detox Program (Continue for as many weeks as needed.)

NOTE: Repeat any of the cleansing programs as needed. Whenever you feel you need a rest, just follow The Acid-Alkaline Balancing Diet. It is best to stay with the program until you are completely well and there is no sign of cancer. Then it is advisable to continue with periodic cleanses to maintain your health and to observe the eating and healthy living habits outlined in this book.

7

SUPPLEMENTING YOUR CLEANSE

Nutritional supplementation is absolutely essential in order to give the body the tools that it needs to fight cancer.

—MURRAY, BIRDSALL, PIZZORNO, RILEY, *How to Prevent and Treat Cancer with Natural Medicine*

The complete cancer cleansing and rebuilding program emphasizes the importance of nourishing the body by thoroughly fueling its natural detoxification pathways with the right nutrients that enable it to achieve optimal metabolic activity. By providing high-quality protein (legumes, whole grains, sprouts, whey protein concentrate), complex carbohydrates (whole grains, legumes, vegetables, fruits), and essential fats (as found in fish oil, flaxseeds, olive oil), the body obtains what is needed to prevent muscle and organ breakdown and depleted energy resources. In addition, vitamins, minerals, enzymes, and phytochemicals are needed to support the functions of the organs that are directly involved in detoxification—the liver, the intestines, the kidneys, and the lungs.

The information in this chapter (as well as the good dietary choices noted in previous chapters) may be particularly important for your recovery from cancer. A survey evaluating sixty-two adult patients with early stages of cancer (six months or less) found substantial dietary deficiencies and a need for dietary supplementation.[1] Supplementing your cleanse with various nutrients can be very helpful in the cleansing process.

WHY SO MANY CONFLICTING STUDIES ABOUT SUPPLEMENTS?

Numerous conflicting reports about antioxidant supplements have appeared in the news in recent years. Vitamin C helps fight cancer, says one researcher. No, it actually interferes with cancer treatment, says another researcher. Beta-carotene is a superhero when it comes to beating cancer, says one study. Another study shows it was actually detrimental. So what is going on?

There are many possibilities as to why we see such conflicting reports. Sometimes studies show a supplement to be ineffective or of no consequence; then a closer look at the study shows that a very low dose (perhaps only 25 milligrams) was used. Sometimes a synthetic form of the nutrient was used, which was actually detrimental, whereas if a natural form of the vitamin had been used, it may have proven quite beneficial. Often only a single nutrient has been studied, which may have value in some instances, but when it comes to the antioxidants beta-carotene, vitamins C and E, and selenium, recent research indicates they work best together. Actually, they may be harmful when administered alone because vitamins too can become oxidized in the process of neutralizing free radicals. These vitamins must be restored to their antioxidant state with the help of other nutrients. For example, vitamin E (tocopherol) when it is oxidized becomes tocopheryl and requires glutathione and vitamin C working together to regenerate it back to its antioxidant status.

Nutrient Support for Organs of Detoxification

The most thorough way to detoxify the body is to fuel its detoxification processes with the nutrients that are necessary to achieve optimal detoxification activity. The list of nutrients following each of the four organs have been shown to assist that organ in its cleansing process.

Intestinal Tract

Zinc, pantothenic acid, L-glutamine (an amino acid), fructooligosaccharides (carbohydrates), and acidophilus and bifidus all help to support detoxification and healthy functioning of the intestinal tract.

Liver

Vitamins A and C, niacin, B_6, beta-carotene, copper, zinc, L-cysteine and L-glutamine (amino acids), glutathione (tri-peptide), and phospholipids (phosphorus-containing lipids) support liver functions and help it transform toxic substances into harmless products that can easily be excreted.

Kidneys

Vitamins A, C, B_6, and the minerals magnesium and potassium are some of the key nutrients that support the kidneys' activity of excreting toxins via the urine.

Lungs

The antioxidants vitamin C and bioflavonoids, vitamin E, beta-carotene, selenium, and glutathione are all protective for the lungs.

NUTRIENTS TO SUPPORT CLEANSING, HEALING, AND REBUILDING

It is typical for us in the West to look for "magic bullets" to cure all our ills. After all, we've grown up on aspirin and antibiotics! If it's not a drug, then we may be tempted to look for the "magic" nutritional bullets we can hang our hopes on. Though some people do claim that it was primarily one intervention, supplement, food, or substance that cured their cancers, most doctors, nutritionists, and researchers have discovered the need for a comprehensive program to facilitate the healing of cancer.

In their book *A Cancer Battle Plan*, Anne and David Frähm say,

> In our fast-paced culture, people typically look for a "quick fix" to their medical problems, something to take—often drugs—to make everything better soon. Reversing degenerative disease, however, is not a quick-fix proposition. It's a matter of an extended period of time spent working to revitalize the entire metabolism and chemistry of the body's system that has been heading downhill for perhaps a very long time.[2]

Though quick fixes and magic bullets rarely exist, opportunities do await us to make profound changes in our health and healing by doing all that we can to change the chemistry of our body, as well as the state of our mind and emotions. Nutritional supplements can be an important part of our detoxification, healing, and revitalization program and can help us restore balance where deficiencies previously existed.

In addition, research indicates that vitamins, minerals, and various phytochemicals may help reduce the toxicity of cancer treatments, such as chemotherapy and radiation. One study has shown that supplementation of high doses of multivitamins improved the survival rate among cancer patients receiving chemotherapy.[3]

The remainder of this chapter is devoted to the supplements that can help detoxify the body, rebuild strength and vitality, and assist in the body's battle with cancer. The following is a list of the nutrients that research studies have determined to be the most helpful in the detoxification and healing process, with an explanation of how these nutrients help cleanse the body and assist it in fighting cancer.

BETA-CAROTENE AND VITAMIN A

Although beta-carotene and other carotenes are often referred to as vitamin A, cancer researchers often use beta-carotene in studies. Pigments known as carotenes give foods their colors of red, green, and orange. Some carotenes are known as provitamin A because they are converted in the body to vitamin A, as needed.

There have been a number of conflicting reports about supplemental beta-carotene and cancer in recent years—some indicating it is helpful in prevention (these results may be attributed to nonsynthetic forms of the vitamin combined with other antioxidants), and others suggesting it might not help at all or even be harmful (these results may be due to the very low doses or to the administration of synthetic forms of beta-carotene usually without the accompanying complementary antioxidants).

One thing is clear: beta-carotene and other carotenes found in plant-based foods have been shown to be cancer preventative in hundreds of studies conducted all over the world; the effectiveness of these carotenes is unquestioned. Scientists suggest that the beta-carotene effect may be accounted for, or enhanced by, other carotenoids in vegetables and fruits such as lutein, zeaxanthin, lycopene, and alpha-carotene.

Here are some of the effects beta-carotene has demonstrated in detoxification of the body and the care and treatment of cancer.

- Helps detoxify carcinogens such as cigarette smoke, industrial waste, and the effects of charbroiled meat. It is a potent quencher of singlet oxygen (free radical).[4]
- Acts as an antioxidant; enhances immune functions.[5]
- Inhibits cancer cell growth and malignant transformation.[6]
- Inhibits the effects of radiation.[7]

Supplements

Apart from what is available in your multivitamin mineral supplements, which is usually about 2,500 to 10,000 IUs (international units) of beta-carotene, I recommend that you get your carotenes primarily from vegetables, fruits, and freshly made juices. I particularly recommend fresh juice, not just because I'm known as the Juice Lady, but because you can juice up more beta-carotene-rich produce than you can probably eat in a day. This ensures that you are getting all the complementary antioxidants, including carotenes and other nutrients that work synergistically with beta-carotene.

Foods Rich in Beta-Carotene

Choose foods that are dark orange, green, red, or yellow. Within these color groups, those highest in beta-carotene include: dandelion greens, carrots, collard greens, kale, sweet potatoes, yams, parsley, spinach, turnips, mustard greens, beet greens, Swiss chard, chives, yellow squashes (such as butternut, Hubbard, and acorn), mangos, sweet peppers (red, yellow, and green), cantaloupe, endive, papayas, broccoli, tomatoes, green onions, and Romaine lettuce.

CALCIUM

Calcium supplementation at 1,200 to 1,500 milligrams per day has been associated with lower rates of colon adenoma polyps (benign tumors that can become malignant).[8] Calcium is thought to help prevent colon cancer by binding with bile salts and fatty acids that can damage the colon's epithelium (lining) and promote rapid multiplication of cells.[9]

A number of studies indicate that we should get our calcium from plant-based foods and supplements, such as calcium citrate, rather than dairy products, because dairy has been associated with cancer risk in some studies. Several studies show dairy food intake associated with prostate cancer risk.[10] An evaluation of 80,326 women in the Nurses' Health Study found that women who consumed the highest amount of dairy (one or more servings per day) had the greater risk for all types of invasive ovarian cancer than those who ate the lowest number of servings (three or fewer servings per month).[11] Other studies have shown a positive result from low-fat dairy products; therefore, the results regarding dairy products are mixed. However, to be on the safe side and for a host of other reasons mentioned throughout this book, dairy products are not part of The Complete Cancer Cleanse Diet.

Supplements

The recommendation for supplemental calcium is 1,200 to 1,500 milligrams daily. The most available form of calcium for absorption is chelated calcium. The best choice is calcium citrate or other soluble forms such as calcium gluconate, calcium lactate, or calcium aspartate. Calcium carbonate has not been shown to be as biologically available. Avoid oyster shell calcium, dolomite, and bone meal; they may have high lead content.

Plant Foods Rich in Calcium

In general, dark leafy greens are an excellent source of calcium. Specific calcium-rich foods include: kelp, greens (such as collard, dandelion, beet, and turnip greens), kale, parsley, watercress, almonds, corn tortillas made with lime, tofu, sunflower seeds, sesame seeds, tahini (sesame butter), and broccoli.

CONJUGATED LINOLEIC ACID (CLA)

A slightly altered form of the essential fatty acid called linoleic acid, conjugated linoleic acid (CLA) arises naturally in animal products of free-range, grazing animals. (*Free range* and *grazing* are key words. No wonder we don't get much CLA in our diets. Very few animals are raised on the range and allowed to eat grass.) CLA was first discovered to have anticancer compounds in 1978 at the University of Wisconsin.[12] Though there does not appear to be research specifically showing it assists in the detoxification process, it is noteworthy that research indicates CLA may offer nutritional support for several forms of cancer—breast, prostate, colorectal, lung, skin, and stomach. The recommendation of CLA is 1 to 3 grams daily.

CLA may be beneficial in that it

- alters a protein in cancer tissue that is essential for its growth; this protein stimulates blood capillaries that supply tumors with nutrients. CLA may cause this protein to be less effective.[13]
- may directly affect the process of carcinogenesis (the production or origin of cancer).[14]
- reduces cachexia (a condition marked by weight loss, muscular wasting, and loss of appetite), which is associated with advanced cancer and certain cancer treatments.[15]
- may inhibit cancer at the initiation, promotion, progression, and metastasis phases.[16]
- acts as an antioxidant and immune regulator.

FLAVONOIDS

Flavonoids refer to a group of plant pigments that give fruits and vegetables their color; they include proanthocyanidins, citrus bioflavonoids (rutin, quercitin, hesperidin, and narigin), quercitin, and green tea polyphenols. These pigments have potent antioxidant action with anticancer properties.

Various flavonoids offer specific benefits:

- Citrus flavonoids have been shown to inhibit certain cytochrome P450 enzymes (liver detoxification enzymes), which can turn cigarette smoke and other carcinogens into forms that promote cancer. Hesperidin has been shown to block a specific enzyme (P450 1B1) from turning toxic substances into carcinogens. The P450 enzyme 1B1 has been shown to be present in high levels in breast and prostate cancer.[17]

- Quercitin has been found in certain animal studies to reduce the number and sites of tumors; it may be beneficial in reducing the risk of stomach cancer. It is abundant in onions.[18]
- Proanthocyanidins have been shown to trap free radicals, delay the onset of lipid peroxidation, and chelate to (combine with) iron molecules, thereby preventing iron-induced lipid peroxidation.[19]
- Flavonoids enhance the effectiveness of vitamin C. It is recommended that they be taken in half to equal amounts with vitamin C.

Supplements

Look for proanthocyanidins (grape seed extract), rutin, hesperidin, and citrus flavonoids. Recommended supplementation may vary depending on the amount of fresh juice you drink and the number of fruit and vegetable servings you eat daily. The recommendation is to consume half to equal amounts of flavonoids to vitamin C. If you are drinking several glasses of fresh vegetable juice each day and eating plenty of fresh vegetables and fruits, you may not need any additional supplementation besides what you are getting from your diet and your multiple vitamin-mineral supplements.

Plant Sources of Flavonoids

In general, flavonoids are found in brightly colored fruits, vegetables, and flowers (choose only edible flower varieties). Some of the best sources of flavonoids are rose hips, parsley, onions, red cabbage, peppers, papaya, cantaloupe, tomato, broccoli, black currents, black cherries, blueberries, raspberries, and blackberries and in small quantities due to their acid content, citrus fruits.

FOLIC ACID

Folic acid (one of the B vitamins) functions in partnership with vitamin B_{12} in many bodily functions. Though we often think of folic acid, also called folate or folacin, as the vitamin that's been newsworthy in the prevention of birth defects, folic acid has been linked to cancer prevention. Scientific research has identified the following benefits:

- Folate along with vitamin B_{12} helps provide correct duplication of DNA. Cancer involves DNA that has "gone awry"—lacking the ability for our cells to replicate correctly and then die at the appropriate time. Studies have found that low folate conditions can trigger "brittle" DNA that fuels cancer metastasis.[20]

- Folate is essential in the synthesis and methlylation of (introduction of the methyl group into) DNA. Low levels of folate may increase the rate of DNA mutations, damage, and replication errors.[21]

- The Nurses' Health Study review of 88,756 women between 1980 and 1984 found that women who had a folate intake of more than 400 mcg (micrograms) daily were less likely to be diagnosed with colon cancer during the study than those who consumed less than 200 mcg daily. Those who took daily multivitamins containing folate for more than fifteen years were 75 percent less likely to develop colon cancer than women who did not use supplements.[22]

- Without optimal amounts of folate within the cells, growth is erratic and prone to errors, such as found in cancer cells. People with low B_{12} and folic acid status present a clinical picture that looks like leukemia.[23] Patrick Quillin, nutritionist and author of *Beating Cancer with Nutrition,* says, "Without adequate folate in the diet, cell growth is like a drunk driver heading down the highway—more likely to do some harm than not."[24] Alcohol is a known folate antagonist, and consumption of alcohol reduces folate's availability.

News about Folic Acid

Research has found that folic acid does not interfere with the effects of the chemotherapy drug methotrexate as once thought; therefore, you can take folic acid.[25]

Supplements

Folinic acid is the most active form of folic acid; the recommended dose is 400 mcg per day. I recommend that folic acid be taken as part of a B-vitamin complex, unless otherwise prescribed by your health-care professional. A high-quality, vitamin-mineral supplement should have adequate amounts of folic acid.

Plant Foods Rich in Folic Acid

Folic acid takes its name from the Latin word *folium,* which means "foliage." No doubt this is due to its high concentration in dark leafy green vegetables (like spinach and kale) and beet and mustard greens. However, folic acid is actually found in highest concentration in brewer's yeast and legumes such as black-eyed peas, beans, lentils, and split peas. Asparagus and broccoli are also good sources of folate along with nuts, especially walnuts and filberts.

GREEN TEA

Green tea originates from an evergreen shrub known as *Camellia sinensis,* from which young leaves are lightly steamed to produce green tea. The powerful antioxidant flavonoids, known as the polyphenols, remain in green tea due to the steaming process. Not only do these polyphenols act as antioxidants, they may also increase the activity of antioxidant enzymes in the small intestine, liver, and lungs. Epidemiological studies indicate that cancer rates are lower in Japan than the United States, believed to be in part due to the traditional three cups or more of green tea the Japanese drink daily.[26]

Research indicates the following benefits from green tea:

- In animal studies, epigallocatechin gallate, the most active of the polyphenols in green tea, was found to inhibit both the activation and promotion phases of cancer development. The green tea polyphenols inhibit the activity of tumor promoters with their receptor sites.[27]

- Green tea has been shown to delay the onset of cancer and prevents secondary primary tumors, recurrence of tumors, and metastasis in those with a history of cancer treatment.[28]

- Chemical carcinogens may be inhibited by green tea polyphenols.[29]

Supplements

Green tea contains less caffeine than coffee—three cups of green tea have about the same dose of caffeine as one cup of coffee. It's easy to add at least one or two cups of green tea to your diet each day. If you are sensitive to caffeine, you may wish to get the decaffeinated tea; always look for naturally decaffeinated tea rather than chemically processed. Many brands offer organically grown green tea and are available at health food stores.

LYCOPENE

Lycopene is the carotene that gives tomatoes their red color. It has powerful antioxidant action that works synergistically with other carotenes such as canthanxanthin, luetin, and alpha-carotene to scavenge free radicals. Lycopene has been shown to have anticarcinogenic and antilipid peroxidation properties. The following are some of lycopene's benefits:

- Phytochemicals such as lycopene can inhibit carcinogenesis (production of cancer cells) by inhibiting Phase I and inducing Phase II enzymes of liver detoxification. This is very important to people who have slower Phase II activity because a slow Phase II allows toxic intermediates opportunity to damage tissues. Lycopene also scavenges DNA-damaging agents and suppresses rapid spread of preneoplastic (tumorous) lesions by inhibiting various properties of cancer cells.[30]

- Lycopene has been shown to accumulate in the prostate. The consumption of tomato products, especially cooked tomatoes (one of the richest sources of lycopene), is associated with reduced risk of prostate cancer.[31]

- For those who have prostate cancer, lycopene supplementation is recommended as one study showed that men taking 15 milligrams of lycopene twice daily had reduced prostate-specific antigens (PSAs) by 18 percent.[32] In another study of twenty-one men with prostate cancer compared to twelve controls, 30 milligrams of lycopene supplement (equivalent to consuming 3 to 4 pounds of tomatoes) that contained a natural tomato-oil resin (which improved lycopene's absorption) was given for three weeks. In just this short time, the men with prostate cancer demonstrated a lower-grade tumor.[33]

- People in the Mediterranean have combined olive oil with tomato sauce (which gives better absorption of lycopene) for generations, and now science has proven their success once again. Not only is their diet heart-healthy, the olive oil improves lycopene's absorption, making it even more cancer-preventative.

Supplements

Lycopene is available in supplement form, which is expensive, but for those with prostate cancer, it may be needed for improved PSA levels. Look for Lyc-o-Mata by LycoRed Natural Products Industries, which contains the natural tomato-oil resin. Take as directed.

Plant Foods Rich in Lycopene

Lycopene is quite stable during cooking and processing. Actually, you will absorb up to five times more lycopene from heat-processed tomato products, such as tomato sauce and canned or bottled tomato juice, as you will from raw tomatoes because processing releases lycopene from the plant's cells.[34] Choose tomato sauce, tomato paste, canned tomatoes, bottled or canned tomato juice, and of course, fresh raw tomatoes as well. Other sources of lycopene include papaya, guava, and watermelon. *Because tomatoes are acidic foods, remember to count them as part of your acid foods in the 25 percent acid-food category for the day.*

SELENIUM

Selenium is among the most thoroughly studied of the micronutrients in relation to cancer. It is a trace mineral that works primarily as a component of the antioxidant enzyme glutathione peroxidase (along with beta-carotene and vitamin E) to prevent free radical damage to cellular membranes. Selenium also enhances an immune response, which has been shown to inhibit cancer growth.[35]

Studies dating back to 1965 have noted that people living in areas where soil and water are rich in selenium show lower cancer rates than the national average.[36] More recent epidemiological studies have confirmed that areas with high selenium content in food and water have shown lower incidence of cancers of the lung, colon, rectum, bladder, esophagus, pancreas, breast, ovary, and cervix.[37] Selenium offers the following benefits:

- Taking supplemental selenium may positively affect the outcome of a cancer treatment plan. For example, some studies have shown a poorer prognosis for cancer patients with lower selenium levels, as measured by blood work.[38] One study has shown that when selenium was given to cancer patients along with beta-carotene and vitamin E, it reduced cancer deaths by 13 percent.[39] Another study showed selenium supplements increased the ability of immune cells to kill tumor cells by 118 percent.[40]

- Selenium is important in detoxification in that it works with the enzyme glutathione peroxidase, which is an antioxidant that neutralizes free radicals that are produced during Phase I of liver detoxification; selenium is also required in a Phase II detoxification process.

Heavy Metals and Selenium

If you have elevated levels of heavy metals such as lead, cadmium, mercury, and arsenic, all of which are selenium antagonists (meaning substances that nullify the effects of another substance), absorption of selenium is adversely affected.[41] Keep in mind that most people in industrialized countries have elevated levels of heavy metals because of industrial and chemical pollution; therefore, it is wise to address detoxification of heavy metals as part of the complete cancer cleansing process.

Supplements

Only small amounts of supplemental selenium are needed daily—between 200 to 400 micrograms. The best form is selenomethionine, extracted from selenium-rich yeast or ocean plants. This is the least toxic and most absorbable form. Vitamin C enhances the absorption of selenium.

Plant Foods Rich in Selenium

Brazil nuts, barley, red Swiss chard, oats, brown rice, turnips, garlic, and radishes are the best plant sources. Keep in mind that cooking reduces selenium significantly and the process of refining strips foods of selenium.

VITAMIN C

Vitamin C (ascorbic acid) is an antioxidant that plays a key role in supporting the immune system by stimulating the production of lymphocytes, which include T cells, B cells, and natural killer cells—the major "attack and destroy unit" that goes after tumor cells. Vitamin C is also required by the thymus gland (the major gland of our immune system). This vitamin is responsible as well for the production of the T lymphocytes that are in charge of cell-mediated immunity. Cell-mediated immunity is critical in fighting cancer cells; and, typically, thymic hormone levels are low in individuals with cancer. Vitamin C increases the mobility of phagocytes, the cells that "chomp up" foreign invaders. It has also been shown to increase levels of interferon (a chemical factor that fights cancer).[42]

Vitamin C is important in fighting cancer as follows:

- Responsible for rejuvenating damaged vitamin E, it also helps the liver deal with pollutants, drugs, and toxic chemicals. It is needed to activate Phase I of liver detoxification.

- Vitamin C is a nitrite scavenger. Nitrites readily form a potentially dangerous, carcinogenic substance known as nitrosamines in the acidic environment of the stomach. As a water-soluble agent (meaning it dissolves in the body's water), vitamin C converts nitroso-compounds to less carcinogenic products, prevents nitrosamine formation in the diet, and converts free radicals to harmless waste in the intestinal tract; vitamin C also detoxifies carcinogenic organic compounds.[43]

- Individuals consuming the typical North American diet have shown mutagens in their feces, which are potential carcinogens. Mutagens have been shown to disappear from the feces when 400 to 1,000 milligrams of vitamin C were added to the diet.[44]

- Research conducted by the distinguished scientist and two-time Nobel Prize–winner Linus Pauling and his associate Dr. Ewan Cameron in Glasgow-area hospitals with one hundred terminally ill cancer patients showed that high doses of vitamin C (10 grams of C per day), given as an adjunct to appropriate conventional therapy, had value for essentially every cancer patient. They lived longer—114 to 435 days longer—than controls. The vitamin C–treated patients also reported feeling better, with increased muscular strength and general vitality. A similar study was carried out in Fukuoka Torikai Hospital, Japan, showing parallel results.[45]

The Great Debate on Vitamin C

Studies on the effectiveness of vitamin C are conflicting, and some argue that it might have adverse effects on chemotherapy or radiation.

Dr. Kedar N. Prasad, professor of radiology at the University of Colorado Health Science Center of Denver, is out to prove differently. Since 1980 Prasad and his colleagues at the University of Colorado have found that high doses of antioxidants, including vitamin C, may not only protect normal cells during cancer treatment but can actually help fight tumors. They have demonstrated that vitamins are selective and inhibit only cancer cell growth; in other words, we can take high doses of antioxidants and our normal cells will only acquire what they need. Cancer cells have lost their mechanism of control, however, and will gobble up antioxidants at a higher level. When vitamin C accumulates in excess, it initiates a series of events that can end in cancer cell death, growth inhibition, or differentiation. Prasad does not recommend vitamins or any other single antioxidant alone, but that vitamins C, E, and beta-carotene always be taken together for their complementary action.[46]

Supplements

Recommended dosage is 500 to 1,000 milligrams, three times a day. Studies show that vitamin C absorption is greatly increased when combined with flavonoids. Flavonoids should be taken in half to equal amounts of vitamin C, and may be obtained in large part from freshly made juices and fresh produce. These foods also provide glutathione, which is necessary to restore oxidized vitamin C (ascorbate, a pro-oxidant) back to an antioxidant. Vitamin E, beta-carotene, and selenium should be taken with vitamin C for best results.

Plant Foods Rich in Vitamin C

It's important to eat fruits and vegetables that are rich in vitamin C when taking supplemental C because they contain complementary nutrients such as beta-carotene, bioflavonoids, and other phytochemicals that work synergistically with this antioxidant. This is also why it is important to drink fresh vegetable juices every day; juicing makes it easy to consume a larger amount of these foods daily than we would normally. Foods highest in vitamin C include: peppers (red chili and sweet), kale, parsley, collard and turnip greens, broccoli, brussels sprouts, watercress, cauliflower, red cabbage, strawberries, papaya, and spinach.

NOTE: All these foods are higher in Vitamin C than orange juice. It may be that orange juice is recommended for vitamin C because it's also loaded with citrus flavonoids, making vitamin C absorption more effective. However, oranges and orange juice are not recommended while battling cancer because of their acidity and higher sugar content.

VITAMIN E

Vitamin E is the premier fat-soluble antioxidant and anticarcinogen. One of its key roles is to protect vitamins A and C from oxidation. Vitamin E protects cell membranes from heavy metals, toxic compounds, drugs, cleaning solvents, radiation, and free-radical damage. It also protects the thymus gland and white blood cells from damage. Vitamin E can help the body in cleansing and fighting cancer as follows:

- Vitamin E functions as a free-radical scavenger. It inhibits lipid (fat) peroxidation by breaking lipid free-radical chain reactions. It protects certain membranes from oxidative damage.[47]

- Vitamin E, like vitamin C, is a nitrite scavenger; it blocks nitrite conversion to nitrosamines (carcinogenic compounds). Fecal mutagens (which cause mutations of cells) were also shown to decrease with vitamin E supplementation.[48]

- Vitamin E has been shown to inhibit highly carcinogenic compounds such as TPA and mezerein.[49]

- A relationship between vitamin E deficiency and cancer has been found in a number of studies. One observational study involving 5,004 women with breast cancer found lower plasma vitamin E levels than were found in control subjects.[50]

- Studies involving animals have shown that those undergoing chemotherapy and radiation showed greater tumor regression when using a combination of vitamins E, C, K, and retinoids (vitamin A).[51]

- Studies have shown that patients receiving chemotherapy that were given 1,600 IU of vitamin E per day experienced less hair loss than usual.[52] One study in 1985 found that 66 percent of the patients undergoing chemotherapy who received 1,600 IU of vitamin E daily did not experience hair loss. The researchers believe that those who did lose hair received the vitamin E too late before beginning chemotherapy.[53]

- Vitamin E, along with other antioxidants, may help stop the downward spiral of wasting (cachexia) experienced by many cancer patients. Here's how it appears to work. The tumor necrosis factor (TNF) alpha prevents the production of albumin. Low levels of albumin (a key protein made in the liver) have been noted in wasting. Researchers have found that one way to halt this process and stop the downward spiral of wasting is to supplement cancer patients' diets with high amounts of vitamin E and the other antioxidants. When oxidative stress is blocked (thanks to the antioxidants!), everything is normalized.[54]

Supplements

The best forms of vitamin E are natural as distinguished by *d* as in *d-alpha-tocopherol;* avoid synthetic forms designated as *dl.* The most active form of vitamin E is d-alpha-tocopherol, with mixed tocopherols being the best choice because that is how they appear in food. Significant increase of vitamin E in the diet is difficult without some supplementation. The risk of toxicity is low at doses between 200 to 800 milligrams daily. More than this amount is not recommended without medical supervision.

Plant Foods Rich in Vitamin E

Vitamin E most often occurs in the fats of plant foods. In general vitamin E is found in whole grains, nuts, seeds, and vegetables. Specific plant foods that are the richest in vitamin E include: sunflower seeds, almonds, spinach, oatmeal, asparagus, and brown rice.

Antioxidant Supplements and Cancer Treatment

Many people have been told to stop taking their antioxidant supplements during cancer treatment, because some people in the health-care profession believe that these supplements may interfere with treatment. At this time, however, research is pointing to the fact that taking all the antioxidants (beta-carotene, vitamins C and E, and selenium) together, rather than any one of them alone, actually supports treatment, protects healthy cells, and helps to reduce some of the devastating side effects of treatment, such as nausea, diarrhea, hair loss, and fatigue.[55]

WHEY PROTEIN

When I think about whey, the first thing that comes to my mind is my grandmother repeating the rhyme about little Miss Muffett eating her curds and whey. Since the day that simple rhyme was written, whey has come a long way—it's been elevated to the realm of high-tech research. One of the areas of focus is its remarkable ability to help fight cancer and support the detoxification process by increasing levels of glutathione—a key component in liver detoxification.

One thing nearly everyone in the field of cancer care and research agrees on is a high probability that you will burn more calories and your need for protein will go up when you have cancer. Your metabolic rate increases on average of 15 percent.[56]

Whey protein concentrates provide quality protein without the animal fat, lactose, hormones, antibiotics, and other undesirable factors associated with animal products. In addition, animal products are not as easy to digest, whereas whey protein is easily digestable and gentle to the system. Whey is the watery liquid that separates from the solid part of milk when it turns sour or when enzymes are added in cheesemaking. Cheesemaking uses the casein (a protein formed in milk), lactose, fat, and minerals, which are filtered out, and pure whey protein is left behind. Whey provides a high-quality protein powder because it is a complete protein, providing all the essential and nonessential amino acids (the building blocks of protein). Whey, when made properly, provides some of the most absorbable and usable protein available.

Weight loss and wasting (known as cachexia and characterized by loss of strength, appetite, energy, and muscle mass) is something many people with cancer experience at some point in their treatments and/or progressions of their disease. This wasting can be attributed to the tumor and metabolic changes and may be compounded by treatments such as chemotherapy or radiation. Cachexia has been likened to a car that burns too much fuel. Tumors have the ability to retain nitrogen (one of the important elements in protein) and undergo cell division at the expense of healthy tissue (known as the "nitrogen trap" concept).[57] In other words, the cancer cells tend to gobble up protein, while the healthy tissues starve.

Studies have shown an increased need for amino acids when you have cancer because cancer cells take more amino acids from the bloodstream than most normal tissues. Simultaneously, synthesis of albumin, one of a group of simple proteins, declines and in some cases breaks down (known as hyoalbuminemia), another characteristic of cancer cachexia.[58]

Some chemotherapy drugs, especially corticosteroids, cause tissue breakdown and promote excessive urinary loss of protein, potassium, and calcium. The lining of the intestines and the digestive process is also adversely affected, altering digestion and absorption of nutrients. Vitamin, protein, and energy metabolism may adversely change as well.[59] If adequate protein is not supplied, the tumor will take protein from the muscles and increase wasting. Therefore, it is very important to increase not only vitamin and mineral intake but also to obtain high-quality protein in an easy-to-digest and easy-to-assimilate form. It is estimated that during illness, treatment, and recovery protein needs almost double.[60]

Research shows these benefits from supplementing whey protein:

- Whey protein appears to inhibit the growth of cancer cells. One study showed that when cancer patients were fed 30 grams of whey protein concentrate per day for six months, some patients' tumors showed regression.[61]

- By raising glutathione levels, whey protein can help to strengthen healthy cells and simultaneously weaken cancer cells. Studies have shown that whey protein does increase glutathione levels.[62] According to the research available to date, here's how it seems to work: Cancer cells appear to have higher levels of glutathione than healthy cells, which makes them stronger. However, when you raise the glutathione level in cancer cells to a point where they "peak out," they will shut off (called feedback inhibition); this causes a reduction of glutathione and weakens cancer cells, making them more susceptible to treatments that destroy them. At the same time healthy cells will take up the glutathione and amino acids they need and become stronger.[63]

Supplementing with Whey Protein

Studies have used 30 grams of whey protein concentrate per day; some doctors recommend 20 to 30 grams of whey protein twice a day.[64] You can mix whey protein in almond milk, rice milk, fresh juice, or water. It also makes a great addition to smoothies and protein shakes, which are delicious.

NOTE: Throughout The Complete Cancer Cleanse Program I have stressed the importance of vegan foods over animal foods for a variety of reasons too numerous to recount here, but whey protein is one exception. In all the research I've reviewed, soy protein has not been the protein of choice for cancer patients because it is harder to digest than whey protein. The benefits of whey protein concentrate appear at this time to greatly outweigh that of soy protein for cancer patients. If you are sensitive to dairy whey, try goat whey protein. If you cannot tolerate either of these, try rice protein.

FACTS ABOUT SUPPLEMENTS AND CLEANSING

Finally as you begin to use supplements, following are a few of the most-asked questions.

WHEN DO I TAKE SUPPLEMENTS?

Unless otherwise directed by your health-care professional or the supplement directions, supplements are best taken with food. Think of your supplements as you would a sandwich. Eat some food, take your supplements somewhere in the middle of your meal or snack, and then finish your food. That way you're giving the supplements the best chance for utilization and yourself the least chance for stomach upset. Some schools of thought say it's best not to drink fluids with meals. It's not only okay to swallow your supplements with water—it's necessary. NOTE: Some supplements should be taken on an empty stomach. Follow the directions accordingly.

WHICH SUPPLEMENTS ARE BEST?

Choose a high-quality line of supplements—the higher the quality the better. You will need to pay more for high-quality nutrients, just as you do for any other quality product. But it's worth it. You're in a battle for your health, and the best is worth the extra money spent. Some of the cheaper brands of supplements use synthetic nutrients or inferior-quality products.

For further recommendations of supplements for cancer, two books that have an extensive list of nutrients for cancer treatment are: *How to Prevent and Treat Cancer with Natural Medicine* by Dr. Michael Murray, Dr. Tim Birdsall, Dr. Joseph E. Pizzorno, and Dr. Paul Reilly (Riverhead Books, 2002); and *Beating Cancer with Nutrition* by Patrick Quillin, Ph.D., R.D., CNS, with Noreen Quillin (Nutrition Times Press, 2001).

SUPPLEMENTING YOUR EASY CLEANSE

If you have limited funds or feel overwhelmed by the thought of taking large numbers of supplements, follow the easy track.

Easy Choice Supplements

Choose a high-quality multiple vitamin-mineral supplement and take the recommended amount each day, which is often two per meal. Or you can get packets of supplements that contain most of the key nutrients and then you don't have to think about what to grab each day. You can tuck the packets in your purse, briefcase, or travel bag.

Easy Choice Protein

Make a smoothie every day with whey protein (goat whey or rice protein if you're sensitive to dairy) for your amino acid supplementation. Smoothies are fun and taste delicious. *The Ultimate Smoothie Book* by Cherie Calbom (Warner, 2001) has 101 delicious and healthy smoothie choices.

8

CLEANSING YOUR ENVIRONMENT

We must use our intelligence, our knowledge, and our wisdom to overcome the negative things in our environment and undertake a healthier way of life.

—BERNARD JENSEN

In many ways our everyday routines are beneficial because they allow us to easily get through our days without having to think and rethink every single detail of our existence. However, when we are recovering from a serious illness, it becomes imperative to live more consciously. Then we must consider how our daily actions and activities affect our health and act in ways that are most conducive to our recovery.

At first glance, it may seem implausible that certain normal activities could be detrimental to our physical well-being. However, if we scrutinize them more closely, with an open mind, it becomes obvious that many conveniences we take for granted are based on the products of technology. Weighed on the larger scale of human history, they are completely new. Yet we feel dependent on a lifestyle that did not even exist two generations ago, one that involves exposure to a myriad of substances that are anything but healthy—and a growing number of which are clearly carcinogenic.

When Rachel Carson wrote *Silent Spring* in 1962, she was a pioneer in the field of ecology. Before then, few people realized that humans were capable of altering their environments in a way that could be detrimental to life. With innocence and optimism we celebrated a technology that, born out of World War II, promised better lives and offered what seemed to be solutions to everything from world hunger to the production of more affordable commodities. Little did we know that these technologies, which relied upon the use of synthetic petrol-chemicals, were releasing substances into the environment that would prove to be deadly. Not only are these byproducts of industry and agriculture toxic, many are also persistent in the environment because they do not break down as do the carbohydrate-based products of the past.

Synthetic chemicals that don't break down are called "Persistent Organic Pollutants" (POPs) or "Persistent Bioaccumalative Toxins" (PBTs). *Bioaccumulative* means that these chemicals are stored faster than they are broken down or excreted when we ingest them from food, air, or water. Prior to 1945, the products of industry were mainly based on plants. For example, from the late nineteenth century to about 1945, even a plastic-like material called celluloid was derived from plants. After 1945 this all changed as our economy "progressed" from carbohydrates to petrol-chemicals.[1]

Each year industries in the United States produce over 250 million tons of hazardous waste, more than one ton per man, woman, and child currently living in America—and the numbers increase each time we use and dispose of these products.[2] These chemicals find their way into our food, our water, our homes, and our bodies. In fact, every person alive today, even children living in remote parts of the world, carries approximately 250 chemicals within his or her body. This is called the "body burden."

Some of these chemicals, such as DDT (dichloro diphenyl thrichloroethane) and PCBs (polychlorinated biphenyls), which are both Persistent Organic Pollutants (POPs), were banned in the United States in the 1970s because they are known carcinogens. In 1994, America exported millions of pounds of unregistered, cancelled, or suspended pesticides to other parts of the world. Many of them then come back to us as residues in our imported foods.[3]

With the increase in environmental pollutants, there has also been an increase in cancer. In 1904, one out of twenty-four Americans had cancer; in the 1950s the cancer rate rose to one in four. By 1999 it was estimated that one in two American men and one in three American women would get cancer in his or her lifetime, and this is not simply because we are living longer.[4] Cancer is also the number one killer of children aside from accidents.[5]

Rachel Carson was not the only scientist to suspect that environmental pollutants may be a cause of cancer. In 1964 Dr. Wilhelm Hueper and Dr. W. C. Conway, both with the National Cancer Institute, wrote, "Cancers of all types and all causes display even under already existing conditions, all the characteristics of an epidemic in slow motion." They said that this epidemic was fueled by the "increasing contamination of the human environment with chemical and physical carcinogens and with chemicals supporting and potentiating their action."[6]

Shortly after the debut of *Silent Spring,* Theron Randolph, M.D., wrote *An Alternative Approach to Allergies,* the first major work relating the indoor environment to human health. Improper ventilation, molds, offgassing (the release of chemicals as a gas into the atmosphere) from synthetic materials, radon gas, wood smoke, and other factors—all contribute to what is known as the "sick building syndrome." This syndrome is far more widespread than people realize, and its effects on human health are almost as varied as the human potential for illness. The sick building syndrome can cause nonspecific symptoms such as headache, swelling, abdominal discomfort, drowsiness, ringing in the ears, fatigue, malaise, and blurred vision.

Indoor pollution can damage DNA and cause neurological problems, birth defects, allergies, asthma, and cancer.[7] If this is true, we may ask why everyone doesn't get sick. Those who suffer these symptoms become ill because their body burden of chemicals is higher from occupational exposure, or from their particular living conditions, or from their nutritional deficiencies, or their impaired ability to detoxify carcinogens. Other individuals are predisposed because of a weakened liver or genetic makeup. Children are more at risk from indoor pollutants than adults because of physical factors, such as higher rates of inhalation and pulse, which allow for more rapid absorption. Even the exposure a mother receives when she is pregnant affects her unborn child.

As our interior air quality worsens, diseases like asthma increase. The prevalence of asthma in the United States increased by almost 40 percent from 1981 to 1988, a trend that is also noticeable in other countries throughout the world. In the case of some toxins, it takes years for an exposed person to become ill. For example, radon accounts for ten thousand to twenty thousand lung cancer deaths per year, and some researchers estimate that the carcinogenic risk of chemicals in residential indoor air is equal to the cancer risk of radon and secondhand tobacco smoke.[8]

The idea that the ordinary, everyday products that most of us grew up with can be harmful is usually met with resistance because it is such a foreign concept. We use such things as bleach, cleaning products, skin lotions, makeup, hair sprays, insect sprays, paints, and varnishes continuously and never consider how they may be affecting our health or our planet. Anyway, we need these products, don't we? No one wants to go back to the pioneer days of "roughing it" *au naturale.* But to go natural, we don't have to live like our ancestors. There are healthful or inert alternatives to every toxic product that we may think we need. We just have to learn what they are and how to use them.

When we make improvements in our personal diet, home and work environment, and lifestyle, our health will improve dramatically. This is a holistic approach to living that not only helps in cancer recovery, it benefits every aspect of our being. By making the effort to follow these suggestions, most people discover that they start feeling better, have more energy, are sick less often, and look better; the obscure little problems they had lived with for so long and thought were simply part of their makeup miraculously disappear. It is true that some people recover from cancer without making major lifestyle changes, but many people do not. And why chance it? Why not put every effort you can into making changes in your favor? It may not be easy—making major lifestyle changes rarely is—but the rewards are well worth the effort.

It's time to get down to business, and the easiest place to embark upon a personal environment cleansing is in the pantry.

CLEANSING YOUR PANTRY

We already know why processed food is inferior to fresh whole food, so let's throw out the junk! To get started, however, it is important to have the complete support of your family and others in your home. This is not a game; your health is on the line, so be a little selfish: let everyone know that *no* junk food can be brought into the house. If they must have it, let them indulge elsewhere.

After being on a fresh, whole foods diet for a period of time, you will lose your taste for processed, unhealthy foods, but in the beginning, before your taste buds become more refined, you will tend to crave what you are accustomed to, even though you know it's bad for you. To keep temptation at bay, get rid of everything that is not life supporting. Of course, no one likes to throw away food, so give it to a local food bank or shelter. Unfortunately, not everyone has the means or desire to buy fresh, unprocessed food.

You Can Become a Fresh-Foods Gourmet

There is a less apparent advantage of getting rid of all that nasty processed food cluttering your pantry and clogging up your body. Such action forces each of us into learning how to cook, and if we go a step further and learn to cook with organic, whole foods, it raises the quality of our lives immeasurably.

In Europe, where high-quality meals shared among family and friends are a daily occurrence, people often speak about what they call "the quality of life," which to most Europeans is almost synonymous with fresh, delicious, well-prepared food. Cooking is not a luxury or drudgery, but a privilege and a pleasure to be enjoyed. This is one of the primary reasons Americans find life in Europe so charming, and although we may not have lunch near the Louvre or enjoy a lovely dinner on the coast of Spain, we can give ourselves the gift of fresh, well-prepared food.

Therefore, rather than thinking of how dreadful it will be to live without hamburgers, frozen pizza, sugary snacks, and chips, why not start thinking about how wonderful it will be to learn to cook with the fresh, luscious ingredients that nature provides? As a fresh-foods gourmet, you will look back on your past as a consumer of the Standard American Diet and cringe.

In the next pages you'll be provided with a list of the eleven categories of food you want to eliminate. Before you panic, I'll let you in on a secret. Your cupboard is not going to be bare, like Old Mother Hubbard's. After you cleanse your pantry, you can restock it with healthful foods.

WHAT TO THROW OUT

1. All Foods Containing Preservatives, Artificial Coloring, Artificial Flavor, or Sweetener

Examples are: cake, biscuit, and pancake mixes; pie fillings; puddings; jelled desserts; soft drinks and fruit drinks; low-fat products with anything imitation, such as cookies, crackers, and some salad dressings. Get in the habit of reading the list of ingredients on the back of packages. If something contains an ingredient that looks like it belongs in a chemistry textbook rather than a cookbook, throw it out.

2. Foods Containing Trans Fatty Acids—Refined Oils, Margarine, Hydrogenated Oil-Containing Products

Trans fatty acids are formed when liquid vegetable oils are processed by hydrogenation to make solid fats, such as in shortening and margarine, and by excessively heating oils. According to S. M. Grundy, director of the Center for Human Nutrition at the University of Texas Health Science Center, "Trans fats do not form part of the normal diet and should not be introduced into the system as they can result in a number of biochemical changes, and . . . can lead to altered membrane structure and concomitant hardening of the arteries." He also says that the free use of extracted, partially hydrogenated oil, rich in linoleic acid, has been associated with cancer promotion.[9] For instance, women with breast cancer have more trans fatty acids stored in their body fat than those without cancer.[10]

Plenty of evidence links high levels of dietary, unhealthy fat to cancer. Therefore, it is important to choose from the most healthful fats for our diet, such as those contained in whole foods, like avocados, nuts, and grains. Extracted oils should be limited to unrefined cold-pressed flaxseed oil, olive oil, and coconut oil. So, when cleaning out the pantry and refrigerator, make sure to get rid of all margarine, vegetable shortening, or foods that contain them, and foods containing hydrogenated oils. Places where trans fatty acids can hide are in baked goods, crackers, cookies, chips, and snack foods. Many brands of peanut butter and other spreads also contain partially hydrogenated oils to keep them from separating.

3. Polyunsaturated Oils

Fats can be described as being saturated, monounsaturated, or polyunsaturated. The extent of saturation depends on what extent its carbon atoms hold hydrogen atoms. In *saturated fatty acids*, each carbon atom has two hydrogen atoms; the carbon atoms are full, or saturated, with hydrogen atoms. In *monounsaturated fats,* one hydrogen atom is missing from each of two adjacent carbon atoms and a double bond replaces the original single bond. *Polyunsaturated fatty acids* have many carbon atoms joined by double or triple bonds, and they lack four or more hydrogen atoms. Polyunsaturated oils are very susceptible to oxidation because of their chemical structure (the bonds can be broken easily), whereas the hydrogen atoms in saturated fats help to protect them from oxidation and rancidity. Because polyunsaturated oils do not have these hydrogen atoms they become rancid more easily than saturated or monounsaturated fats and form trans fatty acids when heated. This produces free radicals, which damage cells and tissues, leading to premature aging and disease. Rancid oils also predispose us to malignancies.[11]

For about two decades, we have been told that polyunsaturated oils are healthier than saturated fats because they help reduce cholesterol. This is true only with oils in their natural state, as in whole foods. However, if the oils are not properly extracted, they become extremely unhealthy. Except for high-quality, cold-pressed flax oil and extra virgin olive oil, the majority of polyunsaturated oils are extracted with the use of high heat and/or chemical solvents, which totally undermines their healthful qualities. On top of that, they are refined and filtered to remove their natural colors and flavors, and this process strips them of antioxidants. This creates an insipid product that bears little resemblance to the original seed, making it more difficult to tell if it's rancid.

That said, let's go to the pantry and get rid of all refined polyunsaturated oils or foods that contain them. These oils include most vegetable oils such as sunflower, safflower, soybean, canola, and corn. Foods that contain these oils include chips, cookies, crackers, and many salad dressings. Only extra virgin olive oil and cold pressed flax oil should be used for salad dressings (flax oil should never be heated). Coconut oil is best for cooking because it has the least chance of forming trans fats.

4. Rancid Nuts and Seeds

Nuts and seeds also contain oils that can easily become rancid. When they are sealed in their shells, they are protected from oxygen and are, therefore, more likely to be fresh. However, when nuts and seeds are shelled, we do not know how long they have been out of the shell, and they are very likely to be rancid, especially when they are not refrigerated. This is particularly true in the summer months and early fall before the fresh crop of nuts is harvested. Walnuts, pecans, and peanuts seem to be more prone to rancidity than almonds.

In mid- to late fall, winter, and early spring it is probably safe to buy shelled nuts and seeds. However, after that, we run the risk of eating rancid nuts and seeds. With a keen sense of smell, it is possible to learn to detect rancid oils in nuts and other foods. To help prevent nuts from becoming rancid you should always keep them in the refrigerator or freezer. Throw out peanuts; they contain aflatoxins, which are carcinogenic.

5. Oils Heated to High Temperatures

When oils and fats are heated to high temperatures, their chemical structure changes to form new compounds such as trans fats, peroxides, aldehydes, ketones, hydroperoxides, and polymers. These compounds can all have detrimental effects on our health. Processed oils are heated to temperatures high enough to render them unhealthy during manufacturing, and when we cook with them, we are getting quite a bit more than we bargained for in the way of toxins.[12] The more an oil is heated, the more toxic compounds are formed. The worst, of course, is deep-frying, especially as in restaurants where the same oil is used over and over. Acrlamides, which are carcinogenic chemicals produced during frying or baking, have been found in high levels in potato chips, French fries, and baked goods.[13] When cleaning out your pantry, it almost goes without saying that all fried foods need to go, along with baked goods, chips, and other snack foods that usually contain oils that are either refined, or have been heated to high temperatures, or both.

During your cancer cleanse, you can stir-fry vegetables in a wok or skillet with a small amount of water (about 1/4 cup) or coconut oil. For more flavor, add a tablespoon of tamari soy sauce and a splash of lemon juice to the water, along with some chopped garlic and grated ginger. If you need some oil for sautéing or baking, pure virgin organic coconut oil is best because its medium chain triglycerides are quite heat-stable. (See Products and Information.)

6. Sugars and Sweetened Food

For decades alternative health proponents of every therapeutic diet from macrobiotic to live foods have repeated the adage "sugar feeds cancer." In most successful alternative cancer treatment diets, even fruit and fruit juice are limited because of their high natural sugar content. Of course, the more a sugar is refined, the unhealthier it becomes, because it has been stripped of the nutrients and fiber that were contained in the plant. Because refined sugar is a highly concentrated substance, it, and foods containing it, are especially harmful. But even if sugar played no role in promoting cancer, there are plenty of other reasons to avoid it.

Refined sugar rapidly passes into the bloodstream, overworking the pancreas, which must produce enough insulin to allow the sugar to enter the cells. When sugar is repeatedly overeaten, normal amounts of insulin become less and less effective and the body must produce more and more insulin. Because the insulin becomes less efficient, sugar builds up in the bloodstream, creating a risk factor for diabetes, heart attack, and stroke. With excess sugar, the body also becomes over-acidified and consumes precious minerals much too quickly in order to balance the pH.

Another harmful consequence of eating too much sugar is that low blood sugar is triggered by the exaggerated insulin response that comes from habitual overindulgence. When this happens, we feel a sudden drop in energy, as if our battery ran down. This, in turn, makes us vulnerable to what can become an addictive cycle of sugar and stimulant use as we try to muster enough energy to function normally.

Many cancer patients exhibit some degree of candidiasis, which is the overgrowth of a yeastlike fungus, *Candida albicans,* in the intestines. Both sugar and fruit aggravate candidiasis; to control it we must stay away from both of these foods. When not controlled, candida can become a serious problem, inhibiting the assimilation of nutrients. In the worst-case scenario, candida can migrate throughout the entire system. This is called *systemic* candidaisis and can be life threatening when left unchecked.[14]

A recent report by Dr. Edward Giovannucci of Harvard Medical School linked high insulin levels to an increased risk of colon cancer.[15] In studies on rats, table sugar caused DNA mutations that have previously been associated with the development of colon cancer.[16] There is also evidence that excess insulin may be related to the development of pancreatic cancer.[17]

High insulin has been implicated in breast cancer as well. In a study from Mount Sinai Hospital in Toronto, 512 women with breast cancer were monitored for four years. By the end of the study the cancer had metastasized in 76 women, and 46 died from the disease. The women who had the highest recurrence and death rate were the most obese women and those who had the highest insulin levels.[18] Therefore, as you diligently go through your pantry, everything containing sweeteners must go.

If you love the taste of sweet foods, this part of your pantry cleanse may be difficult. However, you will find that the overly sweetened commercial products that are so popular rapidly lose their appeal after you have been away from them for a few weeks. If you should go back to them after an extended absence, they do not even taste good.

Once your health is regained, you may be able to introduce the occasional sweet treat made from fruits and unrefined sweeteners back into your diet. But for now, forget they even exist. So, let's get back to the pantry and toss out all candy, cakes, pies, cookies, muffins, puddings, Jell-O, sweetened sauces and salad dressings, sweetened yogurts, sodas, fruit drinks, honey, maple syrup, corn syrup, molasses, brown sugar, brown rice syrup, malt barley syrup, sucanat, "raw sugar," and all artificial sweeteners.

7. Fruits and Fruit Juices

Don't throw these out; just leave them for other members of the family for the time being. If you have a candida problem, most fruits and fruit juices also must be avoided. Otherwise, you can enjoy low-acid fruit, especially papaya and melons. Stevia extract (an herbal sweetener) can be used as a sweetener for homemade lemonade and a cranberry cocktail made with cranberry concentrate, water, and stevia.

8. Flours and Flour Products

Whole grains are all good sources of essential fatty acids because they naturally contain essential fatty acid-rich oils. When a grain is intact, it is protected from rancidity by its outer covering. However, once the grain is ground into flour the oil becomes exposed to oxygen and can easily become rancid. In Chapter Four, we discussed how important it is to eat whole grains, but unless you have a home flourmill, the risk of getting rancid flour is too great. Therefore, it is recommended that you forgo commercially ground flours and flour products while following The Complete Cancer Cleanse Program. Included in this category are breads (whole wheat as well as white), muffins, bagels, pasta, cakes, crackers, cookies, biscuits, couscous, and pretzels.

9. Animal Products

In Chapter Four you learned about the many advantages of a vegan diet for healing, so now is the time to start putting those principles into practice. Say good-bye to milk, cheese, butter, meats, poultry, eggs, and fish and begin to explore all the delicious alternatives. When you regain your health, you may, or may not, wish to occasionally add some organic dairy products, organic poultry, and the safer varieties of fish back into your diet, but during your cleanse it is best to abstain.

10. Moldy Foods

Although common sense tells us that we should avoid moldy food, molds are more prevalent in many foods than we may think. In fact, anything that was once alive has the potential to harbor mold. The obvious molds that we can see, such as moldy bread or grapes, are easy to avoid, but sometimes molds are not easy to spot and sometimes they are not visible at all. Foods especially prone to molding are those kept in airtight packaging or plastic bags, and leftovers. This kind of packaging locks moisture in and allows molds to flourish.

Fresh fruits and vegetables do not harbor invisible molds if you wash the outside, but grains and grain products such as flours, baked goods, pastas, dried beans, dried fruits, and nuts can all conceal invisible molds. Peanuts are especially notorious for harboring the infamous carcinogenic mold *aflatoxin*. Another well-known food mold is *ergot.* This mold is thought of as the one that attacks rye; however, it has also been found in other whole grains, honey, and wine. Ergot is similar in action to LSD. In fact, some historians believe that the strange behavior and confused thinking that precipitated the Salem witch hunts and the strange art of sixteenth-century painters Brueghel and Bosch were due to massive ergot poisoning from moldy rye bread.

Although these two molds are the most well-known, they are not the only potentially hazardous molds. Others include Cytochalasin B, which is found mostly in pasta and attacks the liver, T-2 Toxin, which is present on dried peas and beans, and zearalenone, which is found on popcorn, corn chips, and brown rice. Potentially moldy foods to avoid include store-bought peanut butter, bread that has been wrapped in plastic, crackers, boxed cold cereals, untreated dried fruits, nuts, grains, and beans.[19]

Finally, let me give you a quick way to neutralize food molds.

How to Neutralize Food Molds

Beans and Grains. Wash grains and beans carefully and pick out any discolored, foreign, or broken bits. Soak them for eight hours, or overnight with about 1/4 teaspoon of ascorbic acid powder, which is simply vitamin C, added to the water. Before cooking, drain off the water and rinse. Add fresh water to cook, and to be on the safe side, add another pinch of ascorbic acid (about 1/8 to 1/4 teaspoon) to the cooking water. Presoaking beans and grains also makes them more digestible.

Nuts and Seeds. Soak nuts and seeds in water with a pinch (1/8 to 1/4 teaspoon) of ascorbic acid powder for about ten minutes. Drain them, then either toast them in a 305-degree oven for ten minutes, or dry them in a food dehydrator. (Dehydration better preserves the nutrients.) Store the treated nuts in glass containers in the refrigerator or in the freezer. Homemade nut butter can safely be made with vitamin C-treated nuts in a super blender such as Salton's Complete Health Center or the Vita Mix.

11. Genetically Engineered Foods (GMOs)

Genetic engineering is a process by which genes from two different species that could not be combined naturally by breeding are spliced together in a laboratory to create a totally new life form. The purpose of this is to produce crops with specific traits such as herbicide resistance. This allows the companies that manufacture both the seeds and the herbicides to sell more herbicides.

Other traits that scientists have attempted to engineer into crops are a higher per acre yield and drought or cold tolerance. Plants have also been genetically engineered to make their own built-in insecticides. Some of the more bizarre genetic combinations, such as strawberries with flounder genes, pigs with human genes, and corn with bacteria genes, have earned GMOs the name "Frankenfoods." No studies have linked genetically engineered foods to cancer or to other health problems; however, this is such a new technology that we do not know if problems will arise. If we look at the history of technological innovations, it is pretty safe to say that problems will crop up.

The environmental implications of making such drastic changes to our food supply are largely unknown. Europe has been relatively successful in rejecting genetically engineered foods and keeping them off the market, whereas the United States continues to go blindly into a massive experiment that will radically change our food supply forever. In 2003 the GMO foods on the market in the United States were soybeans (about 60 percent of the total crop), canola (rape seed), cotton (cottonseed oil is used in many processed foods), and corn (even popcorn). Also, a large part of the United States milk supply is from cows treated with a genetically engineered growth hormone (rBGH). The best way to avoid GMO foods is to buy only organic foods, especially when buying the foods just mentioned.[20]

AVOIDING PARASITES

And as you're cleansing your pantry, be wary of parasites on stored food. Parasites are another pathogen that we can ingest through our food. The word *parasite* refers to any organism that lives on or in or at the expense of a host and takes its sustenance from the host. Human parasites are far more common than most of us realize. Some health professionals believe that the combination of parasites and environmental pollutants are the primary cause of cancer.

The foods most likely to be contaminated with parasites are uncooked dairy products and undercooked or uncooked meat, fowl, seafood, and fish.[21] Another way we can pick up parasites is from improperly washed raw vegetables and fruits. Raw walnuts can also transmit parasites. Parasites can be killed by heat, or by soaking produce to be eaten raw in a vinegar/water solution for about ten minutes. Use about 1/4 cup vinegar for a sink full of water, or 1 tablespoon per gallon. Hydrogen peroxide is also effective.[22]

We can contract parasites when we travel outside the United States and by drinking or swimming in contaminated water. Pets, as loveable as they are, are also a primary source of human parasite infestation. Always wash your hands after touching pets and never kiss them or allow them to climb on your kitchen table, counters, or bed. Another source of contamination is the kitchen sponge, especially in households that have pets. Microscopic, airborne parasites can land on the kitchen table or counters, only to be wiped away with a sponge or dishcloth. This damp environment is a perfect place for parasites to grow and be transferred to your food or to other surfaces. Therefore, every day, before food preparation sterilize the kitchen sponge.

An effective and nontoxic way to get rid of bacteria and parasites that lurk around the kitchen is to place your sponge in vinegar water for a few seconds. Every time you wash dishes, put the sponge in the upper rack of the dishwasher and buy a new sponge at least every two weeks. Healthy individuals with strong immune systems can fight off these parasites, but cancer patients should take every precaution to avoid them.

MAKING A WHOLE FOODS SHOPPING LIST

After doing the pantry cleanse, you may panic because there is nothing left in the house to eat. So before fear and hunger set in, replace those foods with fresh, healthy fare. Because you are about to embark on a totally new culinary adventure, you will need a bit of coaching to see you through. In fact, it may be a good idea to buy a good vegan, whole foods cookbook or two as inspiration to get you going.

In a typical supermarket, it is best to avoid most of the aisles, because you will find very little that is life supporting. If your market carries organic produce, this is the first and most important place to look for the staples of a healthy diet. However, apart from the produce, most of the foods we recommend are best purchased in a natural foods store. There you can buy bulk organic grains, beans, herbs, nuts, seeds, and spices that are probably fresher and lower in cost than at the supermarket—a result of products turning over more quickly in natural food stores because shoppers go there specifically to purchase them.

If you are a supermarket customer, the thought of shopping at a natural foods store with its bins of foreign-looking provisions and esoteric, expensive products can be daunting. We all have our shopping routines and to interrupt them can create some temporary havoc in our schedules until we develop new and healthier habits. It doesn't take long, however, to develop a new ritual, and before long, you will be moving through the health food store like you own it.

Tips for Shopping at a Health Food or Natural Food Store

- Stay away from foods not on your list. Except for a few traditionally processed foods, avoid processed "health" foods because they are expensive; although they are perhaps better than their supermarket counterparts, they are unnecessary and not as life supporting as fresh foods.
- Look for local and seasonal produce. If there are organic farms or farmers' markets in your area, make that your primary produce destination during the seasons they are open. Use the supermarket or health food store mainly for items you may need between trips to the farms or farmers' markets and in the seasons when the farmers' markets are closed. In winter, concentrate on vegetables, such as cabbages, onions, garlic, carrots, winter squash, pumpkins, leeks, parsnips, beets, turnips, rutabagas, and hearty greens such as kale and collards. You can supplement your winter vegetables by growing bean, split pea, broccoli, and radish sprouts in your home or by purchasing them at a natural foods store. Summer is the time for tomatoes, green beans, summer squash, tender greens like lettuce, spinach, and arugula, fresh peas, corn, and radishes.
- Don't expect everything you find in a health food store to be healthy. The owners of these stores are in business to make money, so they carry what people want to buy. Be as careful as you are in a supermarket and read the labels.
- Look for foods that are certified organic. If a food is not labeled as such, it is not certified organic.
- Buy in bulk. Beans, grains, herbs, Celtic Sea Salt, and spices are all much better buys if you get them from the bulk bins.
- Check the dates on packaged foods as carefully as you would in the supermarket.

Following is a twelve-item shopping list to replace the eleven food catagories you eliminated.

1. Grains

Start with millet, brown rice, and quinoa. When you are ready to expand your repertoire, try some barley (omit if you are gluten sensitive), buckwheat, amaranth, oat groats, and teff.

2. Legumes

Mung beans, azuki (sometimes called aduki) beans, and green, orange, and brown lentils are all good to start with because they are relatively quick to cook and easy to digest. Other legumes include black beans, chickpeas, black-eyed peas, split peas, pinto beans, Great Northern beans, or any other beans you like.

3. Oils

Extra virgin olive oil and cold-pressed flax oil are the only oils you will need for salad dressings. Look for flax oil in the refrigerator section of your health food store and keep both oils in the refrigerator at home to prevent them from turning rancid. Transfer the olive oil to a wide-mouth jar, so it can easily be spooned out when it gets solid. Date the oils when you purchase them and throw them out after three months.

Pure virgin organic coconut oil is good for sautéing, baking, or any food preparation requiring heat. Because the fat in coconut oil has no double carbon bonds—weak links that are easily broken to form free radicals—they are much more stable under a variety of conditions, such as heat, light, and oxygen, without undergoing any appreciable degree of oxidation or free-radical formation. (See Products and Information for recommendations.)

4. Nuts and Seeds

Almonds, walnuts, pumpkin seeds, flax seeds, sesame seeds, sunflower seeds, and black sesame seeds are best. Make sure to treat them for molds, as mentioned earlier, and then keep them either in the refrigerator or the freezer.

5. Organic Produce

There is no limit for purchasing organic produce; buy everything and anything that appeals to you, only limiting the highly acidic fruits, those high on the glycemic index, and a few of the higher acid vegetables to no more than 25 percent of your diet. Try to emphasize items that are in season.

6. Sweeteners

Liquid or powdered stevia extract is the recommendation for sweetening. Stevia extract comes from a small plant that grows in Latin America, where it has been used as a sweetener for over a hundred years. Liquid stevia comes in a small bottle with a dropper; powdered stevia comes in plastic containers or individual packets. It is about thirty times sweeter than sugar. Stevia extract can be used to sweeten just about anything, but it's best in teas, lemonade, homemade cranberry cocktails, porridge, puddings, and smoothies; in baked desserts stevia does not impart the richness of other sweeteners and can have a mild aftertaste. Stevia is the best sweetener to use while on The Complete Cancer Cleanse Program, because it does not cause the pancreas to produce excess insulin like other natural sweeteners and has never been known to cause any harmful side effects, as artificial sweeteners do. Look for Stevia Plus, which has added fiber that helps to stabilize blood sugar. Stevia can be purchased at most health food stores.

Another sweetener you may want to check out is Birch Sweetener, or Xylitol. Xylitol was discovered in 1891 by a German chemist and has been used for sweetening food since the 1960s. People with diabetes may use it, because it is absorbed slowly and does not create the blood glucose and insulin response of sugar. It has also been shown to be useful in preventing dental cavities, and there are no known detrimental effects. If you choose Xylitol, make sure it is made from birch bark and not another source. When choosing between the two sweeteners, however, it may be best to choose stevia, because it has the longest track record of safe use.

7. Soy Foods

Soymilk, tofu, and tempeh are the best soy foods because they are traditional foods that have been safely used for centuries and are made today in much the same way they always were. Tofu, when you learn how to use it, can work culinary wonders and be the base for everything from delicious meatless loafs to luscious puddings.

Tempeh, which is high in both protein and fiber, is a satisfying addition to oil-less stir-fries and other meatless main dishes. For the sake of convenience, you can buy prebaked, seasoned tofu and precooked and seasoned tempeh burgers. Just cut them into bite-size pieces and add them to vegetable and grain dishes. Avoid any soy products made from genetically modified soybeans. Look for products that say non-GMO.

8. Miscellaneous

Miso, tamari, umeboshi plums, and agar agar flakes are all traditional Japanese foods that are healthful ways to season your vegan meals. Agar agar is a vegan gelatin, which is known to have detoxifying properties. A macrobiotic or good vegan cookbook will be helpful in learning to use these items.

9. Sea Vegetables

Wakame, dulse, and kombu are sea vegetables that are high in minerals, easy to use, and are considered detoxifying in Oriental medicine. They can be added to soups, stews, and bean and vegetable dishes. With a good macrobiotic cookbook, you can quickly learn how to use them.

10. Green Tea, Herbal Tea

Green tea is an antioxidant-rich beverage that can offer a mild pick-me-up without a lot of caffeine. An 8-ounce serving has 30 milligrams of caffeine, compared to brewed coffee, which has 135 milligrams. Some varieties, such as Yogi Super Antioxidant Green Tea, have even less caffeine because of the addition of other herbs. And remember, according to research a cup a day can help keep cancer at bay. Herbal teas are caffeine-free and offer a healthful alternative to coffee.

11. Spices and Herbs

Turmeric, fresh ginger, garlic, cayenne, fennel seed, cinnamon, cumin, basil, tarragon, rosemary, mint, thyme, and bay leaves are among the many spices and herbs that are essential to create flavor-rich healthy meals. Besides providing flavor, most herbs and spices also offer therapeutic benefits.

12. Celtic Sea Salt (sometimes called Gray Salt)

Most sea salts are refined and pure white, but Celtic sea salt is slightly gray and moist looking because of its mineral content. Celtic sea salt beautifully enlivens the flavor of foods. If your health food store does not have Celtic sea salt, it can be ordered by catalogue or on the Internet from The Grain and Salt Society.

SAFE WATER

As you are replacing the foods in your pantry, consider the quality of the water you are drinking. Drinking water helps our body cleanse and detoxify; therefore, it is absolutely essential to have the purest water possible and to drink plenty of it. Unfortunately, this is not as easy as it should be. As our world has become more polluted, our water sources have become tainted. Organic contaminates have been found in drinking water, such as VOCs (volatile organic compounds) and THMs (trihalomethanes), which are byproducts of chlorination. These contaminates, which are considered carcinogenic, are formed by a chemical reaction between chlorine and decomposing leaves, animal matter, or other organic material and are most often found in chlorinated surface waters that are used for public drinking water supplies. Inorganic chemical carcinogens, such as heavy metals like lead, mercury, arsenic, and asbestos, can also contaminate drinking water, as can radioactive chemicals such as radon and radium.[23]

According to the Natural Resources Defense Council (NRDC), arsenic in drinking water causes bladder, lung, and skin cancer. It may also cause kidney and liver cancer, nervous system problems, heart and blood vessel problems, and serious skin problems, as well as birth defects and reproductive difficulties. The NRDC analyzed data compiled by the U.S. Environmental Protection Agency on arsenic in drinking water in twenty-five states. Based on this data, their most conservative estimates indicate that more than thirty-four million Americans drink tap water supplied by systems containing average levels of arsenic that pose unacceptable cancer risks.[24]

Bottled water is not a great solution. Bottled water contributes to the pollution problem by releasing toxic chemicals into the environment during the manufacturing and disposal of the bottles. According to a study by the World Wildlife Fund, 1.5 million tons of plastic are used every year to bottle water.[25]

If bottled water was safer than tap water, the cost and environmental damage might be worth it; however, according to I. H. Suffet, Ph.D., professor of Environmental Science and Engineering at UCLA, "tap water costs less and is at least as safe as bottled water." In fact, in many cases the government standards for tap water are more stringent than those for bottled water.[26]

Another problem with bottled water can be the bottles themselves. The soft plastic bottles and gallon containers often give the water they contain a plastic taste. Some researchers believe that components of these plastic bottles actually leach into the water, creating xenoestrogens in our body when ingested. Polycarbonate, a plastic used in water bottles, has been specifically singled out by California regulations as a problem.[27]

Most experts on water quality agree that the best way to have safe water is a home filtering system. There are many different types, and before you choose one, it may be a good idea to contact your local board of health to find out the particular contaminates in your area. When you have a good water purifier, you can fill your own water bottles, which is a much healthier choice for water on the go. Also consider buying filters for your shower and bath, because some pollutants, such as chlorine, are absorbed through the skin and through inhaling the steam vapors from hot water.

Water Filtering Systems

Some available water filtration systems are as follows:

Sediment Filters. Simple filters that can remove suspended debris, this type is not effective in removing biological contaminants, chlorine, or other VOCs. These filters work best in conjunction with another system.

Distillers. In distillation, water is boiled and the condensed steam is collected, leaving behind the dissolved solids and particulates, and removing microorganisms and most other contaminates. Some health experts do not recommend this method because it removes minerals from the water. If distillation is done at home, problems can arise when volatile chemicals, which were once in the water, escape into the air. Also, the machines are expensive and slow to operate, producing only small amounts of water at a time.[28]

Activated Carbon Filters. These filters do a great job of removing bad tastes and odors from water. They also remove volatile chemicals, such as pesticide residues and chlorine. They do not, however, filter out dissolved solids and particulates, such as nitrates and sodium fluoride; neither do they kill microorganisms. This is their biggest drawback, especially if the water comes from a private water supply, such as a well. With chlorinated city water, a carbon filter is less likely to harbor bacteria, because the chlorine in the water kills most of the bacteria.

It is very important to change carbon filters as often as is recommended. Trying to save money by not changing the filter can cause problems with buildup of both bacteria and toxins. Also, carbon filters should be used daily, which causes the water to flush out bacteria that may have accumulated. Carbon filters are inexpensive and a good solution for homes with a bacteria-free, chlorinated water supply.[29] The Doulton Ceramic Filter is an example of this type of water filter.

KDF Filters. These filters are similar to activated carbon but are more effective at removing chlorine and lead. They do not support bacterial growth and, therefore, are sometimes combined with activated carbon filters. They are considered safe to use on private water supplies.[30]

Reverse Osmosis. This system takes just about all the toxins out of water; however, according to John Bower of the Healthy House Institute, some VOCs do manage to get through. Reverse osmosis filtered water tastes good and has no odor. The main drawback is the expense, and the fact that reverse osmosis systems waste about three gallons of water for every gallon they filter. They also need servicing about once a year.

CLEANSING YOUR COSMETICS AND PERSONAL CARE PRODUCTS

Now that you have cleansed your pantry, it's time to clean out your cosmetics and toss those unhealthy personal care products. Surprisingly, cosmetics and personal care products are another place where carcinogenic substances can lurk. Sometimes called "health and beauty aids," many of the products we regularly use are anything but healthful or beautifying.

Samuel Epstein, M.D., is a professor of environmental medicine at the University of Illinois's School of Public Health in Chicago and one of the world's leading activists working to eliminate carcinogens from consumer products. According to Dr. Epstein and David Steinman, M.D., authors of *The Safe Shopper's Bible*, "Not a single cosmetic company warns consumers of the presence of carcinogens in its products, despite the fact that several common cosmetic ingredients or their contaminants are carcinogenic themselves or are carcinogenic precursors."[31]

You may be wondering how beauty products can be dangerous. After all, we don't eat or drink them. We do, however, apply them to our skin, which is more absorbent than many of us realize. If you doubt this, think of the 1/4 to 1/2 teaspoon of progesterone cream that many women rub onto their skin as hormone replacement therapy, or the nitroglycerine patches worn by heart patients, or the nicotine patches worn by those trying to quit smoking.

The trend toward chemicals in our cosmetics began in the last century when doctors and other medical personnel virtually ceased from making and prescribing beauty creams and lotions, leaving the development and manufacturing open to entrepreneurs. Beauty-oriented consumer services began to prosper, creating new demand for beauty and personal care products, and the petrochemical industry began creating synthetic chemicals for these products.[32] Ease, convenience, and the promise of "A more beautiful you!" drove the industry.

Although most beauty products list the ingredients they contain on their labels, some products, such as perfumes, do not have to list ingredients because these are "trade secrets." For example, laboratory analysis revealed that a popular perfume had forty-one ingredients, some of which are known carcinogens.[33] There is no reason to think that this is the only case. Many chemically sensitive people have adverse reactions to all perfumes and synthetic fragrances.

Kathon GC, a preservative used in certain cosmetics, has been shown to be mutagenic (cancer causing). This preservative is absorbed through the skin and also causes skin-sensitization, which may lead to skin cancer. Although it may be safe at low levels, according to toxicologist Thomas

Connor, Ph.D., "it is probable that a person could use a shampoo, conditioner, styling gel, and skin lotion one or more times in a single day, making the total daily dose substantial."[34]

DEA (diethanolamine) and its fatty acid derivative, cocoaminde-DEA, have been shown to induce liver and kidney cancer in rats. High concentrations of DEA can be found in many shampoos, hair dyes, conditioners, lotions, creams, and bubble baths. This chemical can also be found in dishwashing and laundry soaps. The chemical reaction that takes place when DEA combines with nitrite preservatives or contaminants to create nitrosodiethanolamine (NDELA)[35] further increases the cancer risk.

Hair dyes have been shown to be cancer promoters in certain people. Although this has been disputed in the past, a 2001 study from the Keck School of Medicine at the University of Southern California confirms a link between hair dye and bladder cancer based on individual genetic makeup. Aerylamines are a carcinogen found in hair dyes, and in the USC study it was found that some people can eliminate these carcinogens from their bodies more quickly than others. Persons who eliminate slowly are more at risk of bladder cancer from hair dye.[36]

There are many other harmful substances to look for in cosmetics and even in some popular brands sold in health food stores:[37]

- Antiperspirants contain aluminum; rocks sold as aluminum-free natural deodorants contain magnesium-aluminum silicate
- Hair color containing lead
- Lipsticks and lip liners containing barium, aluminum, titanium, and red dye
- Eyeliners and shadows that contain chromium and cobalt
- Hair spray, shampoos, and face creams that contain isopropyl alcohol and PCBs
- Toothpastes and shampoos with sodium lauryl sulfate/sodium laureth sulfate (SLS); the label says "from coconut oil," but these chemicals are synthetically produced and rarely come from coconuts

- Shampoos with imidazolidinyl urea
- Perfumes, soaps, and shampoos with benzyl alcohol
- Perfumes, hand lotions, nail enamel remover, hair spray, and laundry detergent with linalool
- After-shave, deodorants, and bleach with terpineol

These are just a few examples of the common body care ingredients known to be toxic; unfortunately some product ingredients have never been studied, so we know little about them. When it comes to cosmetics and personal care products, you can be fairly safe in assuming that if you cannot pronounce the names of the ingredients on the label, it is best to avoid them.

To learn more about the health hazards of cosmetics and personal care products, you can read *The Safe Shopper's Bible* by Samuel Epstein, M.D., and David Steinman, M.D., *The Take Charge Beauty Book* by Aubrey Hampton and Susan Hussey, and *The Consumer's Dictionary of Cosmetic Ingredients* by Ruth Winter.

Some products that you should avoid are listed as follows, along with suggestions for safe alternatives:

Deodorants and antiperspirants. Don't buy antiperspirants that contain aluminum. Believe it or not, baking soda, applied under the arm like powder, is an excellent, nontoxic deodorant. Health food stores also carry many brands of natural deodorants that do not contain harmful ingredients.

Hair color. Try natural henna as a hair color and conditioner, but make sure to carefully read the label for added ingredients. If you have gray hair, try getting a very good, stylish short cut. With the right cut, gray hair can be stunning.

Hair gel. Aubrey Organics makes a good hair gel with high-quality safe ingredients.

Hair spray. There are no safe alternatives exactly like the commercial products; however, Aubrey Organics does have some good styling products.

Shampoo. Aubrey Organics makes several different safe shampoos; also Soignee MSM shampoo is one of our favorites.

Hair conditioners. Some of the best hair conditioners are in your kitchen. Apple cider vinegar is great for red or dark hair. Lemon juice brings out the highlights in light brown or blond hair. A beaten egg added to your shampoo is a hair-beautifying trick from our grandmother's time, and a treatment of homemade mayonnaise or mashed avocado left on the hair for an hour or more and then carefully washed out is great for dry hair. Aubrey Organics' GPB is a good conditioner.

Makeup. It is best to stay away from makeup as often as possible for the time being; however, if you just can't go without it, look for brands such as Eco Bella (found at health food stores). Dr. Hauschka makes a Toned Day Cream that is very good. Organic Beauty and Gabriel make lip glosses, lipsticks, and powders with safe ingredients, and Burt's Bees makes lipstick.

Perfume. Use natural essential oils such as rose or jasmine or any other wonderfully fragrant oil available from health food stores. These oils are nicer than perfume and can even have a therapeutic effect, such as calming, invigorating, or detoxifying. Find a book about the properties of essential oils and experiment. It can be fun.

Toothpaste. Even many of the health food store brands contain ingredients that are questionable, such as sodium lauryl sulfate/sodium laureth sulfate (SLS), but baking soda, diluted into a paste with a little water, is excellent. The taste may take some getting used to, but it really leaves your mouth feeling clean and fresh. If this is too much of a stretch for you, look for a health food store brand that does not contain fluoride or sodium lauryl sulfate (SLS).

Soap. Traditionally made olive oil soap from France is excellent, but not easy to find. Organic Beauty makes many wonderful, safe products. For the shower, Dr. Bonner's Pure Castile Liquid Soap is good (found at most health food stores).

Face creams and lotions. Olive oil and coconut oil are fabulous for dry skin. Add a few drops of your favorite essential oil for a nice scent. Dr. Hauschka makes a great eye cream and rose oil day cream. Health food stores carry a variety of natural products.

Cleansing creams and face wash. Dr. Hauschka makes a good cleansing milk, and Aubrey Organics makes a good foaming facial cleanser.

Giving up your favorite perfume, shampoo, or body lotion may be challenging, and some of the safe alternatives may take some time to find and get accustomed to, but this is another important way to limit your exposure to toxins. It is worth the effort. By switching to safer body care products, you may even notice that allergies and other chronic problems disappear or improve and that your skin looks better, even younger. Another benefit may be a fresher, more natural look that will earn you unexpected compliments.

CLEANSING YOUR HOME

Most of us never imagine that something inside our homes might be making us sick. We've heard that the outdoor air is often unhealthy—laden with sulfur oxides, carbon monoxide, industrial chemicals, pesticides, and more. We look out over many of our cities and see the brown, hazy smog that hangs over them like a dirty blanket. But what we may not be aware of is that indoor air pollution can be as bad, if not worse. According to the American College of Allergies, 50 percent of all allergies are aggravated or caused by polluted indoor air.

Materials used in construction, decoration, and furnishings all have the potential to be extremely hazardous to our health because they are made with or contain materials that outgas volatile organic compounds (VOCs). VOCs, being volatile, evaporate easily and, being organic, contain carbon. Some VOCs, such as the scent from oranges or garlic, are harmless or may even be beneficial, but others, especially synthetics, can be highly dangerous.

Indoor air usually contains anywhere between thirty to one hundred easily measurable VOCs. Other hazards can include radiation, electromagnetic fields, ozone, molds, mildew, dust mites, asbestos, airborne particulates, heavy metals, gasses from combustion appliances, pesticides, and natural radon gas. Any one of these pollutants may be enough to make us sick, and some are known carcinogens, but mix them all together and we have a highly toxic "soup" in our indoor air. When two or more of these pollutants are combined, as is the case in most of our homes, the synergistic effect is thought to be many times more harmful than any one pollutant on its own. Unfortunately this synergistic effect has not been the focus of much study.[38]

When we consider that unless we work out-of-doors, we spend most of our time in an office building or our home, the importance of a healthy indoor environment cannot be stressed enough for those seeking to regain or maintain their health. This subject, however, is so vast that whole books are written on any one of its many facets. This section offers an introduction with enough information to motivate you to begin creating the home environment that is the most conducive to your recovery. A good, all-around book to consult for more information is *The Healthy House* by John Bower, published by the Healthy House Institute. The institute also offers a very informative thirteen-episode video.

Many of the suggestions made here may seem extreme at first, but the more you explore this subject, the more you will become convinced that your indoor living and working environments play a major role in either supporting or damaging your health.

According to Jean Renoux, a provider of continuing education on the subject of healthy building and design to architects and interior designers, the first and foremost issue to consider when accessing an indoor environment is air quality. The 1970s energy crisis initiated the trend of super-insulated homes; although this energy-conserving measure cuts down on heating and cooling bills, it simultaneously traps toxins inside the house. This, combined with the fact that we use more noxious synthetic materials in construction, decoration, and home maintenance than we did in the past, can make our indoors a toxic place containing literally hundreds of VOCs and other pollutants.[39]

IMPROVING AIR QUALITY

There are two ways to improve indoor air quality. The first, and most obvious, is to keep toxins out of the house; the second is to remove them once they are in the air by filtration and improved ventilation. According to John Bower of the Healthy House Institute, the three most offensive materials commonly found in our homes are carpets, particleboard, and combustion appliances.

If you happen to be getting ready to build a new house or to do extensive remodeling, it may be beneficial to engage a consultant, architect, or contractor who is a specialist in healthy construction. This person will have the best ideas about important issues such as ventilation and insulation.

Let's look at the seven home and garden materials that can be harmful to us.

1. Carpet

Getting rid of carpet is one of the easiest things we can do to improve the air quality in our homes. Synthetic, wall-to-wall carpeting can release large amounts of VOCs, including benzene, toluene, xylene, trichlorethylene, and formaldehyde, all of which are cancer promoters—and some can actually induce cancer.[40]

For weeks after the installation of new carpet, numerous chemicals can linger in the air. They come from the carpet itself, the glues, the padding, the dyes, and the backing. In a laboratory study, mice actually died after exposure to new carpeting.[41] Even though the chemicals given off by new carpet dissipate with time, old carpet can also create a problem because it tends to absorb biological contaminants such as bacteria, molds, yeast, dust, animal dander, and VOCs from other sources. The fibers of older carpet can also deteriorate, contributing to dust, and when this dust enters the home's heating system it can burn, giving off additional fumes.[42] Safe alternatives to carpet are ceramic tile, terrazzo, stone, slate, marble, linoleum (not vinyl), tile, hardwood, bamboo, and cork.

2. Manufactured Wood Products and Other Sources of Formaldehyde

Formaldehyde (also known as formic aldehyde or methyl aldehyde), one of the most insidious of all VOCs, is colorless and odorless in the concentrations found in wood products in our homes. Although the time it takes for formaldehyde to outgas is dependent on the particular product and the temperature of its location, it is usually said that in six years the outgassing will be half of what it was in the beginning.[43] Exposure to formaldehyde can cause watery eyes, nausea, coughing, chest tightness, wheezing, skin rashes, allergic reactions, and burning sensations in the eyes, nose, and throat. It has been shown to cause cancer in laboratory animals and may cause cancer in humans. Formaldehyde is also a possible mutagen and teratogen, causing birth defects.[44]

Permanent press fabrics, which are used for clothing, upholstery, and draperies, are other sources of formaldehyde in our home. Formaldehyde is also used in certain types of insulation and some paper products.

3. Combustion Pollutants

Inside our homes, the most prevalent combustion pollutants are from our heating systems: gases and particles such as carbon monoxide, nitrogen dioxide, and polycyclic aromatic hydrocarbons, which are made by burning any fuel such as wood, natural gas, kerosene, charcoal, or tobacco. Carbon monoxide is an especially serious concern because it is odorless, colorless, and tasteless and can cause death at high levels of exposure. Indoor carbon monoxide pollution can come from unvented combustion appliances, such as gas stoves, kerosene heaters, and charcoal grills. Even vented combustion appliances, such as furnaces, wood stoves, fireplaces, gas water heaters, and gas clothes dryers, can be possible sources if the ventilation system is malfunctioning or improperly designed.

Besides carbon monoxide, other combustion pollutants to be aware of are PAHs and particles PM10, which are small, inhalable particles that arise from tobacco smoke, wood-burning stoves, kerosene heaters, charcoal grills, scented candles, candles with metal wicks, incense burning, and certain hobby materials. Self-cleaning ovens, as well as the forementioned appliances, give off both particles PM10 and aromatic hydrocarbons (PAHs), which are known carcinogens.[45]

To avoid pollution from combustion sources, avoid any unvented heaters and have your furnace checked and serviced regularly. Also make sure flues, chimneys, and vents on wood stoves are working properly. This hopefully goes without saying, but *never allow anyone to smoke inside your house or outdoors by an open window.*

4. Paints

Many products we use for routine house maintenance and cleaning can also contribute significantly to indoor pollution. Paints, varnishes, sealers, paint strippers, polyurethane, and solvents such as mineral spirits, acetone, and turpentine can all be quite toxic. Chronic exposure to these substances may increase cancer risk.[46] Professional painters who have had long exposure to paint vapors have demonstrated nervous system, liver, and kidney damage.[47]

Never use paint, varnish, and strippers or make arts or crafts involving solvents in the same house with a cancer patient, and if you have cancer, never use these products. Also, care should be taken when sanding a surface to prepare for painting because the dust may contain lead particles if the surface contains lead-base paint. When a house must be painted, vacate for a few days, ventilate carefully, and use special, less-toxic, low-VOC water-based paints.

5. Cleaning Supplies

Most cleaning supplies are very strong, containing potent chemicals that emit VOCs. Lysol contains phenols and dioxin (agent orange). Bleach is so toxic that OSHSA requires workers in industrial areas to wear impervious protective clothing—hard hats, boots, aprons or coveralls, and chemical goggles or full face shields; bleach can only be used in well-ventilated areas.[48] Ralph W. Moss, Ph.D., recommends that we use the safer cleaning products sold in health food stores, such as Ecover Brand.[49] Products that we should avoid are chlorine bleach, disinfectants, toilet cleaners, air fresheners, potpourri, oven cleaners, ammonia, most scouring powders, window cleaners, spray cleaners, laundry detergents, and dishwashing detergents.[50]

6. Pesticides

We spoke of the dangers of pesticide use in Chapter Four when we covered the importance of organic food. Food and agriculture is not the only source of pesticide exposure; home and garden pesticide use flourishes in the United States in spite of the serious health and ecological risks. How many of us have regular treatments of our homes and lawns by pest control companies or, worse yet, do it ourselves?

Because pesticide use is so common, it is crucial to emphasize again that pesticides are chemicals or biological substances designed to kill living organisms. They are *poisonous.* Just because pesticides are registered with the EPA does not mean they are safe.[51] Epidemiological studies have shown that as children's exposures to home and garden pesticides increase, so does their risk of non-Hodgkin's lymphoma, brain cancer, and leukemia. A study in southern California found that children who live in homes treated by pesticides have seven times the risk of non-Hodgkin's lymphoma. Multiple myceloma, a bone marrow cancer, is also associated with toxic chemicals.[52]

A study published in the July 1987 issue of the *Journal of the National Cancer Institute* showed that children living in pesticide-treated homes had nearly four times the risk of developing leukemia than children living in untreated homes. If the garden was treated as well, the risk of developing leukemia was 6.5 times greater.[53] Golf course superintendents, who work with pesticides intensively, have double the rate of deaths due to non-Hodgkin's lymphoma and brain cancer than the general public.

For some reason, even people who are aware of the dangers of insecticides do not always have a healthy fear of herbicides, thinking that they just kill weeds, not people. A study by oncologists Dr. Lennart Hardell and Dr. Mikael Eriksson of Sweden revealed clear links between a popular garden weed killer and non-Hodgkin's lymphoma.[54]

Products never to have in or around your house include insect sprays, bombs and foggers, herbicides, flea and tick collars, flea sprays and flea shampoos, rat poison, and pest strips.

7. Electromagnetic Fields (EMFs)

Electromagnetic fields (EMFs) are invisible lines of force, which are manifested in the spaces around any mechanism that is powered by electric currents. All power lines, electrical appliances, power tools, and household wiring create EMFs. Some examples of EMF sources are computers, hair dryers, electric drills, and radio towers.

Many of us have heard stories about leukemia rates being higher in children living near power lines and stories about the harmful consequences of electric blankets, but is there any truth to this? As with many subjects pertaining to health, technology, and consumer products, this area needs further research because data on EMFs is conflicting. However, epidemiological studies of children living near power lines do suggest a correlation between EMFs and leukemia. Laboratory studies also suggest that EMFs may promote the development of cancers by suppressing the production of melatonin; this in turn may weaken the body's immune response to cancer.[55] Even weak electromagnetic fields can affect us biologically. There is evidence that a 50-hertz electrical field can have an effect on chromosome segregation that could lead to mutation.[56]

IT'S A MATTER OF CHOICE

Robert A. Mendelssohn, M.D., says, "Health is a matter of choice, not a mystery of chance." The action steps noted in this chapter offer each of us an opportunity to choose a healthier personal environment in the areas we can control. Perhaps you feel overwhelmed thinking about all the things you need to change in your life to create healthier surroundings. Let me reassure you that you don't have to do everything all at once. Nor do you need to hire a work crew and start tearing out carpeting or remodeling your home tomorrow.

Start where you can and tackle the most obvious things that need changing. Most people feel they can make an immediate difference by cleaning out their pantries and choosing nontoxic personal care and household cleaning items. You may not have the energy right now to move a computer or television out of your bedroom to avoid EMFs while you sleep, but you could unplug your electric blanket and get an inexpensive, non-electric clock. Every choice you make to cleanse your environment is a positive step in the right direction.

Detoxifying your body in the ways suggested will take time and energy. And maybe many weeks and months. As you work through this process, you might want to begin your emotional, mental, and spiritual cleansing. My husband, John, will work you through those steps in the next three chapters.

9

EMOTIONAL CLEANSING

Holding on to anger is like drinking poison and hoping the other person will die.

—ANONYMOUS

Many people are aware of the connection between stress and their health because the news media has faithfully reported the latest findings concerning stress and heart disease. We know that the driven, Type-A personality is much more likely to suffer a heart attack than others in the general population. However, many folks are not aware of the connection between their mental and emotional attitudes and their health. A compelling body of research shows how unmanaged stress and toxic emotions are as destructive to our health as poor food choices and polluted air.

A conservative estimate is that 75 percent of all visits to primary care physicians are due to stress-related disorders. Simply stated, scientific research is showing that anger (expressed and repressed), anxiety, and worry significantly increase the risk of diseases such as cardiovascular disease and cancer. Even more sobering is that a recent number of landmark studies have revealed that emotional stress is more predictive of death from cancer and cardiovascular disease than smoking. This is so important it needs to be stated again: our emotional state may be even more important to our survival from cancer than quitting smoking, yet no one would suggest that a person with cancer should not quit smoking.[1]

We are learning that our ability to heal and remain free from cancer is connected to our ability to manage our levels of stress, heal our emotional wounds, and release emotional toxicity. The cleansing of these destructive emotions will significantly help in the healing process.

Though such healing and release may seem a daunting task, there is hope! It is not only possible to identify toxic emotions and old wounds, it is possible to release them. We can go so far as to cleanse our negative emotions and heal old wounds. Deeply held beliefs may cause all kinds of havoc in our lives; childhood traumas may still significantly shape who we think we are and how we present ourselves to the world. And the pain from old wounds may be stored in the cavities of our soul.

We are embarking on a new journey! This journey may not always be easy. Many of our emotions and ways of thinking have been entrenched over a lifetime. But we can decide to slay the dragons of our soul. We have an opportunity to grow in *love* and move toward *wholeness*.

The first step is to see if our personality is leading us to create negative emotions that are harmful to our recovery.

THE CANCER PERSONALITY

Over the years, doctors and researchers have talked of a relationship between cancer and a patient's personality type. Overall, cancer patients seem to have similar behavioral and emotional patterns, which is known as the "Type-C Personality."

This personality often shares the following traits and experiences:

- Very often there has been an experience of loss: loss of a loved one or loss of hope. There may have been an unwanted divorce; the death of a child, a spouse, or a beloved pet; the loss of career; or a loss of faith in God or in others. Whatever the situation, the individual feels a sense of hopelessness and despair.
- A sense of hopelessness and despair often is deeply associated with questions about the meaning of one's existence. Many Type Cs have questioned their right to be on earth or to be alive from as far back as they can remember.
- Another common trait among people with cancer is the suppression of emotions. Anger is the emotion most often suppressed, along with resentment and hostility. Cancer

patients generally have not learned to express their anger and have refrained from communicating their feelings. This generally is a lifelong habit.

- Often, people with cancer experience loneliness. Feelings of loneliness frequently began in childhood with a lack of closeness with one or both parents. They continued into adulthood with a lack of close friendships and fulfilling relationships.[2] Many times the loneliness culminated with a loss of a spouse or significant person.
- Often cancer patients are those who carry other people's burdens and take on extra obligations; they may have a tendency to worry for others.
- There appears to be a great need for approval among Type Cs. They need to make people happy and are usually "People Pleasers."

Do you see yourself in these descriptions? Not all people with cancer have all of these characteristics, but most people share a pattern of being conscientious, caring, and hard working. They have been unable to communicate their negative feelings and emotions, which are poisonous to the body and create an atmosphere where cancer can grow.

The next step is to understand our emotions so we can cleanse our body of the ones that are toxic.

WHAT ARE EMOTIONS?

The word *emotion* literally means "energy in motion." It is derived from the Latin verb meaning " to move." An emotion is a strong feeling, such as love, joy, sorrow, or anger. Our emotional experiences are imprinted in our brain cells and memory, where they form patterns that influence our behavior.

Emotional energy functions at a higher speed than thought, because the world of emotions operates at a higher speed than the mind. Repeatedly, scientists have confirmed that our emotional reactions are recorded in brain activity before we even have time to think about them.[3]

Learning how to manage this flood of energy called emotions is essential for our healing. Love, forgiveness, and letting go of our demands that the world or reality be different from what it is—these are keys to neutralizing the effects of toxic emotions in our bodies.

EMOTIONS AND THEIR ROLE IN CANCER

Christiane Northrup, M.D., a renowned physician and women's health expert, has noted that "toxic emotions" influence the body, because thoughts and emotions are mediated via the immune, endocrine, and nervous systems. They are, in fact, biochemical events. She believes that our physical, emotional, and spiritual aspects are intertwined and cannot be separated.[4]

Others in the health professions also believe that "under emotional distress, the brain may signal the adrenal glands to produce chemicals called corticosteroids—hormones that weaken the immune response. Cancer-related processes are accelerated in the presence of these chemicals as well as other stress hormones like prolactin."[5]

Recent findings in psychoneuroimmunology (PNI) explain the connection between emotional stress and cancer survival. This research suggests that the growth of cancer cells depends in part on internal body controls that retrain or stimulate tissue growth. Psychological factors appear to regulate these controls through neurological, hormonal, and immunological (immune system) pathways. These and other mind/body links could play a major role in determining a person's ability to survive cancer.[6]

Our emotions can cause chemical events in our body that create an environment where cancer can thrive. Toxic emotions can greatly affect our ability to heal. We simply cannot ignore the role of our emotions, especially if we want to regain our health and remain cancer free.

MOLECULES OF EMOTION

One of the foremost neurobiologists of our time is Candace B. Pert, Ph.D., a former chief of brain chemistry at the National Institute of Mental Health. Her book *Molecules of Emotion* chronicles her groundbreaking research into opiate receptor sites on cells, the discovery of endorphins (the body's natural opiate), and how emotions affect our health.[7]

Dr. Pert discovered that peptides are made up of a string of amino acids, joined together by strings of carbon and nitrogen; this bond is so strong it sometimes takes days of boiling them in strong acid to break them down. Her research has shown that neuropeptides (chemicals secreted by the brain) affect our mood and behavior. They are responsible for "signaling cancer cells via their receptors (opiate receptor sites on cells), causing them to grow and travel, or metastasize to different parts of the body."

These neuropeptides are chemical messengers that go between our different cells, influencing the digestive system, the immune system, and the neurological system. The neuropeptides, or molecules of emotion, can generate activity in that system or decrease activity, slowing it down.[8]

Some neuropeptides trigger cancer cells to metastasize, and others help keep our body healthy and cancer cells in check. Pert's belief, proven by her scientific experiments, is that neuropeptides carry emotions that flow through the body, influencing its systems for good or for ill. Our emotional expressions are always tied to a specific flow of peptides. When we suppress our emotions, we are creating a massive disturbance in our psychosomatic network. Being in touch with our emotions and learning to channel (not stuff) them in healthy ways will lead to cellular and system health.

If we accept the premise that peptides and other informational substances are the molecules of emotion, then we can accept the belief that the body expresses the unconsciousness mind. Repressed traumas caused by overwhelming emotions can be stored in a body part, thereby affecting our ability to feel that part or even move it—as well as affecting this body part's ability to function.[9]

Trauma produces intense emotions that can become stuck on the cellular level. Much has been written about sexual abuse and its effect on adults who were molested as children. The same goes for physical abuse, verbal abuse, abandonment, rape, abortions, and many other traumas. What we know is that any form of trauma, emotional or physical, is stored in the body.

Linda Marks, M.S.M., has written about a particular trauma that she calls "neglect trauma." This trauma generally occurs with newborns through children twenty-two months of age. These children may have parents who have set times for feeding, ignoring the infant's biological needs. They also let their children cry and cry without attending to them because they do not want the child to be spoiled. To that I would add the classic cases of incubator babies who are restricted from touch and attention. These traumatic moments are stored in the child's body and can cause the child to grow into an isolated adult who has problems forming emotional attachments and bonds with other people. These unhealed events are ticking time bombs, just waiting for the right moment to explode within our emotions and body as adults.[10]

Because these events are stored in the body on a cellular level, it is very helpful to find a health practitioner who specializes in releasing such traumas via loving touch. We are seeing marvelous results with body therapies such as massage, Touch for Health, and Body-Centered Psychotherapy.[11]

The last step in this process is to cleanse our toxic emotions.

CLEANSING TOXIC EMOTIONS

Pure emotions such as anger or fear are not good or bad in themselves. We all need to feel fear so that we won't walk out in front of a speeding automobile. Sometimes we need to feel anger so that we can rise to the defense of someone in need, such as a child who is being mistreated. But we also need to let these emotions go. And we must be aware that the mutated emotions such as bitterness, resentment, blame, or dislike are always toxic. Holding on to the events that spawned such emotions causes illness within our body. And as I mentioned earlier, stuffing these emotions only creates havoc in our body because these emotions are stored on the cellular level and in the tissues, and they can direct cancer cells to reproduce. They need to be thoroughly cleansed from our body so that we can be healthy and whole.

FORGIVENESS

All toxic emotions block the flow of energy in our body. Blocked or stagnant energy drains the body and taxes the immune system. Though we may hold such emotions because we believe the offender must pay, and we'll not let him go until there is justice, our body pays the price. At times we may feel in control when we hold a grudge, but the truth is that attempting to control another person or situation makes us powerless.

If unresolved anger and resentment are toxic, forgiveness is the antidote. We must be willing to let go of all stored bitterness, blame, grief, animosity, or any other toxic emotion. Hillary Stokes and Kim Ward of Sanoviv Medical Institute say that "sweet forgiveness cannot hold any taste of bitterness. They are mutually exclusive."[12]

When the apostle Peter asked Jesus, "Lord, how many times shall I forgive my brother when he sins against me? Up to seven times?" Jesus answered, "I tell you not seven times, but seventy-seven times'" (Matt. 18:21–22 NIV). This was a symbol of infinite forgiveness. Jesus also instructed His disciples after the Lord's Prayer, "For if you forgive men when they sin against you, your heavenly Father will also forgive you. But if you do not forgive men their sins, your Father will not forgive your sins" (Matt. 6:14–15 NIV).

Over and over we are taught to love one another and the Christian tradition teaches us to pray for those who offend us and to forgive them. Most other religious traditions agree: forgiveness is the path to wholeness. There simply is no other way.

Throughout our life we come in contact with many people. Some pass through our life without leaving any effects on us; others leave deep scars or joyous memories. It is easy to say that we have forgiven, when in fact deep within our tissues lie the residue of rage, hurt, bitterness, sadness, or other harmful emotions.

Here is a partial list of people who may have left scars in your life. I invite you to place a check or mark by every person toward whom you may have negative emotions. Read through the list from left to right, starting with your immediate family and extending to those who are more distant from you. I have left blank spaces at the end for you to add someone who is not mentioned in the list.

____ Mother	____ Father	____ Stepmother
____ Stepfather	____ Sister	____ Brother
____ Foster parent	____ Aunt	____ Uncle

___ Grandmother	___ Grandfather	___ Husband or Ex-husband
___ Wife or Ex-wife	___ Daughter	___ Son
___ Mother-in-law	___ Father-in-law	___ Daughter-in-law
___ Son-in-law	___ Neighbor	___ Pastor
___ Priest/Minister	___ Teacher	___ Boss
___ Friend	___ Girlfriend	___ Boyfriend
___ Coworker	___ Yourself	___ God
___ Sunday school teachers	___ School principal	___ Jesus
___ Coach	___ Spiritual teacher	___ Attorney
___	___	___
___	___	___
___	___	___

The list could go on and on. So please feel free to add any other names that need to be there for you. I have found that nearly all people need to forgive themselves, so please do not leave yourself out.

Letters of Forgiveness

If you read my wife's story in Chapter One, you know that Cherie's mother died of breast cancer when she was six years old. Her father was very angry about his loss, and he took that anger out on Cherie verbally. Her childhood was hard. Later in her life she sat down and wrote him a letter. Her inner-healing class instructor had suggested this step for everyone who wanted to be emotionally healed. Cherie included the hurts she had stored up in her heart concerning her childhood and her father's treatment of her. She told him she forgave him for his actions and asked his forgiveness for the bitterness she held in her heart toward him. She said she realized that her bitterness had fostered passive/aggressive behavior on her part. She said that she wanted to have an open channel of love once more. And she mailed the letter.

What Cherie didn't know was that her father was very ill, in fact, near death. When he received the letter and phoned her, the first thing she heard was his sobs. Throughout the conversation he sobbed and sobbed, and she cried as well. By the end of the conversation their relationship had been restored. One month later he died. And Cherie was able to continue her life without the deep wounds and old hurtful emotions she had been carrying. A year later we met and married. I do not believe this was a coincidence since her instructor had encouraged everyone who was single to attend to old wounds with their parents if they wanted to break their patterns of attracting people who weren't right for them and instead find a healthy relationship.

Are there people to whom you need to write letters of forgiveness? Some may now be deceased. That does not matter. The letter still needs to be written. (Cherie wrote a letter to her deceased mother at the same time she wrote to her father.) Some are estranged. Some are alive and very much need to hear from you. In some instances you need to write the letter, but it is not appropriate to mail it (such as to an employer). Use good judgment in these cases.

I recommend using discretion. Do not place yourself in a position where you will receive more abuse or later regret what you have expressed. Focus on what your heart says and receive an affirmative answer from within before you mail any of the letters. Some letters will need to be torn up or burned. Some will need to be rewritten so they are more loving. The important step is for you to write the letter and release the emotions stored inside.

When you are satisfied with the contents of the letter, I suggest that you read the letter out loud. Stand in front of a mirror where you can watch your body language and facial expressions. Are your eyes tearing? Is your voice shaky? How are you feeling? Have you really forgiven the individual or is there still an emotional charge?

Over the next few days or even weeks continue this exercise in front of the mirror until you can read the letter without any negative emotion. At some moment you will know you are free. That is the time to mail the letter, or to burn it if it should not be sent.

CLEANSING EXERCISES

I have found the following exercise to be very effective for my wife and myself, and I have also used this method with countless numbers of clients. This technique can help you deal with harmful emotions and release or transform them.

LETTING GO: "THE SEDONA METHOD®"

The Sedona Method is a simple, extremely powerful process that helps us release unwanted emotions that may be poisoning our body and soul. I have personally found this method to be very powerful and have used it over and over again in my consulting practice.

The creator of The Sedona Method, Lester Levenson, nearly died of a massive heart attack and was given just weeks to live. During an intense period of self-examination, he came to believe that it was not the world or the people in it that were the cause of his problems. Instead he acknowledged that his own emotional responses to events in his life had caused his health issues. Levenson discovered that he was capable of completely discharging all his negative emotions. As a result his health and life blossomed, and The Sedona Method was born.

This technique has undergone numerous scientific studies. Dr. Richard Davidson of the Laboratory of Cognitive Psychobiology at the State University of New York and Dr. David McClelland of the Department of Psychology and Social Relations at Harvard University conducted one such study. Dr. Davidson concluded that "The Sedona Method is indeed a highly effective stress antidote procedure." In a three-and-a-half month follow-up study, dramatic reductions in stress were still present.[13]

According to Levenson, people have three ways in which they deal with a feeling: they *suppress* it, they *express* it, or they *escape*.

When we *suppress* a feeling, we create an environment in which tension, anxiety, depression, and many other problems may fester. This is very toxic to the body, and the most harmful way to deal with the emotions. These suppressed emotions create behavior that is unhealthy. This is a characteristic of the Type-C personality.

The second way people deal with an emotion is *expressing* or *venting* it. All of us have blown up at one time or another. Although the emotion is vented, it does not go away. The emotion is still there, needing to be dealt with, but now there is often an accompanying emotion—guilt. We usually are remorseful for our lack of control and for our unkind words. All in all, *expressing* our emotions is not the best way to deal with them.

The third way people deal with their emotions is that of *escape*. We may watch television, read a book, eat, call a friend on the phone, go shopping, drink alcohol, gamble, use recreational or prescription drugs, have sex, or smoke. But the emotions are still causing stress in our body. Like the other two ways of dealing with emotions, *escape* does not work.

There is a healthy way to handle our emotions that has been taught by many teachers throughout time: *release the feeling and simply let it go*. Most of us have experienced arguments in which all of a sudden we realize how silly the whole thing is—and sometimes we burst into laughter. The emotion is no longer in our body tissues, neither is it contaminating our dialogue.

Levenson has found that *discharging* the feeling is the healthiest way to deal with our emotions. When put into use, this technique has a cumulative effect. We are more clear-headed, productive, and calm. Over time we can reach a state of imperturbability in which nothing or no one can throw us off center. We will be more productive on the job and happier in other areas of our life. Here is how the technique is done.

Step One: Focus

Select a problem area in your life. For instance, people I counsel might mention, "My boss doesn't seem to appreciate my work," or "I'm overwhelmed by the stress of trying to fight cancer." Choose something with a lot of "emotional juice." Now allow yourself to become relaxed and calm.

Step Two: Feel

Ask yourself, "What am I feeling right now?" It really is important to tell the truth about your feelings. Levenson has broken feelings down into nine categories in his workbook. Of the nine, six are considered to be toxic.[14]

These six feelings are called root feelings. The emotions listed after them are other expressions of the root feeling, just as leaves of a plant are outgrowths of their roots.

As you read through these six, place a check mark by the feeling or feelings that might be holding you captive.

_____ *Anger.* Other emotions that fall under anger are feeling: aggressive, annoyed, argumentative, defiant, demanding, disgusted, frustrated, furious, hateful, impatient, jealous, mad, mean, outraged, resentful, spiteful, stubborn, sullen, vengeful, vicious, and violent.

_____ *Apathy.* Many other emotions fall under the category of apathy, which includes being: bored, careless, defeated, depressed, discouraged, disillusioned, drained, futile, hopeless, overwhelmed, powerless, resigned, wasted, and worthless.

_____ *Fear.* Feelings subtyped under fear include being: anxious, apprehensive, cautious, cowardly, doubtful, foreboding, inhibited, insecure, nervous, panicky, scared, shaky, trapped, and worried.

_____ *Grief.* Some types of grief are feeling: abandoned, abused, accused, anguished, ashamed, betrayed, cheated, embarrassed, helpless, hurt, ignored, left-out, misunderstood, neglected, rejected, and sad.

_____ *Lust.* This emotion yells, "I want." Offshoot emotions are: anticipation, craving, demanding, desiring; feeling devious, driven, envious, frustrated, greedy, manipulating, obsessive, ruthless, selfish, and wicked.

_____ *Pride.* Some other associated emotions are feeling: aloof, arrogant, boastful, clever, contemptuous, cool, critical, judgmental, righteous, rigid, self-satisfied, snobbish, spoiled, superior, selfish, unforgiving, and vain.[15]

Focus on what you are feeling as you think about what has caused you hurt, fear, loss, rejection, or any other harmful response. Watch your body and see what it is doing. Is your heart beating rapidly? Are your eyes tearing? Is there a nauseous feeling in your gut? Tension in your muscles? Whatever is happening in your body is a clue to the strength of that particular emotion.

Levenson has found that the process of release is far more effective and powerful when the *root* feeling is released in its purest form. For instance, it is more efficient and dramatic to release the root of anger than it is to release the feeling of being annoyed. This release is like pulling a weed out by its roots, rather than just pulling the leaves off the plant. When the root has been removed, the weed is gone as well.

Step Three: Feel Your Feeling

Allow yourself to become emotional. Perhaps you are angry. Allow yourself to be enraged. Or perhaps you have uncovered deep feelings of grief or sorrow. Allow yourself to feel the sadness; you may find yourself crying or sobbing. That is exactly what needs to happen at this time. It is okay to allow your feelings to permeate your body. This is not the time to stuff them.

Step Four: Could You Let Go?

As you are feeling the feeling, ask yourself the simple question, "Could I let this feeling go?" One of the most freeing aspects of being an adult is being able to differentiate between our emotions and our true self. Our emotions are not who we are. They are simply energy moving through our body. Each of us has a "Watcher of True Self" who can observe the emotions as they flow through our body. This "Watcher" is asking the question, "Could I let go of this particular feeling?" We can view the emotion as a *shadow image* that has superimposed itself over who we really are.

Once you realize you can feel the feeling and your True Self can ask a question at the very same time, you are able to see the possibility of releasing the feeling.

Step Five: Would You?

You can release this feeling by asking yourself, "Would I let it go?" This is where you need to be very honest. Sometimes you are still simply too angry or upset to let the feeling go. In that case you need to allow yourself to continue to feel this emotion, rather than trying to intellectualize or escape from it. Eventually you will be tired of the harmful effects of this emotion and the mind chatter that goes with it. When this happens you can truthfully say, "Yes, I can let this feeling go."

Step Six: When?

Once you have acknowledged the possibility of releasing this feeling, the next question is, "When? Am I ready to let it go now, in ten minutes, tomorrow, next week? When am I going to let this feeling go?" At some point in time the answer will be, "Now! I am willing to let this feeling go now! I don't want it anymore."

The next step is simply to release the feeling—let it go!

Step Seven: Release

Releasing your emotions will bring a wave of relief to your body. You may find yourself laughing or crying or having a sensation of chills up and down your spine. Whatever the sensation, you will feel lighter, as if a heavy burden has just been lifted from your body.

You may find that other emotions need to be released. Simply go through the process as many times as needed. It's like peeling an onion. When one layer is gone, you may find more to peel. Be patient with yourself and continue on. It may take a period of time to completely cleanse yourself of all destructive emotions. The most important thing is not to give up. This process creates a clean slate for you to begin the next phase in your healing. (This information is copyrighted by Sedona Training Associates. See endnote for contact information.[16])

Most people who use this technique find that their energy skyrockets, their bodies are less tense, and they are more at peace with themselves and the world. The more the technique is used, the easier it gets. Practitioners of this technique find that they are able to release emotions as they arise in the morning, making their family lives or work environments much more congenial and peaceful.

The state of *imperturbability* (a state where bad feelings like resentment, bitterness, and anger are not allowed to remain in our consciousness) is the result of releasing these underlying emotions and wants. In this state of serenity and peace, our body can mend and heal from the onslaught of cancer or any other illness or disease.[17]

Another way to cleanse negative emotions is through laughter.

> **I let go of all demands for a better past.**
>
> **—Chuck Sorenson, my mentor**

THE LAUGHTER CLEANSE

Humor is a great stress reducer. No other immune booster compares with laughter, which can increase the flow of blood to the extremities of the body. Laughter improves the function of our cardiovascular system. Laughter enhances the body's release of endorphins and other chemicals that elevate mood and kill pain. Laughter also helps with the transfer of needed nutrients and oxygen to internal organs.[18]

You may have heard of Norman Cousins's remarkable healing experience with laughter. In 1964 he moved into a hotel room across the street from the hospital where he was being treated for a life-threatening disease. He rented comedy movies and literally laughed his way back to health. He later wrote the book *Anatomy of an Illness* about this experience. He said laughter "serves as a blocking agent. Like a bulletproof vest, it may help you against the ravages of negative emotions that can assault you in disease."[19]

Here are some ways to bring more laughter into your life:

- Spend time laughing with children. They have such contagious laughter that it is easy to be joyous with them. Whether or not you have children, you may want to volunteer. Numerous organizations, from church Sunday schools to day care centers to Boy Scouts and Girl Scouts, need adults to help.
- Make reading comics a daily habit. Many comic strip authors have published books of their work. See if your local library has any of these books. If not, purchase them. They will bring hours of comic relief and laughter to you and others in your household.
- Learn how to tell jokes. Find a good joke book and learn how to inject laughter into your conversations. Charlie Chaplin said, "To truly laugh, you must be able to take your pain and play with it!"
- Watch the newspapers and find out where the latest comedies are playing. Then call up a friend and go together. If you've seen *My Big Fat Greek Wedding* or other good comedies, you

know how a theater full of laughing people primes the laughter pump.

- Comedy audiotapes or CDs can make traveling or driving a light-hearted event.
- Think about some of the funniest moments in your past. Which ones make you smile just thinking about them? Get together with friends or relatives who can share the humor of those moments and laugh together.

We all need to bring more laughter into our lives, our homes, our workplaces, and our churches or synagogues. Laughter may well be the "Miracle Medicine" of the twenty-first century.[20] Learn to laugh at yourself. Not taking yourself or your circumstances so seriously is good for your health.

AN ANTIDOTE FOR THE LONELINESS OF CANCER

Sandra Steingraber, author of *Living Downstream*, experienced the loneliness that many find comes once a person has been diagnosed with cancer. When she was discharged from the hospital, she arrived home to find that her roommate had moved out—unable to live with a cancer patient. It was a redefining moment in Sandra's life. Even fifteen years later, she still bursts into tears when she sees a bare mattress.[21]

Take care of yourself. If friends or family have emotionally or physically moved out on you because they don't know how to deal with your cancer, or because they are afraid they will lose you and they do not know how to deal with that pain, you can create a new network of friends. Perhaps you can find a cancer support group. Or make friends with another cancer patient who's on the journey, as Sandra Steingraber did. Be vocal about your needs to your family and friends who want to listen. This is not the time to be isolated or stoic. It's a time to be nurtured and loved. And most of all—forgive. To forgive those who are not emotionally or physically capable of being there for you is an important step you can take toward wholeness.

10

MENTAL CLEANSING

For as [a man] thinks in his heart, so is he.

—PROVERBS 23:7

Each of us has a private world, made up of our thoughts and perspectives, invisible to others. This secret place is uniquely shaped by our environment—our parents, our siblings, our spouse, our children, and our friends—and by our school, our neighborhood, our religious affiliations, the media, and so much more. Some of our respective private worlds are dark and depressing, some are violent and filled with hostility and rage, some are filled with creativity and benevolence, and some with laughter and love.

If others could see our private world, they might be shocked. There are places in our mind that need cleansing—attitudes, beliefs, judgments, vows, negative thinking, which cause us disease. We may feel victimized by our past or by what is happening in the present. We may have reoccurring thoughts that seem to loop through our heads, never ceasing long enough to give us a moment's peace. We must remove toxicity from our mind, as well as our emotions and our body, if we are to be well. This is good news because we are the painter on the canvas of our mind, and every moment we are painting new strokes on that canvas, choosing the colors and the illustrations.

In this chapter we will explore how our mind affects our body and our health. Then we will look at the heart's role in our healing. Yes, our hearts control more than our relationship with others. Our heart can make a significant contribution to our healing. I'll show you why. Finally we will consider the impact our inappropriate demands have on our health.

THE MIND: ITS ROLE IN CANCER

Two recent studies of breast cancer patients published in *Lancet* and *Women's Health and Primary Care* are providing us with evidence about our mind's role in cancer. Both studies demonstrate similar conclusions: a correlation between depression, helplessness, and hopelessness and a higher risk of cancer relapse or death. One study found that having a high score for depression, helplessness, and hopelessness is linked to a significantly reduced chance of survival in breast cancer patients.[1]

TOXIC THINKING: HOW IT AFFECTS OUR BODY

Our body is made up of an intricate network of systems designed to work harmoniously and efficiently. Just as our emotions affect the health of our body, toxic thoughts negatively affect the body, making it sick and preventing it from healing. Our thoughts also shape our future. Therefore, it is imperative that we recognize and discard habitual toxic thinking.

> While most of the population reports experiencing personal or emotional problems in the course of a year, about 50% of these people say that they are unable to solve their problems and about one-third state that they are unable to do anything to make their problems more bearable. —HeartMath[2]

Our negative thoughts, which we may have entertained for years, might have become so habitual that we are unaware of them; they may even seem "normal." Scientists have found that they actually promote negative physical reactions. For instance, when we think about a situation that makes us angry, our blood pressure can rise. Often our heart beats faster and our jaws clench. Such physical reactions are caused by thoughts that trigger emotions, and vice versa. "This vicious self-reinforcing cycle will eventually bring itself graphically to your attention as physical symptoms," says Barbara Hoberman Levine in *Your Body Believes Every Word You Say*.[3]

How does one get rid of toxic thoughts? The first step is to identify them. Examples of toxic thinking follow. Place a check by those that apply to you and add to the list as other negative thoughts come to mind.

_____ *I hate my body. I'm too short, too fat, too skinny.*

_____ *I hate my life.*

_____ *Nobody loves me.*

_____ *I'm never going to get well.*

_____ *I have only a few months/years to live; the doctor said so.*

_____ *Nobody cares about me.*

_____ *I've had a terrible childhood.*

_____ *I had/have a rotten marriage.*

_____ *I can't stand my job.*

_____ *There's never enough money to pay the bills.*

_____ *My life has no meaning, no purpose.*

_____ *I'm so lonely.*

_____ *I don't like where I live.*

_____ *I've never done anything exciting in my life.*

_____ *My mother/father treats/treated me terribly.*

_____ *What's the use of trying to overcome the cancer? I can't really make a difference anyway.*

_____ *Nothing ever works out for me.*

_____ *I've always been sickly.*

_____

_____

_____

_____

_____

_____

This list could go on and on; the important thing is that we recognize that thoughts are either life enhancing or self-poisoning. Our inner dialog either helps to promote healing or contributes to disease.

My wife, Cherie, is a good example. Her loving maternal grandmother raised her after her mother died. Very concerned about Cherie's health, her grandmother repeatedly said to her, "You are a sickly child and must take it easy." Therefore, Cherie started thinking of herself as a sickly person. When she experienced her health crisis, she had to reprogram her thinking. Repeatedly, she stated out loud, with conviction, "I am healthy! My body is healthy! My body vibrates with health and wholeness." She no longer wanted "sickly" to be a definition of who she was. This was a struggle. Thoughts of illness were deeply entrenched. Yet she was able to create a new inner environment for herself, in which vibrant health was expected and experienced. Today she seems to have endless energy, exercising strenuously and working almost nonstop. To get to this place she had to change her negative thought patterns to those that were life giving and health affirming.

The same is true for each of us. We must dissolve old negative thoughts and replace them with positive ones that will help us win our battle with cancer. Rather than affirming our illness, we can affirm our health!

Let's begin by looking at the sources of our negative thoughts: judgments with bitter roots, inner vows, and shock, trauma, and cancer.

Judgments with Bitter Roots

Our mind reasons by making distinctions. We naturally evaluate people, events, and situations for the purpose of understanding and forming judgments. But judgments can create stress, incoherence, and toxicity. In fact, when we judge others, we are often the one hurt the most. And when we make a mistake and judge ourselves too harshly, we limit our ability to grow.

The most toxic judgments are those that have bitter roots, which are characterized by bitterness or unforgiveness. Just as a tiny mustard seed grows into a large tree, we may sow a tiny seed of judgment and reap a large, destructive harvest. A law of physics says, "For every action there must be an equal and opposite reaction." In the moral and spiritual realm this is expressed as, "Whatever a man sows, that he will also reap" (Gal. 6:7). The longer a seed of judgment remains in the soul, the greater its increase, and the greater the toxicity to the soul.[4]

Inner Vows

An inner vow is a *determination* that we set into our heart and mind as a child in reaction to something that has happened to us. We usually forget these vows as an adult. Yet our inner being remembers these vows and continues to act on them. Examples of inner vows are: *I will* never *be loved by anyone. I will* always *be sickly. There* never *is enough money.* These vows become the rudder that guides our life. Even if we change our mind and heart later, these inner vows continue to be played out, resisting the normal maturation process.[5] One way to cleanse the soul of inner vows is through prayer.

Examine, in particular, anything you may have vowed as a child that could have affected your health. For instance, the child of an alcoholic father might vow, *I will never trust men again.*

If you have identified something that appears to be a vow, or you even suspect something, you can pray the following prayer:

> I acknowledge a vow I made (or may have made) to ______________.
> I choose to release it. I break this vow, now, in Jesus' name.

Shock, Trauma, and Cancer

Many health-care professionals have observed that cancer is often preceded by a shock or traumatic experience six to eighteen months prior to diagnosis. We need to look at what was happening in our life prior to our cancer. If we have experienced a traumatic event, we can "reframe" the incident and take the sting out of it. Reframing is important; it's one of the reasons some people who experience shocking or traumatic events don't get cancer, whereas others do. What we tell ourselves about the event, how we choose to view it, and our daily thoughts about it can make the difference between healing and disease.

One physician noted that he contracted cancer after his son was shot and killed, and that his wife died within a few months of his son's death.

He soon discovered that many of his cancer patients also had gone through a severe shock.

Throughout life we are going to be shocked and disappointed. Deaths, accidents, and losses disrupt our life and destroy our equilibrium. We are betrayed and devastated by each other, often unintentionally. Yet we can reframe these negative experiences.

HOW TO CHANGE NEGATIVE ATTITUDES INTO POSITIVE ACTIONS

In my counseling with cancer patients, I suggest that they take five positive steps to reframe their negative experiences.

Step One: Identify the behavior, attitude, or symptom (the message your body is trying to send to your mind, like a headache or fatigue) you want to change.

Think about your own life. What negative behaviors, attitudes, or symptoms do you want to change? For instance you may be thinking, *I'm never going to get well* or *I've always been sickly*. List them on a blank piece of paper.

Step Two: Ask yourself what is the reason (the experience that caused this negative behavior, attitude, or symptom) for your behavior, attitude, or symptom.

For instance, the experience that led you to think, *I'm never going to get well,* could have been the day the doctor diagnosed your cancer. At that moment you probably thought, *People with cancer usually die*. List your own experience on that piece of paper.

Step Three: Know that even most of the behaviors that make you miserable have a "positive intention."

In order to change the behavior, you must find out the purpose or positive intention of these behaviors or attitudes. If you thought, *I've always been sickly,* you probably want desperately to change this weakness, but you don't know how. Or you now realize that being sickly meant that people gave you extra attention or consideration. Write the positive intention of your behavior on that piece of paper.

Step Four: Change that positive intention into a new, conscious intention.

Create conscious intentions like *I will concentrate my thoughts on activities that will help me to heal* (the proper diet, exercise, juicing), *rather than continually thinking about my cancer.* Write your new intention on that piece of paper.

Step Five: Ask yourself to come up with three new ways to satisfy your new intention effectively.

If your new intention was concentrating on activities that help you get well, three ways to satisfy that intention might be to buy organic foods, eliminate sugar in your diet, and walk a few more minutes each day. Write three ways to satisfy your new intention on that piece of paper.

Step Six: Make a commitment to begin the new behaviors now.

Start practicing one of the new behaviors today, then add the second behavior, and incorporate the third change as appropriate. When you fall short of your goals, don't give up. Keep at it. You'll soon be on your way to new, more effective behaviors.

Now that we've changed our toxic thinking, let's look at the impact our heart can have on disease.

THE HEART: ITS ROLE IN OUR LIFE AND IN CANCER

Many questions have arisen about the heart: "Does the heart think? Can it speak to us? Can we hear from our heart?" Proverbs 23:7 alludes to the heart's intelligence and its influence on us: "As [a man] thinks in his heart, so is he."

Recent scientific research backs up this Scripture, showing that the heart "is a highly complex, self-organized information-processing center with its own functional 'brain' that influences and communicates with the cranial brain via the nervous system, hormonal system, and other pathways. These influences profoundly affect brain function and most of the body's major organs, and ultimately determine our quality of life."[6]

THE HEART-BRAIN CONNECTION

Two researchers, John and Beatrice Lacey, were light years ahead of their colleagues during the 1960s and '70s. They found that the heart seemed to have its own peculiar logic, which was different from that of the autonomic nervous system. In fact, the heart was actually sending messages to the brain that the brain understood and obeyed. And these messages appeared to affect a person's behavior. No longer could scientists claim that the heart and nervous system were simply following orders from the brain.[7] The Laceys' research into the heart and its function was met with skepticism until other researchers, like Dr. J. Andrew Armour, verified their findings.

Armour revealed that the heart has its own nervous system, which is sophisticated enough to qualify as a "little brain," an intricate network of proteins, support cells, neurons, and neurotransmitters. These cells, which are similar to those found in the cranial brain, enable the heart to learn, remember, feel, and sense. The heart is able to operate and process information independently of the cranial brain or nervous system, which is brought about by approximately forty thousand neurons called sensory neurites that detect circulating hormones and neurochemicals and sense heart rate and heart pressure. The heart's nervous system translates this information into neurological impulses, which are then sent on to the brain. These signals help to regulate the autonomic nervous system, as well as the higher centers of the brain where they affect perception, decision making, and other cognitive processes. In many ways our heart's brain is independent of our cranial brain, directing behavior and organ functions.[8]

> **The heart directs the entire organism, and when grace gains possession of the heart, it reigns over all the thoughts.**
>
> **—SAINT MAKARIOS**

The Institute of HeartMath (a research and educational organization that has developed simple user-friendly tools to relieve stress) has shown through their experimentation that negative emotions lead to increased disorder in our heart rhythms and autonomic nervous system. And balance is achieved in heart rhythms and the autonomic nervous system when we create positive thoughts and emotions. Dr. Armour and his colleagues have shown that the heart's nervous system is vital for the proper functioning and stability of our cardiovascular system, and without the heart's little brain, the heart cannot operate properly—and neither can we.[9]

The heart produces and releases a hormone called ANF (atrial natriuretic factor) that affects blood vessels, kidneys, adrenal glands, and a large number of regulatory regions located in the cranial brain. It also secretes oxytocin, which is commonly referred to as the "love" or "bonding" hormone and is vital to our psychological well-being. Researchers have found that concentrations of oxytocin in the heart are equal to those in the brain.

HeartMath researchers have found that the heart responds faster than the brain and can interrupt emotional impulses before they reach the brain and cause adverse behavior. So many of us have had experiences where we just "felt" something wasn't right and ignored the impulse. We should have listened to our heart, rather than our brain, which was overriding the heart's wisdom. It is my belief that the heart is also where our body receives the frequencies of love sent out by our Creator.

Our heart can lead us step by step out of dark and desperate thinking, into the frequency of love. A simple technique can help us tap into the wisdom of our heart so we can cleanse our mind. The Institute of HeartMath offers this simple exercise to help increase stability and health in both body and mind. This is the ultimate cleanse for the mind—choosing to listen to our heart, instead of our mental chatter.

> **Descend from the head into the heart. Then you will see all thoughts clearly, as they move before the eye of your sharp-sighted mind. But until you descend into the heart, do not expect to have due discrimination of thoughts.**
>
> —BISHOP IGNATII

ATTITUDE BREATHING[10]

Attitude Breathing helps to soothe and disperse anxious feelings, bringing you back into balance.

Step One: Shift your attention to your heart and solar plexus/stomach area.

As I tell my cancer patients to work through this step, I ask them to think about their situation as they live each day with the threat of cancer in their bodies. Please do this now. How do you feel when you think about this cancer? Write your attitudes and feelings on a piece of paper.

Step Two: Ask yourself, "What would be a better attitude for me to maintain in this situation?"

Now I ask my patients to set up an inner attitude, like *Stay calm.* Again, please do this now. One way to do so might be to put your life in God's hands. You are feeling helpless because you fear you have little control over this disease. Why not trust a Higher Power (God)? Write the best attitude to help you face your cancer on that piece of paper.

Step Three: Gently and sincerely pretend to breathe the new attitude you want in through your heart. Then breathe it out through the solar plexus and stomach to anchor it.

As my patients take this step, I ask them to feel more emotionally balanced. "Pretend to breathe the feeling of balance through the area of tension," I say. Please do this now.

Then listen to what your heart wants to tell you. Most of us have never realized our heart's influence or intelligence. You might want to look for this direction in the days ahead. Now might be the time to access the wisdom of your heart.

This heart focus exercise increases stability. Heart focusing allows you to access the wisdom of your heart and the wisdom of God. With practice, you will find yourself accessing your heart throughout the day.

Appreciation: A Power Tool for Cleansing "The Little Brain" (The Heart)

Appreciation has a highly beneficial effect on your body. It is easy to activate and can shift your attitudes and perspective quickly.

- Make a conscious effort to look for things in your life you can appreciate; remember these when times get tough.
- Write an appreciation list. What are you thankful for?
- Stay on the lookout for areas in your life where you take things or people for granted. Make an effort to appreciate these people and things. Say "Thank you!" often.

GUARDING THE HEART

Many of us have driven by vacant land where the owner created a private garbage dump of his own. Rusty cars and trucks, old farm implements, tires, and garbage of all kinds litter the site; birds and other wild animals pick through the refuse. Often there is a stench, and we feel sad at such a disregard for the earth.

We can pollute and poison our heart and mind just as we do the earth. In fact, many of us are doing this every day by watching violent television and movies, engaging in gossip, listening to graphic and ear-splitting music, frequenting harmful Internet sites, speaking foul language, and scores of other activities. God has given us this marvelous gift called the heart, which began beating of its own volition when we were just twenty-five days old, in our mother's womb. Yet every day, without realizing it, we throw garbage and refuse into it.

Proverbs 4:23 says, "Above all else, guard your heart, for it is the well-spring of life" (NIV). We can do many things to protect our heart. We can read uplifting literature, watch heart-warming movies and television programs, spend quality time with supportive friends, listen to inspiring music, spend time in nature, cook a wholesome meal, walk our dog, volunteer, or choose activities that add to our enjoyment of life.

Now that we have cleansed our mind and our heart, we need to overcome our inappropriate demands.

A FINAL CLEANSING: OVERCOMING OUR INAPPROPRIATE DEMANDS

Why is it that we can get up in the morning feeling positive and happy and two hours later become so tied up in knots, angry, and irritable that some may say we are a "poor excuse for a human being"? Unfortunately most of us are trying to find happiness in things we believe will give us security, power, or sensation (sex, food, drugs, television).

In the process of growing up, we have programmed into our bio-computer (our brain) beliefs that we have decided will bring us happiness. Many of these beliefs become addictions, because when they are not fulfilled, we automatically experience pain, fear, or anger. In other words, *they control us: we don't control them.*

When this happens, our reticular activating system (the alerting system of the brain) only selects the stimuli or information picked up from our senses that is compatible with what we have previously programmed into our brain. That is to say, we see what we want to see, based upon how we believe our world to be.

The three lower levels of consciousness, the ways in which we have programmed ourselves to achieve happiness, are known as security, sensation, and power centers. Ironically, the end result of focusing on any of these three areas is that we set ourselves up for the very thing we are trying to avoid—unhappiness. If we tell ourselves that in order to be happy we must be *secure*, we program our brains to be preoccupied or dominated with having enough of what we perceive will make us feel secure—peace at all costs, job security at the expense of true fulfillment, or perhaps a predictably boring life.

If our focus is on experiencing happiness by having pleasurable *sensations*, our life will be centered on getting more and more sensation—food, sex, drugs, visual stimuli such as pornography, or any other pleasurable input. If our focus is on getting *power*, we will find ourselves automatically trying to control people and situations for the purpose of getting more wealth, prestige, or success.

Let's look at three individuals who typify an addiction to power, to security, or to sensation, respectively. The first is Alan, a small-business owner who suffered from hypertension and was referred to a counselor so he could learn more effective ways of dealing with his emotions. Alan owned his own business and considered that to be a major source of his problems. Alan had decided early in life that the way to happiness was to control everyone and everything around him. At work, this philosophy created a lot of problems for Alan. He was continually angry and frustrated when he perceived his authority to be challenged. He was not able to let go of control enough to allow his employees to make their own decisions and independently solve problems.

Alan was often critical and demeaning to those who worked for him. When an employee had a differing opinion, he would frequently get angry. Alan was unable to keep employees, so his business had a high rate of turnover, which caused him considerable financial loss because he constantly needed to train new employees and much of his time was focused there. This caused a "fight or flight" response (a typical reaction to stress), which contributed to his hypertension. Alan was addicted to power.

Annette decided that in order to be happy, she had to feel secure. Her criteria for security was harmony at all cost, a steady, dependable income, and an environment where little changed. Her marriage relationship caused her a great deal of stress because her husband seemed very unpredictable; he loved change, displayed a variety of emotions, and enjoyed spending money spontaneously. Every time she and her husband disagreed, she became fearful and anxious that he would reject her. This caused her to "clam up" more and more, even though her husband valued lively discussions and honest communication. Therefore, in response to her silence he became angry, which caused her to withdraw further. She seemed to have a constant fear of loss, not only regarding her marriage, but everything she was sure she couldn't live without if she were to feel secure. Eventually Annette began to experience migraine headaches, and her family physician could not help her. Finally, he referred her for counseling. Annette was addicted to security.

Phillip had learned that happiness was equated with pleasurable sensations. He was a connoisseur of good food, fine wine, and chocolate. Phillip discovered that certain foods gave him more pleasure than others, and the more of them he ate, the more pleasure he received. Eventually, his whole day was centered on his next meal or snack. When he was sad, anxious, or depressed, he ate chocolate for comfort. When he was happy and wanted to celebrate, he drank expensive wine and prepared his favorite meal. When he was bored, he snacked on junk food. When he was excited about new possibilities, he ate desserts. When he was feeling nostalgic, he ate ice cream and cookies.

Within three years, Philip gained a hundred pounds. He had developed an appetite he could no longer control. No matter how much he ate, he always wanted more. Eventually he was diagnosed with adult-onset diabetes, which was directly related to his weight gain and overconsumption of sweets. His doctor put him on a strict diet, which caused him considerable anxiety and depression. Finally, he sought help from a counselor. Philip was addicted to pleasurable sensations.

All of these persons held inappropriate demands for their lives. These beliefs controlled Alan, Annette, and Phillip. If these demands for power, security, or sensation sound familiar to you, I recommend you practice the following exercise daily.

REPROGRAMMING THE MIND

Step One: Explore what's bothering you.

Close your eyes, take several deep breaths, tune into how you feel right now, and let yourself really experience your deepest feelings. Picture what you were doing just before you experienced your most intense emotions. Who is there? (For instance, Annette might picture her husband returning from one of his spontaneous buying sprees.) Describe that person or situation on a piece of paper.

What is happening and what is being said? (Annette might write a few words that showed her anxiety and the realization that she soon clammed up.) Write your own description on that piece of paper.

What emotions are you feeling now? Describe how your body feels. What emotions are you experiencing? (Annette would be feeling anxious and insecure.)

Now look at how you have interpreted the incident. What words went through your mind? What is it that bothers you the most? What is the worst thing that can happen? (Annette would have to admit that she feared being in debt, losing the home she enjoyed, or being abandoned by her husband.)

Step Two: Pinpoint your addiction.

At the time of the incident in which your desire for power, security, or sensation manifested itself, what did you want to happen? What should someone else have done? What should you have done? (This was easy for Annette. Jim never should have bought that new car.) Write those thoughts on that piece of paper.

To discover your underlying addictive demands, ask yourself, "If I don't get what I want, and things don't go the way I want them to, what does that mean to me?" "How do I feel about myself?" To pinpoint your primary demand, ask yourself, "What do I think I need to be happy?" (Annette had to admit she liked her predictable life. She wanted security more than bright lights and faraway places.)

Step Three: Select phrases to renew your mind.

Do you see how the addiction to power, security, or sensation makes you suffer or keeps you from enjoying life? Are you tired of suffering? Are you willing to let go of your demands? Get in touch with all the pain your addictions have caused you and really determine to get free. Let your discomfort drive you to freedom.

To change the old programming, choose one or two ideas to reprogram your thoughts about what will make you happy. For example, *I don't always have to please people to be loved and accepted,* or *My happiness doesn't come from food.* (Annette might think, *I will extend my boundaries a little. I will take a few risks and see what happens.*) These are your reprogramming phrases. Write them on that piece of paper.

Step Four: Focus on reprogramming.

Keep your reprogramming phrases in mind and practice them with determination until you sense you have made a difference in your brain. Now put yourself back in the same scene that started your pain. Reaffirm your new programmable phrases. (Annette decided to react with less emotion the next time Jim overspent. And she suggested that they take a vacation to the Caribbean, even though her insecurity after the 9/11 attacks had kept her from any airplane travel.) Write that description down now on that piece of paper.

Finally, see yourself in a new situation with positive responses and feelings based on your new programming. Reaffirm that you can be free of old programming—of old addictions. You can enjoy life without these obstacles.[11]

Hopefully you have been able to reconsider the messages your mind has been sending to your body. And you have been awakened to your heart's wisdom and influence. The Scripture verse that began this chapter is so true: "As [a man] thinks in his heart, so is he." Cancer patients need to enlist every part of their being so they can overcome this unwelcome invader—negative, toxic thinking.

11

SPIRITUAL CLEANSING

When we live in love,
we are no longer driven by a determination to prove
something to others or to beat someone else's record.
In love, our deepening being is
glad to be true to itself.

—REVEREND TOMMY TYSON
(1922–2002)

Spirituality is multifaceted; it reaches far beyond the finite and defies description. It is personal, ever unfolding, and is shaped by our particular path of life. Each of us experiences spirituality and spiritual growth in different ways; each of us has our unique perception of God. There are attributes of God, however, that nearly all of us can agree on: God is love, goodness, wholeness, and beauty. There are truths most of us share, such as the belief that we can have a relationship with God. Most of us know it is important to nurture our spirit. And most of us have found the way to communicate with God through prayer.

But some of us have not been able to take advantage of sacred practices such as prayer because of traumatic, harsh, or cruel experiences associated with religion. Therefore, we will begin by looking at religious abuses that we may have experienced through religious leaders, family members, or religious organizations. These abuses may have caused us to confuse unloving actions with God. Let's start our journey of spiritual cleansing by taking a look at where we may have been "turned off" or hurt spiritually so we can let go of anything that stands in our way of healing.

RELIGIOUS AND SPIRITUAL ABUSE

In the last ten years we have seen the bloodshed in Northern Ireland between Protestants and Catholics and been bombarded with images of the Muslim suicide bombers and their victims. These actions have one thing in common: religious leaders justifying hatred as holy, using their religious position to manipulate individuals. Most of us can recognize the sickness of these extreme "religious" acts. We can see the insanity of burning someone at the stake, of the apartheid's repression, or of the killing of innocent civilians through terrorism. What we may not recognize are the abusive and toxic religious activities that surrounded us in our childhood, former years, or that are a part of our life today.

In order to cleanse our body of cancer, we also need to cleanse our soul of toxic religious wounds and beliefs. And we need to replace them with spiritual exercises and beliefs that are life giving and nurturing.

Has your relationship with God been damaged by spiritual abuse? To help you identify toxicity in your spiritual life, check the following statements that might apply to you:

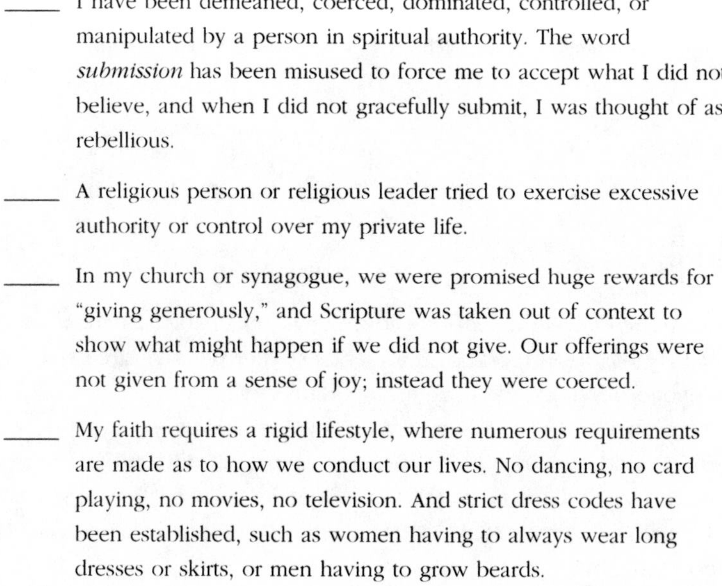

_____ I have been demeaned, coerced, dominated, controlled, or manipulated by a person in spiritual authority. The word *submission* has been misused to force me to accept what I did not believe, and when I did not gracefully submit, I was thought of as rebellious.

_____ A religious person or religious leader tried to exercise excessive authority or control over my private life.

_____ In my church or synagogue, we were promised huge rewards for "giving generously," and Scripture was taken out of context to show what might happen if we did not give. Our offerings were not given from a sense of joy; instead they were coerced.

_____ My faith requires a rigid lifestyle, where numerous requirements are made as to how we conduct our lives. No dancing, no card playing, no movies, no television. And strict dress codes have been established, such as women having to always wear long dresses or skirts, or men having to grow beards.

_____ Some members of my church, synagogue, or mosque feel they are superior. They seem to believe they have a clearer or higher understanding of the truth.

_____ When I left my old place of worship, I was shunned and demeaned by people I was once close to. My entire social circle disappeared, as my "friends" no longer wanted to associate with me. This was extremely painful, as I had few other friends.

_____ My feelings of anger, grief, or sadness were thought of as sin, rather than as legitimate feelings people have from time to time.

_____ My personal needs were thought of as selfish or unrighteous. I was told to "act right" so I could be worthy to be loved and accepted.

_____ I was sexually abused by a priest, minister, rabbi, mullah, or a person with religious authority.

_____ My faith promises rewards in an afterlife for violent behavior in the present life.

_____ Our church council, elders, or prominent givers decided to change our church structure or beliefs or methods of functioning to do things their way. The rest of us were forced to comply.

_____

I have tried to list the most conspicuous forms of spiritual abuse, but this list may have spurred you to remember other types of abuse you have experienced. If so, add those in the blank space.

Spiritual abuse is insidious because the abusers claim to be representing God; victims of this abuse feel alienated from God and unable to call out to Him for help. In these instances, our relationship with our Creator has been broken, so the healing process is often more painful and protracted.

Instead, God calls us to healthy spirituality.

HEALTHY SPIRITUALITY

Our definition of healthy spirituality is "showing or encouraging moral or psychological soundness." Healthy spirituality is both morally sound and psychologically whole, and it is characterized by love. I have stated earlier that God is love, and when we are experiencing love, we are experiencing God. Jesus said to His disciples, "'You shall love the LORD your God with all your heart, with all your soul, and with all your mind.' This is the first and great commandment. And the second is like it: 'You shall love your neighbor as yourself'" (Matt. 22:37–39). Any religion that does not have love at the core is toxic. Any action by those in spiritual authority that is not loving is toxic. Any action that claims to be love but is experienced as abuse or manipulation is toxic.

What some people have experienced in churches, synagogues, mosques, and spiritual groups is totally alien to what we know about God. Jesus told His disciples, "A new commandment I give to you, that you love one another; as I have loved you, that you also love one another. By this all will know that you are My disciples, if you have love for one another" (John 13:34–35). The apostle John told the early Christians, "He who does not love does not know God" (1 John 4:8). Any religion that does not encourage us to cultivate love within our home and heart and to extend the love of God to others in tangible ways is toxic. The heart and core of the gospel is *love*. Jesus reached out in love to the poor and to the wealthy, to the educated and uneducated. He lived among us modeling selfless love, care, healing, and compassion. He is our example of spiritual wholeness and health.

Cleansing our heart is vital to our emotional, mental, spiritual, and physical health. It is essential for us to remove the pain and heal the wounds that we have received at the hands of spiritual leaders and/or members of our religious affiliation. As we heal from spiritual abuse, we need to allow time to take small steps of faith and forgiveness. We are on a journey to reconnect with God and a sense of love and joy.[1]

I know that forgiveness is not easy, yet God calls us to radical forgiveness.

RADICAL FORGIVENESS

In the past we may have been pressured by someone's admonition to hurry up and "forgive and forget." We may have been shamed into thinking that unless we let go of our hurts, our anger, and our pain quickly, we are being stubborn and unforgiving. We may have been counseled to grant forgiveness preemptively, without appropriately processing the event(s) needing to be forgiven. If we do this, we experience a distorted forgiveness that is actually just a mental or verbal assent. Instead we need to wrestle with our hurt, so that when forgiveness takes place, it is legitimate and real.

Think about the ways you have been abused or hurt in any religious context. Write them on a piece of paper.

Forgiveness is not about being a patsy so that others can walk all over us. Forgiveness is gutsy, confrontational, and truthful. You will need to wrestle with your feelings. Try to look at the situation as objectively as possible. Ask yourself, "What was my part in this situation? Do I need to apologize and make amends? What is the other person's part in the situation? Did that person's behavior cause my pain, or did some other unresolved situation from my childhood get triggered?" These questions are not easy and need time and often distance to sort through. Write your initial answer to these questions on that piece of paper.

In their workbook *The Choosing to Forgive Workbook,* Les Carter, Ph.D., and Frank Minirth, M.D., walk readers through the questions they ask patients to answer when they are trying to forgive. You might want to answer these questions as you attempt to personalize your choice to drop your bitterness.

First, be honest and ask yourself, "Why would I want to remain bitter?" (For instance, "It makes me feel powerful" might be an answer, or "It gives me the excuse I need to withdraw from this relationship.") Write the reason(s) on that piece of paper.

To forgive this person you don't need to excuse his or her behavior. But you do need to forgive that person. Even though your anger is justified, Scripture says, "If you do not forgive men their trespasses, neither will your Father forgive your trespasses" (Matt. 6:15).

Sometimes we compare our sins to other people's and say, "Mine aren't so bad," but God says all sin is harmful. Remember, forgiveness doesn't make the other person right; it makes us free. When we forgive, we make a choice to no longer allow other people's shortcomings to dictate how we feel or what we do.

Now ask yourself, "What would be the likely consequences of clinging to bitterness?" (For instance, a possible answer might be "I am not able to ask God to heal my cancer or to walk through it with me," or "It could become a habit that would eat away at my energy to fight the cancer.") Remember, answer from your heart. Write your answer(s) on that piece of paper.

Often we are harmed by our anger, resentment, and hostility. These emotions were all in the list of cancer personality (Type C) traits on pages 228–29. In his letter to the Ephesians, the apostle Paul tells the early Christians, "Let all bitterness, wrath, anger, clamor, and evil speaking be put away from you, with all malice" (4:31).

In their years of counseling people for depression, anger, and anxiety, Dr. Minirth and Dr. Carter say they have never encountered anyone who ultimately experienced pleasant consequences from holding on to bitterness. It is doubtful that you will find the consequences of bitterness to be life giving either.

Realizing that holding on to your pain and bitterness is a choice and its consequences are not desirable, move on to one final question: "Why might forgiveness be a better option than bitterness?" (For instance, an answer might be "I'd be choosing not to live in the past, which would free me to be more effective in my fight against cancer," or "I can redirect this emotional energy toward my healing.") Write your answer(s) on that piece of paper.

Les Carter and Frank Minirth admit that no one is duty bound to forgive. People are free to choose, they say, even if it means they might make poor choices. Are you willing to forgive the person or persons who hurt you? If so, put him or them in God's hands. And pray for that person (or those persons) daily for at least a week.[2]

Scripture says that this person in a position of authority will be strictly judged for the harm he or she has caused anyone: "Not many of you should presume to be teachers, my brothers, because you know that we who teach will be judged more strictly" (James 3:1 NIV).

Forgiveness doesn't require that everything be the same as it was before the offense. It doesn't require that you continue associating with the other individual if there is no change in behavior. It does require that you come to peace with the situation, so that you no longer hold bitterness and resentment against the other person or hurt and pain in your soul.

Now that you have forgiven your abuser, let's replace the negative experiences of the past with the scriptural practices that will connect you to the God of love. Three cleansing medicines that can help in healing spiritual abuse are prayer, Scripture, and music. These same prescriptions have been proven to be good medicine for those who are ill.

PRAYER AS CLEANSING MEDICINE

In the past scientists and some doctors were contemptuous of prayer, seeing it as an escape with no scientific basis to support its helpfulness. However, within the last twenty years scientists have rolled up their sleeves and put prayer to the test in the laboratory. David D. Larson, M.D., of the National Institute of Healthcare Research in Rockville, Maryland, explored the relationship between one's spiritual beliefs and health. A former senior researcher at the National Institute of Mental Health, Larson states,

> Statistically, God is good for you. I was told by my [medical school] professors that religion is harmful. Then I looked at the research, and religion is actually highly beneficial. If you go to church or pray regularly, it's very beneficial in terms of preventing illness, mental and physical, and helps you cope with illness much more effectively. If you look at the research, in area after area, it's 80 percent beneficial. I was shocked.

Larson went on to learn that 43 percent of American physicians pray for their patients on a regular basis. Recent surveys reveal that 75 percent of patients believe their physicians should address spiritual matters as part of their medical care, and 50 percent would like their doctors to pray with them.[3]

It is "good medicine," says Larry Dossey, M.D., and renowned researcher on prayer. "It helps us become warriors, not worriers." When Dr. Dossey began to explore double-blind studies utilizing prayer, he was astonished to find over 130 had been conducted, and over half of them *strongly* indicate that prayer works. Another 250 studies have indicated that when prayer is included in religious practices, prayer promotes health. Dossey came to believe that prayer is one of the best-kept secrets in modern medicine. He discovered that religious faith is associated with a faster recovery rate after surgery. And prayer, even offered from a distance, increases the healing rate of surgical wounds. Cardiologist Randolph Byrd studied prayer with 393 patients in the coronary care unit of San Francisco General Hospital. This was a double-blind study—no one knew who was being prayed for from a distance. All other treatments being equal, Byrd found that the prayed-for patients did significantly better on several outcome measures.

Psychiatrist Thomas Oxman and his colleagues at Dartmouth Medical School also studied the role of "religious feeling and activity" in 232 patients undergoing cardiac surgery. These patients were all over fifty-five years of age. They discovered that the patients without hope derived from religion had lower survival rates than those who believed in a Higher Power. Faith has been shown to assist a person in getting well by mobilizing his or her immune system and other defense systems.[4]

The most important aspect of successful prayer is *love* and *compassion*. Scientific studies have shown that when love and compassion are not present, prayers have little effect. Dossey states, "In its simplest form, *prayer is an attitude of the heart*—an attitude of *being*, not doing. Prayer is the desire to contact the Absolute, however . . . conceived. When we experience the need to enact this connection, we are praying, whether or not we use words. Prayer transcends our definitions, as it is our heart speaking and crying out to God's heart. And if we are at a place where we can pray, *Thy will be done*, we can enter into a place of peace, hope, and rests."[5]

We can utilize prayer when we are cleansing our body, emotions, and mind. We can call on God to help us in our battle with cancer. And we can ask others to pray for us. When we pray and when we seek out others to pray for us, keep in mind that it is okay to ask and keep on asking. Francis MacNutt, founding director of Christian Healing Ministries, says "soaking prayer"—praying over and over again, often with laying on of hands—is often needed. In the years that Francis MacNutt has been involved in praying for the sick, he has observed that repetitive prayer often brings about results. Each time a person is prayed for, he or she may get a little better, until the condition is greatly improved or that person is completely well. Reverend Tommy Tyson says, "Soaking people with prayer is somewhat like soaking clothes to get them clean; some of them need to stay in the water longer to get the job done."

Because research has shown that prayer is an aid in our journey to wholeness—a powerful tool not to be ignored—you may want to pray the following prayer every day for yourself.

A Daily Prayer for Physical Healing

This prayer is adapted from one written by Sister Jean Hill, a Benedictine Oblate. She suggests you start by laying your hands on your head each time you say this prayer.

> Jesus, I thank You for the light of Your life now coming into my head. May the chemistry of my brain, my electrical impulses, and my entire circulatory system come under Your Lordship so that my body might function in perfect health. Let Your light permeate the entire chemistry of my body, drawing all my fluids and tissues, the functioning of my every organ and system into perfect order. I command my blood to take to every cell all that I need to be in perfect health so that my whole body will be in harmony.
>
> Let the light of Your loving presence spread to all the unhealed areas of my being; into the places of my deepest fears, angers, and unforgiveness, and into any dark areas of guilt that need Your cleansing grace and wisdom.
>
> Keep me today in Your Truth, and in Your perfect love. In the name of the Father, Son, and Holy Spirit. Amen.

Another prescription for spiritual abuse and good medicine for illness is Scripture.

SCRIPTURE AS CLEANSING MEDICINE

Meditating on Scripture is an excellent way to bring about deep, lasting change to our heart, emotions, and mind. When we read Scripture we are placing living, life-giving spiritual food into our mind and heart. But that by itself is not enough. In order for true spiritual cleansing to occur,

Scripture needs to be "chewed"—meditated and prayed—so it can enter the deepest regions of our subconscious mind, replacing old, defunct programming that is still running our life.

If you are unfamiliar with the Bible, the fourth book in the New Testament, the gospel of John, which is called the "Gospel of Love" by many, is a wonderful way to begin. The book of Acts and the book of Luke were written by a Greek physician named Luke, as letters to a friend. In recent years Luke has become recognized as one of the most accurate historians of ancient times. In these two books he lists over two hundred governmental officials and their offices, and recent archeological finds have confirmed all but a handful of those listed. Luke diligently interviewed hundreds of people as he wrote histories of what had occurred in Israel surrounding the birth, life, and death of Jesus.

In the Old Testament, many of the Psalms, originally sung as songs by King David, and Proverbs, written as a book of instruction, are very nurturing and life giving. Before becoming king, David was a fugitive, hunted by a jealous King Saul. David poured out his feelings in his songs, which provide us with examples of how "real" we can be with our Creator about our illness and current situation.

MUSIC AND SOUND AS CLEANSING MEDICINE

A final cleansing medicine I suggest is music. Diverse branches of science are investigating the effects music and sound have on the human body as well as surfaces such as water, sand, and gels. Music therapists have documented the soothing effects music has on cancer patients suffering from chronic pain.[6]

In 1787 musician and physicist Ernst Chladni demonstrated that sound does affect physical matter. Chladni drew a violin bow perpendicularly across the outer edge of flat plates covered with sand and created geometric shapes in the sand, even though he had not directly touched the particles. These figures are known as Chladni Figures. In 1967, a Swiss physician, artist, and researcher named Hans Jenny, M.D., demonstrated that materials such as sand, spores, iron filings, water, and other viscous substances created shapes and motion patterns when they were exposed to sounds. When Dr. Jenny changed the frequency and amplitude, the shapes would also change.[7] Recently, Dr. Masaru Emoto has photographed the molecular structure of water that has been altered by music and other human vibrations created by such expressions as hate, love, and appreciation. His photos provide a visual proof that music, sound, and emotions can alter physical substance.[8]

From this research we can gain some exciting insights regarding our health and healing. About 75 percent of our body is made up of water; each of us is like a large, wet (or dehydrated) sponge. The water in our body is continually carrying nutrients to each cell and removing toxic waste materials. Because our body is so porous, the sounds and vibrations that make up our world affect it. Not only does music and sound affect our mood; it appears that it also affects the molecular structure of water within our body.[9]

A French ear, nose, and throat specialist, Dr. Alfred Tomatis, became very interested in the process of hearing and listening and the ways our brain processes incoming sounds.[10] His work resulted in fourteen books and numerous journal articles, two prestigious European Medical Awards, and the establishment of medical treatment centers throughout the world.[11]

One of his studies involved a group of monks in a Benedictine monastery. The monks had become listless and fatigued, and Tomatis was asked to find out why. He soon learned that the new abbot had eliminated their six to eight hours of daily chanting. His research indicated that this chanting was an excellent source of high-frequency overtones, which Tomatis believes are as important to health and wellness as proper nutrition, because they provide electroneural stimulation to the brain. Tomatis's solution was to instruct the monks to resume chanting, and they quickly regained their vitality. He concluded that Gregorian chants are "a fantastic energy source," due to their multitude of high-frequency sounds.[12] These sounds seem to recharge our body and brain to the same degree that batteries are recharged. Unfortunately, due to stress and environmental noises, most of us have lost the ability to hear these energizing frequencies.

From all of this research we can conclude that certain sounds are helpful to our body, while other sounds are depressing and life draining. Swearing or cussing, critical words, or depressing statements affect our body in a negative way. Heavy metal and rock music or any discordant sound has a detrimental effect on our body as well. Dr. Masaru Emoto has photographed water crystals that have been subjected to heavy metal music and negative language. The crystals are ugly and deformed. On the other hand, water molecules placed between stereo speakers playing classical music have lovely crystalline shapes.[13] Evidence suggests that the following types of music have positive effects on the brain and body: classical, baroque, Gregorian chants, romantic, certain types of jazz, and relaxing instrumental music.[14] From my own experience I can also suggest that uplifting sacred music has a positive effect.

I'd now like to challenge you to see your cancer as a health opportunity.

SEEING YOUR CANCER AS A HEALTH OPPORTUNITY

When attendees arrive at the Optimum Health Institute (OHI: a center for alternative health education and raw foods cleansing), they are instructed not to discuss their illness while at OHI, but to refer to their condition as a "health opportunity." They are encouraged to speak only positive, life-affirming words to everyone in the course of their stay. Although some people are very ill, the Institute pulsates with life, healing, and hope. Some people who arrive with what appears to be "hopeless situations" are often healed and return home to live out their unfulfilled dreams.

Calling cancer a "health opportunity" may at first cause you to pause. But truly, it is an opportunity to uncover and release toxicity in all aspects of your being—body, soul, and spirit. Now is the time to set yourself free to live—really live. You can create your own hope-filled future.

SEEING YOURSELF WELL

In their book *Getting Well Again*, O. Carl Simonton, M.D., and his psychologist wife, Stephanie, said that a person's will to live is very important to his or her recovery. They found that two people with the same diagnosis would often experience very different outcomes. Those who said they couldn't die until they had completed something or because they were greatly needed often had better outcomes than those who did not have a compelling reason to live. These people said such things as "I can't die until my son graduates from college," or "They need me too much at work." Those with no reason to live more often had a negative outcome. The Simontons found those who believed "that they exerted some influence over the course of their disease" took a stance toward life and had a much better chance for survival. Choosing to live is very powerful.[15]

The Simontons also found that imagery was very helpful. They had their patients draw pictures of cancer cells, then add white blood cells with large teeth that would begin to gobble up the cancer cells. These pictures would progress until the patient would see the white cells victorious and the cancer cells dead and eliminated from the body. Patients undergoing chemotherapy or radiation drew pictures of the radiation hitting the cancer cells and avoiding the other healthy cells in their bodies. Patients were encouraged to picture these positive results frequently during the day until their recovery was complete. This proved to be powerful for their patients and seemed to lessen the side effects of the radiation and chemotherapy.[16]

Quantum physics is helping to explain the dynamics of our energy field. Scientists propose that when we create pictures in our mind, our imaginings become electronically charged with energy. This energy field draws people and situations to us that align with our energy field and repel that which is not aligned with it. Dr. Karl Pribram, renowned neurosurgeon and psychologist at Stanford University, drawing on the work of Nobel Prize–winner Dennis Gabor, believes the brain energizes our pictures. When our eyes see an image, they act like a camera. The image is changed into wave storage, and then into images in our mind. The mind then radiates these images out into the atmosphere. According to this theory, these waves draw the pictured result to us and repel those things that are different from our internal pictures.

Images of Hope

Find a picture where you were really healthy and happy. Place that picture on your refrigerator, bathroom mirror, or a place where you can see it frequently. Whenever you look at it, tell yourself, "My body is becoming just as healthy as it is in this picture. My future is filled with health and promise!"

We are at the edge of the scientific frontier in understanding the dynamic of our body's energy fields and how these fields impact our health. Understanding quantum physics helps us to see how vital it is to hold positive images of health and healing in our mind. We may have images of X-rays showing tumors, or mental tapes of medical doctors gravely speaking a life-shattering diagnosis. These images and words have their own negative energy and magnetic power that need to be transformed into something more positive and life promoting.[17]

Are there things you really want to do? Perhaps you want to go on a missions trip, swim with dolphins, help build a Habitat for Humanity home, visit Europe, help the homeless, or learn a foreign language. Whatever your dreams may be, focus on one that requires that you be in better health to fulfill it.

The following exercise can help you see yourself as well.

A HEALING EXERCISE

Step One: Secure a quiet place.

Decide on a time each day when you can focus your attention on images of vibrant health and healing and on the dream you really want to experience. You need to unplug the phone so you will not be interrupted. You may need to place a note on your door, asking to be left alone during this time. Whatever it takes, it's important that you be undisturbed and comfortable with the place you choose to do this exercise.

Step Two: See yourself as healthy.

Imagine a scene in which you are extremely healthy and happy. Choose one image that has a very positive, emotional feeling attached to it. This is the picture you want to recreate. You want to be as vibrantly healthy again as you are in this picture. Quiet any thoughts that may interfere with what you are presently doing; any negative thoughts that may want to crush your hopes for a better future.

As you imagine the scene, you can pretend that you have a magnifying glass with a light attached to it in your hand. Now go over each detail of your dream. Focus all your attention on the healthy, happy person you intend to become.

As you hold the scene in your mind's eye, you need to hold this image in your heart. Feel how excited, joyous, accomplished, exuberant, and satisfied you are once you have accomplished your goal of regaining your health. You need to hold these feelings for at least *thirty seconds*, as this triggers an image in your imagination. The more you experience feelings of desire around this healthy image, the more your image is changed into a magnetic waveform. Your feeling energy now catapults these waves inside and outside your body. The greater the desire, the more energy is propelled within and beyond your body.

Step Three: Speak affirmations of your healing.

Now you can say your healing affirmations *out loud* with *enthusiasm:* "I am vibrantly healthy! My body pulsates with health and wholeness! I see myself swimming with dolphins! I see myself visiting Europe!" (Avoid any reference to your health challenge and only affirm what you want to create.) By speaking *out loud* with *animation,* you are seeing results and vibrating the pictures away from yourself where others can help you achieve your goals. Imagine that the image you sent out loops back to you in the tangible form you envisioned. Feel joyful and healthy and allow yourself to bask in the feeling of your achieved desire.

Healing Words

These are examples of statements you can say to yourself that will bring healing into your body. You may want to stand in front of a mirror and read these words out loud several times a day. Hearing your own voice speak words of hope is very powerful.

- I am strong.
- I am healthy.
- I am very grateful to be alive.
- I am very hopeful about my future.
- I am getting better each day.
- I am grateful for my friends and family.
- I am now willing to forgive myself and others.

- I give up all demands for a better past.
- I listen with love to my body's messages.
- I can overcome this cancer. My thoughts and feelings do influence my body.
- My immune system is strong.
- Everything in me cooperates with my healing.
- I trust God with my future.
- Each day is a gift from God: that's why we call it *the present.*

Step Four: Listen to your heart.

Once you have energized your desired result, sit quietly for a while. This is when your heart may want to speak to you, giving you direction as to what to do next. You may receive a hunch that you need to visit a certain health practitioner, or perhaps someone is brought to your mind whom you need to forgive.

When you feel complete with this exercise, promise yourself that you will do this everyday on a regular basis. It is very important that you not share this goal or dream with others. This is your secret. Even your most positive friend or your mate may unknowingly discourage you from achieving your dreams. You do not need their negativity at this time![18]

There Is No Reason to Fear

As you read Michael Mahaffey's story, you'll discover what the Twenty-third Psalm meant to him as he battled life-threatening leukemia. Cherie and I have written our own version of the Twenty-third Psalm as a prayer for you. You might want to write this prayer on a piece of paper that you can take with you wherever you go. Read it often. We pray it will encourage you when the days are tough.

The Twenty-third Psalm as a Prayer

The Lord is my shepherd; I shall not fear cancer.
He makes me to lie down in peace.
He leads me to health and wholeness for His name's sake.

> Yea, though I walk through the valley of despair,
> I will not be discouraged,
> For You are with me.
> Your love and strength comfort me.
> You prepare a table before me of wisdom, knowledge, and guidance
> in the presence of discouraging diagnoses.
> You anoint my head with the oil of healing;
> My cup is full of joy.
> Surely goodness and mercy shall follow me all the days of my life;
> And I will dwell in trust and hope forever.

Many cancer survivors have conveyed their discovery that having cancer was the best thing that ever happened to them. They were forced to grow and change in ways they would not have considered without their health challenge. In Part Two, Michael Mahaffey shares his astounding story of healing. His diagnosis of leukemia was the beginning of a journey that is still unfolding.

PART TWO

A Renewal of Your Body, Your Mind, and Your Spirit

12

ONLY THIRTY DAYS TO LIVE

Giver of life, creator of all that is lovely,
teach me to sing the words of your song . . .
help me to try to follow your leading.

—ANONYMOUS

On February 16 of 1983, as Kathy and I drove the final straightaway to our ranch from the doctor's office, tears returned to stream down our cheeks. The finality of the doctor's pronouncement seemed to echo around us. This crisis of cancer was pulling the strings tight around my remaining life. Thirty days to live offered me few possibilities, with nothing to grab on to and no place from which to negotiate. I could not talk my way through this. I was trapped. It didn't matter what I had in material possessions, who I thought I was, or what I had done in my professional career. Ironically my survival up to now had been based on being in control. Now, the cancer had complete control. I was helpless.

Where has the time gone? I asked myself. *What do I have to show for my life?*

As we pulled into our driveway at our ranch, my friend Rudy Kopfer drove up next to us. I had called Rudy, a practicing oral surgeon in San Francisco, after talking to Tom Dolkas about the appointment to draw my bone marrow. Rudy had called and talked with my doctor shortly after we had left his office. Being the friend he was, he canceled his appointments for the rest of the afternoon and immediately came to offer his support and assistance. Kathy went into the house as I shuffled across the parking area and into his comforting bear hug.

"Michael, I am not sure you can beat this even if you want to," Rudy said tearfully. "But, if you and I put together a game plan and work the plan, it may happen."

Just a short while ago, I had been told that my life was over, and now my friend and I were going to make the plans that would keep me alive.

Rudy drove me back into Auburn where I bought over five hundred dollars' worth of vitamin supplements. Then it was back through the canyon to my dream home on the hill. Together we formulated a scheme to deal with the leukemia. Rudy's deal for his professional services was this: if I smoked even one cigarette, he would get back in his car and head home to the Bay Area. I had been going through two to three packs a day. The cigarette I had in my hand as we made the bargain was the last one I've had.

Sitting and planning our attack together, Rudy and I became co-conspirators, teammates, teacher and student, and I had no adequate words of gratitude. At that time, he was my only hope. Rudy, Dr. Rudolph Kopfer, had been my close friend for over ten years. I never held it against him that he is tall and good-looking. He, quite possibly, is about five years older than I, but I never asked him. Our families—his wife, Donna, and their three girls, and Kathy and my kids—did lots of things together. Kathy and Donna were very close, almost like sisters. Rudy lived and practiced in the Bay Area so I saw him quite often, as often as my business took me there.

By the time Rudy left, Kathy had the five kids assembled around the kitchen table, where we normally held our family meetings. During the ride home, Kathy and I had talked about breaking the news to them. We knew they already suspected something was wrong. Their concern had grown as I, who never missed a day of work in my life, had stayed in bed throughout the week, complaining of nothing more specific than "feeling awful all over." Kathy had been making frantic phone calls throughout the afternoon to locate everybody, and judging by the nervous silence that filled the room, I could tell my "secret" was no longer private information.

They were all there: Colleen, my oldest, nineteen and a recent high school graduate. Short and blonde like her mother, she had a curious smile that always seemed to be asking a question. Possessing a tremendous amount of energy, she would soon put together a drive that prompted donors to give up to five hundred units of blood. Shana, in her senior year and eighteen, was creative and fiery with a smile that kindled my heart. Brendan, our youngest, was a seventeen-year-old junior, also an athlete, a dreamer, and a friend to many. Completing our immediate family circle were our two foster sons, Jeff and Brian. Both boys had been living in our home for the past several years.

Now we were ready to experience the shock together and prepare as best we could for the disruptive days ahead. Colleen, who is normally very outgoing, was atypically quiet. Shana, along with Jeff and Brian, looked nervous. Our son, Brendan, had rushed in late and sat at the far end of the table.

"Your father has a very advanced case of acute leukemia," Kathy told the children, struggling to remain calm. "The doctors don't give him a chance."

For a while no one spoke. As I sat there avoiding eye contact with them, I felt detached, as if Kathleen, the children, and I were delivering tear-jerking lines in a B-grade movie. Finally Jeff, who's usually quiet and shy, spoke up. "Well, if I were God and wanted to grab Dad's attention, I would use this illness to do it. But I know, from the bottom of my heart, that Dad isn't going to die."

What did he mean: God's grabbing my attention through leukemia? It was an odd idea—so odd that in that moment it flew right by me.

In true macho fashion, I was desperately holding in my emotions. I think I was trying to preserve my position of patriarchal strength. I kept thinking, *I've got to get this right. I need to be brave.*

I had never cried in front of my children. Actually, I had never shown any form of emotion at all—except violent, abusive anger that made the kids fearful.

Suddenly it dawned on me. My children and I had no real relationship at all. Unlike Kathy, I had devoted practically no time to my family. They were "little business," and I was, after all, a "big businessman." This realization was so devastating I found it difficult to even think about it.

In bed, later that night, I thought back to Jeff's cryptic words: "If I were God and wanted to grab Dad's attention, I would use this illness to do it." God? Up to this point I had no room for God in my life. Material wealth was the only god I was acquainted with. Nevertheless, feeling that the ordeal ahead might be so gruesome that dying might be preferable to sticking it out, I made a feeble attempt at prayer. Given my nonexistent state of spiritual development, it was an exercise in futility. I cried and cried until dawn.

That next morning I experienced aloneness and emptiness. In the past I had chosen to not discuss finances with Kathy. I talked a lot but rarely let anyone into my heart. I had said, "I do" and "till death do us part" to this woman twenty-one years before. We had a relationship that was more than that of strangers, but I still had not let her into my innermost secrets.

What am I afraid of? I asked myself. *What blocks me from confiding in her?* I wanted to hold her and tell her I was sorry. I wanted to confide in her my fears of dying. I wanted her to know I felt insecure thinking that she would marry again. I wanted to tell her, "I love you."

I saw how I was still struggling with my inability to express those feelings. Looking back, I find it incredible! She and I had shared a life together, made love, argued, laughed; and still, I was trapped in my fear that she might see the real me.

What a deal! I was dying. Yet I had created a chasm so wide and deep that I could not share my thoughts and feelings concerning cancer, chemotherapy, death, or the children. The aloneness and despair I felt in that moment was overwhelming. In fact, in those few moments I would have been willing to trade my remaining thirty days to clean the slate with her and to have her and our children know how much I loved them. I heard myself utter a prayer: "Lord, I haven't talked to you much, hardly at all, but I need more time. I cannot die until I make peace. Please, Lord, have mercy on me and my family."[1]

I felt like a hypocrite. Like a fraud. Certainly God would want nothing to do with the likes of me. *Besides,* I thought, *my family would be better off with me gone.* The businessman side of me knew that Kathy would cry, collect herself, and proceed to do what needed to be done. She was pretty simple and direct about being responsible. I knew she would not leave me; out of love or out of a sense of duty she would stay by me until I was gone.

After four days Rudy was able to make contact with Dr. Cecil Pitard at the University of Tennessee in Knoxville. Cecil had lymphoma and was successfully treating himself with a combination of natural products that he felt would benefit me. By running blood tests daily, it quickly became apparent to Rudy that my situation was rapidly deteriorating. We made the decision to go to Tennessee right away and work with Pitard.

Rudy and I and our wives flew into the Knoxville airport at midnight and were met by Dr. Cecil Pitard, a strange little man, very studious looking with wiry, white hair. When he spoke he seemed more like one of my college professors than a doctor of medicine. All four of us were drawn to his generous personality and his quick sense of humor. It must have looked like a comedy act at the circus when the five of us climbed into his tiny BMW, which was already filled with a thousand audio tapes.

As soon as we were crammed into his car, Cecil Pitard turned to me and asked, "Michael, when do you want to get started?"

"Now!" I responded.

He drove us directly to his office, and we got started. Pitard's treatments stopped the stage-four blast crisis I was experiencing (this is as close as you get to dying without crossing over), but the leukemia was stationary, ready to break loose any minute. At the end of eight days of daily therapy, the three of us talked—Cecil, Rudy, and I. Cecil was crying as he advised me to have chemotherapy or elect to die.

For two weeks, Rudy and I had tried to find a miracle. We had called doctors and laymen, dedicated healers and quacks. We had read books and medical journals, seeking a fix to cancer. I had popped vitamins and minerals, been injected with illegal drugs, more vitamins, and harmless but helpful herbs. I was sore and heartsick, and so were Kathy, Rudy, and Donna.

Now another decision was reached. I had been away from home many times through the years, for much greater lengths of time, but this time I missed my kids deeply. I did not want to die away from home and family, and death seemed to be just around the corner.

The very next morning we were in the air, headed home. And soon after that the trip to the hospital became a reality. The physical pain had become intolerable. Prior to this I had prided myself on possessing a high tolerance for pain, but I had never experienced the internal physical agony that permeated my entire body. My bones and joints felt as if they were going to explode.

In my youth I had learned to divorce myself from the hurting by focusing on another area of my body that was without pain. Or I could simply create a picture of some future event that represented pleasure, and that would sustain me until my pain eased. But not now. This pain was everywhere, especially in my mind. The intensity was so great, I couldn't take the time for my mind to find an oasis. I needed to be present in the pain just to survive it.

Sitting beside my wife in the hospital admitting room, I felt very dependent, helpless, and slow-witted. In the few short weeks since the diagnosis, the power had shifted. Kathy was the strong one, someone to lean on, and I was desperately weak and needed to lean.

I struggled to think positively but also battled with strong feelings that I was not worthy to live any longer. I felt that my pain was my punishment from God. At that time the pain was so excruciating I only wanted relief, and if that meant death, so be it.

Realizing the critical nature of my situation, I could not help but reflect on my past life. I had persisted in thinking life was forever and that I was indestructible. I had drowned in booze, tarnished myself with indiscriminate sexual encounters, and deliberately buried myself under countless hours of work. My way of minimizing my fear was to deny it, to act as if things didn't matter. Or I had let my fear come out as anger, accompanied by rage and violent, verbal outbursts. I had manipulated people into doing what I wanted with my intimidating behavior and physical size.

I watched as Kathy methodically went through the insurance forms with the admittance people. I sensed her anxiety as her voice rose. There seemed to be a problem, something about unpaid premiums. She looked my way and assured me she would handle it. I didn't have to worry. I was so grateful I was not checking into the hospital alone.

The eighth floor cancer ward was the perfect place for me to see the reality of my situation. Here the mortality rate was high and the odds of surviving the cure were slim.

I walked the standard hospital circular-floor route and looked about at the others, the dying and those who loved them. I saw a weary, older woman who looked as if she were afraid to leave her husband for a minute for fear he would die in her absence. A family gathered in a football-type huddle outside a room discussing a doctor's last update. A young, totally bald woman sat beside her husband watching television.

Death and its companions, pain and despair, were everywhere. If it weren't for the intense aching of my body I would not have stayed in the hospital. My thoughts kept jumping from *I won't die, and it will be all right* to *Okay, Michael, breathe the air and look around because it may be the last time you get a chance.* These two views warred with each other for my attention, and I felt myself leaning toward death.

Admitting personnel led me to a room that had been totally sterilized. Everything—the brown linoleum floor, the cream-colored walls, two metal chairs, the sink, the mirror, the small closet, and even the television mounted from the ceiling—had been sanitized for the health of the occupant; in this case, me. Without any thought to personality or warmth, the room was designed to provide an antiseptic environment for cancer patients. The only thing they couldn't remove was the smell of cancer. It dominated the entire floor. Near panic, I briefly thought of others who had stayed in this disinfected room of silence.

Then everyone left me alone. I felt abandoned by the world and incredibly frightened.

Early the next morning, I was wheeled into surgery. Just the day before I had been scared and powerless, but now I knew that the depth of those feelings had been minuscule compared to what I was feeling this day: frantic, trapped, dying, despairing, deserted by my loved ones. This was fear beyond fear.

In the operating room I acquired a new and unsightly orifice. They inserted a device into my chest called a Hickman catheter, which allowed the doctors and nurses to inject fluids, blood, platelets, and the chemotherapy treatments directly into my bloodstream without having to inject me each time. It would also permit them to draw blood without inserting a needle each time, so I would become grateful for its presence.

Back in my adult-size isolation I was suspicious of every twitch in my body and of everyone who entered my germ-free space.

The hopelessness I was feeling in the hospital was similar to the feelings I had experienced a couple of months before when I had made the decision to stop drinking. I had been a practicing alcoholic for twenty-two years. I had practiced so often that I was a very accomplished drunk. The end to my boozing happened like this: I awoke after a hard night of drinking and looked around the room. The empty bottles filled me with disgust for myself and for my behavior. After all the times I had promised myself and my family that I would quit drinking, I knew on that morning I was through with alcohol. Somehow, for some reason, I realized that particular moment that I had put myself and others in jeopardy with my habit. As a self-proclaimed "good guy" I knew I could not stand the inner condemnation I would inflict on myself if I continued to imbibe. I was an alcoholic and could not drink ever again. So with that resolve I quit the boozing.

Now lying in this hospital room, connected to all these tubes and machines, I thought about my life and in particular my drinking. Why had I quit drinking just to die some other way?

Faithfully, Kathy came to stay with me all day, every day, but her presence did not interfere with my reflections.

I was not in that hospital being a model patient, contemplating my life and my limited future. I was giving the nurses and doctors a rough time. If they wanted me to do one thing, I demanded to do something else or at least do it my way. Against the advice of everybody, I made a lot of business and personal calls from that room. I tried salvaging the business, tried to make sure there was enough money for Kathy and the kids—all by phone from my hospital bed. These interactions with others occurred before Kathy got there or after she left. When she came, we talked about little things that really didn't matter.

Sometime during the week after I entered the hospital, one of my nurses suggested that I might like to talk to the priest who visited the floor. I think he had stopped in my room a couple of times those first few days, but I had been too sick and scared to even acknowledge him. Well, a week is a lot of time to think about dying, and I knew that I was dying without anyplace to go. For some people there was heaven, but not for me. As much as I had tried to clean up my act, inside myself I knew I wasn't acceptable to God. I thought that "they"—those folks who knew God—had figured something out I wasn't able to comprehend. So, just maybe, this priest could tell me. I agreed to talk to him.

Initially, Father Pete came two or three times a day, and we talked about his hospital experiences or, sometimes, about me. He looked like many other medium-built, graying men of sixty-something until I looked into his eyes. The depth of his blue eyes told me that he knew things I wanted—no, *needed*—to know. Serenity and comfort entered the room with him.

After a few days more, I began to ask questions. About the hereafter, about heaven and hell. By this time, I was convinced he had some secret answers that would ease my feeling of hopelessness.

As I lay in that sterile bed in that totally disinfected cubicle of a room, questions rose in my mind and in my heart. I couldn't help reflecting on what I had and what I felt I had missed. My feelings of loss, regret, and grief were overwhelming. Hoping to find some comfort, I opened up to this old priest and finally found the courage to ask him my main question: "Tell me what God truly is and how I get to know Him in the few days I have left?"

He studied me before he answered. "Michael, I'm not sure what God is. I'm not sure He is anything, although I experience Him as everything. If you want to know God, you must be willing to see Him with a childlike mind. Simplicity is the answer. You were born already in relationship with God from above. It is His gift to mankind. You cannot will or demand a relationship with the Lord. It just is."

I asked him what he meant when he said "from above."

Laughing, he replied, " I do not mean 'from above' as if it were a physical place. I mean 'from above' your limited thinking. An active relationship with God is preceded by rising above your current, limited way of reasoning."

The priest's uniquely blue eyes reached directly into my heart when he asked, "Do you want to be in relationship with God? Do you want to experience inner peace? Then you must be willing to think God! You must be willing to forget all you know and all that you think you know and trust that God will open your eyes. Raise your consciousness. You must know that you are in Him and He in you. You must be willing to hold God as the most powerful Presence there is. You must be willing to believe that nothing is impossible to God."

Passion and power flowed from him as he continued, sparking hope within me. "To let Him reveal to you what is next, you have to be willing to surrender every moment of your remaining life, knowing that He is leading you on the path chosen for you, His friend."

Only half in jest, I said, "Dying might be easier." I knew intuitively that he was asking me to surrender at a depth that I was unable to, one that I felt was impossible.

At that point death still seemed to be the only option. Not that I was consciously choosing to die, but it was so close I could feel myself giving into it. I had lost over two pounds a day and my hair was falling out in clumps. I was living in constant terror that each day would be my last, and I began to be angry. I directed this anger toward my doctors and accused them of not telling me the full story of my illness.

In the middle of the night I could feel death approaching. Yet there were two distinct feelings within me. Part of me wanted to hide, to stop fighting life, to die. Yet my passive inner nature wanted another shot at participating in the world: to be a contributor to society, to be a good husband and father. This side of my persona had been like my silent observer, my conscience, and had forever tugged at me regarding poor decisions and behaviors. Now this self was suddenly becoming stronger. Somehow the conversations with the priest were inspiring that part of my spirit to come alive.

During one of our talks Father Pete suddenly and uncharacteristically became very silent. The intensity of the silence seemed to be an invitation for me to stretch beyond my limited thinking and understanding. Something was about to happen. I was nervous, and just a bit concerned.

It took awhile before I was finally able to quiet my busy mind, but when I became still I surrendered to the peace in the room. I wanted it to last for an eternity. In that moment of surrender my feelings slipped away to an unknown destination and were replaced by a promise of life and the peace I saw mirrored in the old man's face. He had somehow helped me to experience the Sacred Presence. In that void of thought, yet filled with feelings, I recognized the nature of my longing. There was now a bridge across the gap between the god in my mind and the God who lived in my heart.

In that instant the priest became recognizable to me. He was the Christ Spirit. Alive! In my room. I felt scared, and unworthy, and joyful.

When the old priest next visited I told him about my experience of seeing him as Christ. He assured me that what I felt and what I thought I saw was within myself; he was just an old priest long overdue to retire. I told him I knew that the vision had precipitated a shift in my life. I explained to him that when I was quiet, I was also aware of a sense of aliveness, which was beckoning me to question the diagnosis and the prognosis of only thirty to ninety days to go. Anxiously, I asked him if it could be a sign from God.

Father Pete laughed and assured me that it was my longing for divine presence and for spiritual nurturing that had allowed me to see and experience God's compassion and love. "Michael, the crisis of your impending death has rendered you broken. Without the ability to be in control you have had time to listen to your inner voices. You are recognizing that your feelings and thoughts about 'being separate' from God were only beliefs that were solely in your head."

Flat on my back in the ICU, with tubes running in and out of my weakened body, I had countless hours to contemplate and meditate on the priest's uplifting words. I determined that even though I had chosen a path contrary to God's, He had not abandoned me. With deep humility, and desperate need for something, someone to turn to, I opened my heart, just a bit, to God.

At that point I did not consider myself changed, nor did I start acting like a loving person. Being on the eighth floor had its small privileges, of which I took complete advantage. No one cared what you ate, so I demanded lots and lots of ice cream. I pitched a fuss each time a nurse interrupted one of my visits with Kathy or the old priest.

I got it into my head that I would feel better if I could have a daily soak in the hot tub in physical therapy. I drove the doctor and nurses nuts until they agreed that I could use the spa. My use of this facility had many stipulations, but I met them all, and for the last two weeks of my hospital stay, I immersed myself in hot, soothing water every day.

A few days before I got the "bug" about the hot tub, the old priest and I were deep in another one of our conversations about God. He suggested that I become willing to have God in my life rather than continue to seek His Presence. "God's Spirit will continue to draw you upward and closer if you just remain willing," he said.

He then gave me something that I treasure to this day. He had written the Twenty-third Psalm on a small piece of paper for me.

Father Pete instructed me to read this five times a day for seven days. He encouraged me to make the prayer a part of my daily life for as many days as God gave me. I was not to memorize the psalm, but to read it. I was to be willing to think about each verse as I allowed sufficient time for the words to come alive within my heart.

In the quiet of that night a question emerged from all that had happened and all that I had discussed with the wise old priest. Could it be that the death I feared had nothing to do with my body dying? Maybe it had something to do with facing my innermost fears. The mere thought of addressing these feelings and thoughts caused my heart to pound loudly in my chest.

Late that same evening I began running a very high fever, an expected condition in leukemia patients, usually followed closely by death. As the fever continued to rise I knew I was dying. My body was on fire, and my bedclothes were wet with my sweat. Everything my eyes tried to focus on looked blurry. I wanted to press the call button to alert the nurses' station, but I feared all the commotion. I knew the second I pressed it people, shots, machines, and noise would follow almost immediately. For a moment I thought if I didn't signal them maybe it wouldn't be real.

My God, my life is going to end right here. With my heart beating frantically with fear and anxiety, I held the call button in my hand. Why would this be happening now? Why had I opened my heart to God if I was going to die?

With complete terror, I remembered overhearing Richard, the young intern assigned to me, explain how sometimes leukemia patients get spiking fevers, and if the fever is not quickly arrested the patient dies. As my body began trembling with the fever, I heard Richard outside in the hall. The sound of his voice released me from my inertia and allowed me to press my call button. In an instant Richard was in my room, and after one look at me he called for immediate assistance.

Within seconds, an entire crew of nurses swooped in, gave me several shots, and then, as quickly, they all left—all but Richard. He held my hand and said he would remain with me as long as I needed him.

Struggling to overcome the nausea and nearly delirious with fever, I cried out to God, "Oh Lord, hold me, love me, and nurture me."

Then complete darkness overcame me, and I knew I had died.

Suddenly, there was light. God was there, in my sterile hospital room. I felt His Presence.

Slowly, I realized I was up in the corner of the room, looking back at myself lying in bed with Richard standing beside me holding my hands. The light's glare was like a stadium, alight for a Friday night football game, only more intense. The brilliance seemed to have a center, and my eyes were focused on this central illumination.

A figure emerged out of the brightness. I knew it was God coming to retrieve my soul.

And then I saw Christ.

From my vantage point in the upper corner of the room I saw Him put His arms around me, and as though I were in two places at one time, I could feel His mighty arms around my physical body. Even though I was not in my body I felt the joy and peace of His comforting touch. He was cloaked in brilliant light and fully visible to me. I was enfolded in His power. Had I wanted to turn away, I would not have been able to.

Jesus lifted my spirit out of my physical body, and I watched His light flood every cell of my being. My body glowed with the outpouring of His love. I knew then that some part of me would always be alive. The cancer had driven me to an unceasing prayer: "God, please hold me, nurture me, and, God, please love me."

In that moment I experienced a death. Old beliefs and perceptions that had influenced my life, and ones that had left me feeling alone, unloved, and angry at everything would now begin to die. I wasn't sure what would happen next, but I felt that God would not create this miracle and then abandon me. I was given life. I now had hope.

Early the next morning, I was still alive. The disinfected cell of a room no longer seemed stark and dreary. Everything in and around me glowed.

My fever was totally gone.

I had been with God! He had held me and filled me with His light. I knew it was not a dream. I felt like a kid who had discovered something wonderful but didn't know who to trust with my discovery.

Soon, Richard came in to do a blood draw. For the first time, I truly looked at him. I saw a young man, about twenty-five, medium height, with dark hair. A skinny guy, with bulging gray eyes, someone whom I would not have even acknowledged at any other time in my life. Now I saw him as my friend.

Wearing a smile he crossed the room to my bedside. He stood there looking at me, then placed his hand on my shoulder, saying, "Michael, you are on your way. The first day I saw you, I realized you knew little about being alive, but in being around you the past few weeks I have seen that you have the capacity to demonstrate tremendous spiritual power. If you could somehow access that power, you possibly could move through this crisis." He paused before continuing, "You probably don't have any idea of what I am talking about, do you? Last night when your physical crisis seemed to peak, you let go of control. I suspect in so doing you accessed a holy part of your being. The Presence, God, lives in each of us and is always longing to be acknowledged and to be able to express Himself through us. Last night, when you cried out to God for help, I experienced you not as an adult but as a lost child."

I interrupted him, "Richard, stop! I am at a loss to explain why or how last night happened. All I know is that Jesus was here for me and held me in His arms, in this very room."

Richard looked at me in a way that resembled the old priest. "I know. I was here with you, remember?"

He said that as he was working on me, I had suddenly screamed out, "Lord Jesus Christ, have mercy on me!"[1]

I recounted my version of the night's events as Richard listened. I told him I remembered crying out, and that I remembered being out of my body watching Jesus hold me. With a happiness I hadn't felt in years, I told him I would never forget the brilliance of the light and how God flooded me with it until my whole body was filled with that bright energy.

Later that day, Richard encouraged me to consider studying the life of Jesus. It was a recommendation I would have ignored a few short months before. He suggested that Jesus coming to me in my crisis was a beckoning, and that God, through Jesus, was leading me forward.

"Have you seen Father Pete in the last few days?" Richard asked.

I was puzzled at his inquiry. I asked him what he knew about the old priest. He laughed as he said that he personally held Father Pete in high regard, even though they did not really know one another. Richard went on to tell me of his own spiritual path and of a time he had spent with a spiritual teacher similar to Father Pete. He wanted to know if I had been reading the Twenty-third Psalm five times per day.

"Yes," I answered with surprise. I was astonished to find out that Richard had been watching over me.

I went on to share with Richard how earlier in my life I had felt called to become a minister. But on both occasions, I had suppressed my feelings, quickly gathered myself together, and gone right back to living as before. After last night's experience, I knew I was clean, whole, loved, and forgiven of all that I had been that was hurtful to myself and others.

When Richard left, I began repeating the Twenty-third Psalm over and over again, like a chant. I would rotate between reciting the psalm and the Lord's Prayer. Meaningful phrases from these prayers became my companions and my assurance when I needed positive affirmation. I would chant silently to myself before going to sleep, rarely ever missing a phrase, continue the process while sleeping, and wake up to repeat the same prayer, all without skipping a beat! I would isolate *He restores my soul* in my mind and have it churning through my consciousness while sleeping, then pick up its thread in the morning when I awoke. Slowly, my attitude began to improve.

I had been in the hospital for three weeks when the doctors unplugged my I-Med machine, a device that fed me the chemotherapy. They said it would give my body, by now weakened to its limits, a chance to regenerate. The machine vanished; the tubes to my chest were removed, and the opening to the Hickman capped off.

Because my immune system was still nonexistent, I lay defenseless in critical isolation. While the tubes had been connected to me and the chemotherapy was flowing I had felt I was doing all I could. Now lying there just waiting, I missed the reassurance and sense of purpose that the gurgles and noises of the machine had provided.

Richard continued to spend long hours at my bedside. After taking what care he could of my physical needs, he would make suggestions on how I could improve my thoughts and attitudes, which, in turn, would improve my health. Richard advised me that concentrating on solving my personal problems depleted my physical and emotional energies, energies that I needed to challenge the cancer. "Survive first, concentrate on what's right before you. I promise that the other issues will take care of themselves.

"Think about remission. Put all your efforts into focusing on health for the next week and then the week thereafter. Until a remission turns into a cure, stop thinking about your tomorrows or your colorful past. Simply and purposefully live to live."

Father Pete was at my bedside when my doctor came in to speak to me about going home. "Mr. Mahaffey (he never once called me Michael), your body has responded well to the chemotherapy. When the leukemia returns we can easily pop you back here for more treatments."

I barely controlled an instant and intense desire to rage and throw things (including the doctor) when I said, "You have no idea what went on here. You don't know where the cancer came from and you don't know where it went. It really is a mystery to you."

My eyes sought Father Pete's. "My friend, you don't know either. But then you never pretended to know."

The old priest acknowledged my statement with an affirming smile. He was letting me know that I had learned this one lesson: reject the negatives. For just a fraction of a second, the huge, schoolroom-type clock caught my attention. As I watched the dial snap to record the next minute, I knew I had also learned a truth: only God provides the next moment!

Right then and there I made up my mind to get myself a new doctor. This one's attitude accepted, maybe even encouraged, disease, not health. I didn't need or want his negative thoughts directed at me. After all the long, cold nights I lay in this bed on the eighth floor cancer ward, wondering if the next twitch of my body would be my last, this doctor had the gall to say that it would be okay for me to do it all over again.

Thirty-seven days after I was admitted to the sterile world of isolation, it was time for me to leave. My weight had dropped from 275 to 198, and my clothes hung off me like grandpa's nightshirt on one of my kids. Most of my hair was gone, and I was embarrassed by the few little hunks scattered across my scalp.

Though I was incredibly weak, I had walked the halls often enough that I had the strength to get myself out of bed and dressed. But my muscles had atrophied so that my walk was a mere shuffle. I felt old. I looked old. But it didn't matter how I looked. It didn't matter that I still had the catheter in my chest. I was going home, out of that room, off the eighth floor, away from the hospital, and away from the smell of cancer.

As Richard assisted me to the car he said, "Michael, you are a perpetual learner, and just a beginner. Wherever you go you will meet other teachers, other mentors, who will see you through various stages of your growth. Remember that your passport to this new awareness is patience and willingness. Your restoration has begun. You are not the person I first met here thirty-seven days ago. Go in peace!"

During the ride to the ranch, Kathy and I were each locked into our separate thoughts and talking was kept to a minimum. Generously, Kathy had chosen to drive me home the back way, a small road winding through the foothills of the Sierras. I had traveled this road hundreds of times before, but never had I experienced such intensity of colors and light. I saw the beauty in every flower, every rock, every cow, and every tree.

Even though I was still very close to physical death I felt alive. I cried! I was so glad to be out of confinement and to be in the countryside I loved. Being alive in that car, that morning, was a miracle to me, and the world exposed itself to me in a glory I had never seen before.

13

NO LONGER SEPARATE AND ALONE

Trust in the L*ORD with all your heart,*
and lean not on your own understanding.
In all your ways acknowledge Him,
and He shall direct your paths.

—PROVERBS 3:5–6

I had only been home from the hospital for twenty-four hours when my attorney called to advise me that a meeting had been called by one of our Vancouver, British Columbia, partners. Surprisingly, fourteen of my business associates had agreed to come to the ranch to discuss our situation. Four of them were my main investors; the other ten people were representatives from companies who were thought to have an interest in purchasing our business.

Scheduling the meeting provided me with a familiar sense of purpose and power. It felt good to be in control again. Members of the partnership were holding out for the possibility of striking a deal that would save the company and my family's personal holdings. I felt I needed to be an active participant at the meeting, because I wasn't willing to trust anyone else to pull it off. In addition, I had invested a considerable amount of time and money courting a company from Italy with the hope that they might purchase the partnership interests completely.

Kathy was worried. She asked me to conserve my strength, to focus on my health, to let it go, and to not worry, but I was not ready to let go of the reins yet. Even though I was still reading the Twenty-third Psalm and spending some part of each day reflecting on my relationship with God, it was very easy to slip back into old habits and deeds.

During the next few days, everyone at the ranch began to realize that our way of life was in jeopardy. Until now, I had held our world together and provided a materially abundant life for us all. The kids had concerns about where we were going to live and if they could continue in college. I had very few solutions to offer, and I couldn't bring myself to make any empty promises.

All fourteen associates, briefcases bulging with documents, came to support their individual interests on May 8, 1983. Frustrated and fearful, I listened to the politicking and maneuvering for position. I had gone into the meeting with the hope that the ranch could be removed from the negotiations and left unencumbered for my family. It was not to be. Each partner and associate was trying to get what he could out of the deal. After listening to two hours of haggling and arguing about possible deals, I lost my temper and asked everybody to leave.

On his way out one partner told me that the group had decided to meet in town the next morning, and he offered to call me with the results. I suggested that he come back to the ranch after the meeting. He declined. Exhausted as I was, I was relieved, but at the same time sad and disappointed to be losing everything. As much as I felt I should continue the battle to save the ranch, I knew that ultimately I had to let go.

After the family breakfast the following morning, Shana said, "Dad, I know you can find a way to keep the ranch. You have always solved all the problems."

That one, short sentence had such an impact on me. I felt totally defeated because I knew there was no hope that our home could be salvaged; ultimately, the bank would have to foreclose. My mind and body felt lifeless, without spirit or the will to continue. Letting go of the last ray of hope was the final blow. Everything we had would soon belong to someone else. In my heart I knew I didn't have anything left to fight this battle. Shana didn't realize that I was no longer the same man she knew as her dad. And it didn't enter my mind to try and let her know how I was feeling.

Barely a week passed before it became an accepted fact that we were losing our home. We began to pare down our possessions, hoping to draw in as much cash as possible. The ranch was bustling with folks wanting to help and with other people looking for what they could steal. It was a sad time, a time to develop new insights. Some of our best friends, people I had counted on to help the most, didn't help at all. Some neighbors, folks who had not been in our tight circle, provided untiring help, aiding us like we were their family.

While I had been in the hospital, Kathy had shut down the office. She had let all eight employees go, cancelled the lease, and set up a small office in the house. Now she began liquidating furniture, office equipment, horses, trailers, and anything else of value. During this period I got up after the kids were off to school and went for walks on the property; in this way, I was able to find some peace for a while. These walks were usually between the barn and the house, just a short quarter of a mile. Because my stamina was gone, I had to force myself to walk up the road without stopping, and often I ended up collapsing alongside the path. I'd find a tree to lean against and look out over the world that had been mine. I was a weary spectator of my own life. In this time, between coming home and moving out, I spent a considerable amount of time alone. No longer needing to search for ways to rescue my finances, I was able to return to the thoughts and practices begun at the urgings of Father Pete and Richard.

I had spent hundreds of thousands of dollars in one of the finest medical centers in the world. There I had discovered that despite all the doctors' scientific knowledge and their noble intentions to contribute to the health and well-being of the people they serve, doctors knew little more about this disease than I did. They knew how to identify the leukemia, how the disease reacts to chemical invasion, and how a human body might respond. In short, all they could do was present a lot of maybes and offer hope. But they didn't offer enough.

I began to realize that my responsibility was to take care of myself and to find the places and people who would support me. My health and well-being were uppermost in my mind. I spent less time with family members and spoke very little to anyone. On these journeys and in my periods of rest, I began to learn more and more about contemplation and prayer. Prior to the diagnosis I had avoided being alone; now I cherished these quiet, still moments. A deeply personal spiritual journey was taking place within me. I was beginning to develop a relationship with God. This growing relationship provided me with the strength to survive my losses.

> **How would I have known that I was lost**
> **Had You not searched and found me?**
> **How would I have known my bleeding**
> **'Til You bound Your love around me?**
> **—Beth Moore, *Breaking Free***

During the next years I went through a journey that I now call PurposeFull Living, which is the process I use with the patients I counsel at the Cedar Springs Renewal Center. This is the process that I will work you through in this chapter and the next one so you can begin a journey of your own. We will begin with a Focusing Your Vision exercise and then consider our Spiritual Purpose.

FOCUSING YOUR VISION

Back in the hospital when I was meeting with Father Pete, he encouraged me to override my mind, which was telling me that I had less than thirty days to live. He knew I just wasn't able to exist with that thought. The old priest asked me to focus on shutting off my mind. That would become my vision, my specific goal for the time I was in the hospital.

I ask patients to write down the three most important specific accomplishments they want to make in their lives. I then ask them to work on those visions during the weeks they are with us (this could be one week or twelve weeks). "We're the only ones who stop us from getting where we want to go," I say. These three visions must be measurable and attainable. One participant's answers were:

1. To continue not smoking and not using caffeine.
2. To pray each day, first thing.
3. To develop and deepen my support relationships.

Write your specific visions on a piece of paper.

Now think about what you might have to give up to make these visions a reality. Obviously this one participant had to give up cigarettes and coffee. He had to allow the wall he had built around himself to tumble down so he could deepen his support relationships. Finally he had to give some time each morning to prayer. Write what you need to give up on that piece of paper.

Once you have written out your three visions, you need to develop a spiritual purpose to help you accomplish these visions. At this moment we're setting up a road to make your visions come true.

PUTTING YOUR SPIRITUAL PURPOSE AND VISIONS TOGETHER

DEFINING YOUR SPIRITUAL PURPOSE

During my first month or so at home, I continued to defer to the wisdom of the old priest. He had instructed me, "Think God, seek God, expect God, and God will not only make His presence known, He will light the way to wholeness as He has since the beginning."

Now I wanted the Lord to hear me, to hold me, to love me, to tell me I mattered, and to confirm that I had been blessed with a vivid experience of Him. *The Lord is my shepherd; I shall not want* had been beyond my belief system, but now I began to accept these words. I made the decision to try to live like I truly believed and see what happened.

Most of us know how to live socially correct, to present our good side to others while inside our world may be falling a part. Desperation can be an instigator to break the mold. When cancer patients are truly honest with themselves, they usually admit they want to live and do not know how to share that degree of desperation.

I ask our participants, "Can you change the circumstances in your life? What influence do you personally have over these circumstances?"

Most cancer patients will then admit that they have no control over their circumstances. That's the frightening part about having cancer, or any life-threatening illness for that matter. There's really not much people can physically do. But, they can address the beliefs and attitudes that can influence their health and well-being.

I certainly know how they feel. Father Pete asked me these same questions and encouraged me to think about my spiritual purpose. During the time I was in the hospital, my spiritual purpose was: How do I take my fear to God? How do I rely on Him to get me through this period of time?

As I had struggled with that purpose, the old priest told me, "That's too big for you at this moment. Let's not do that. Let's take your vision of overriding your mind and give you something you can do instead of the vision."

That was the moment he wrote the Twenty-third Psalm on a piece of paper and told me to repeat it every time my mind went off. This would remind me that there was a God.

Take a moment right now to think about a purpose that will serve your highest good. If that's to survive your cancer, then that's your purpose. Your purpose should drive you beyond your mortal and physical limitations and be the source of your inspiration. Through this insight you can redirect your life away from culturally conditioned ends toward higher, more fulfilling ones. Many cancer patients say that their purpose is to be free of cancer. Write your purpose on that piece of paper.

Now I want you to draw every vision you have through this spiritual purpose.

Go back to the three visions you mentioned earlier. How would they relate to your spiritual purpose? For instance, that one participant's three visions were: to continue not smoking and not use caffeine, to pray each day, first thing, and to develop and deepen his support relationships. Ultimately he will have to take these three visions to God because he's going to find that he doesn't pray every morning, and he's going to do his relationships as he's always done them. This man needs help with these things. He's always needed help with them. Once he admits this, his spiritual purpose is to surrender these visions to God and enlist Him as an ally to accomplish these three visions.

Some people submit to cancer. Others surrender to it. The difference? If you are submitting to cancer, you think, *I've got cancer. Now I've got to do this and this and* . . . Submitting is an act you do because something's in your way and you have to do such-and-such to get rid of it. However, if you surrender to cancer, you think, *I've got cancer. It's here. Now what kind of an influence can I have over it?* It's not such drudgery anymore. It doesn't keep you focusing on your illness. This step invites you to bring God into your situation, praying to Him, talking to Him, being in an intimate personal relationship with Him.

Now you can go to the Lord and say, *I need Your help with this.* Then you begin to filter it through God's perspective and purposes.

Once you've filtered your three visions through your spiritual purpose, decide which of your visions needs the most attention. Many months after I left the hospital, I decided that the most important of my three visions was to see myself cancer free.

> **We are wired to believe in something beyond us. We are wired for God. And that is very good for us.**
>
> **—Dr. Herbert Benson, Founder and Associate Professor of Medicine, Mind/Body Institute, Harvard Medical School**

DECIDE WHICH OF YOUR VISIONS NEEDS THE MOST ATTENTION

One of my visions was a vision of being alive and having healthy, cancer-free cells. About three months after I left the hospital, Kathy and I decided that I should go to the Bio Med Clinic in Tijuana, Mexico, which had been recommended to me. Kathy had already begun a life separate from mine. She had opened an office in town where she was working out the details of the bankruptcy. In partnership with my ex-secretary, Kathy was attempting to build an accounting business. Each day she left early in the morning and worked until late in the evening.

Now I would be moving to a place where cancer and pain, death and life were constantly discussed and experienced. With other cancer patients, I could talk about my fears of dying and of my relationship with God. It would be a place where I could be free and open with my thoughts and my expression. I was eager to learn to live moment by moment with God as my partner.

My doctor and his associates were not happy that I had chosen alternative medications and practices as a way to get well. Never wanting to be dependent upon doctors and their system, I had pulled away from them as soon as I was able. I, alone, watched my body for the clues that would signal a need for a transfusion. The medical world continued to remind me that I could exit this state of remission at any time. It felt to me that they were ready to pounce, just waiting to begin their treatments all over again. What they didn't know was that I had vowed to never return to the cancer ward. This was my own decision, not one that I am recommending to you.

I felt blessed to be in this state of health. I was grateful that medicine had done its work for me, and my body had miraculously and gloriously responded. Now I sought answers to the questions concerning my mortality, my feelings of separateness, the nature of God, my purpose on this planet, and how I might create a life different than the one I had known. I had grown to view the cancer as a part of me, not as my enemy. Before it left my body, I wanted to understand the message it carried.

And I intuitively knew that I needed to be open to a relationship with it. In my prayers I saw how the cancer was like a rebellious child acting out against the established order of my body and to ignore its demand would mean certain death. I asked God to show me how to be in a loving relationship with this aspect of my personality.

God had allowed me to see clearly, but I was grossly inadequate to put a plan in motion based on that knowledge. I wanted to explore my choices. I had to determine what I was willing to commit my life to. I was hopeful that if I spent time with others like me, I might find some of the answers. Initially I intended to stay for a couple of weeks or a month. I ended up staying for the better part of two years.

As a part of my vision of being alive and having healthy, cancer-free cells, I decided to be vigilant about what I ate. I was a real meat eater. I decided to cut back on the amount of meat I would eat and to specifically stay away from white sugar, white flour, and milk. I decided to juice and to eat lots of raw vegetables. And I decided to buy organic produce so I could avoid pesticides.

My Organic Diet

The diet I have followed throughout these years is very similar to The Cancer Cleanse Diet. I called Cherie Calbom when I was changing my eating habits so I could learn about juicing. This was the beginning of a lifestyle change for me, and the start of a great friendship with the Calboms. Here is the simple diet I have followed:

10 percent animal protein
30 percent cooked foods (cooked above 105 degrees Fahrenheit)
60 percent raw or juiced foods
16 ounces of Spirulina daily

Now think about your own life. Decide which of your visions needs the most attention and write that on your paper. Think through whether this vision will need a couple of steps to accomplish it, just as my vision to have healthy, cancer-free cells involved a couple of steps, like juicing.

The next step is to bring your spiritual purpose into every moment of your life.

BRING YOUR PURPOSE INTO EVERY MOMENT OF YOUR LIFE

Try to bring your purpose into every moment of your life. Use it as a filter. That's what I did during those two years at Bio Med.

At first Mildred Nelson, the director, suggested that I spend time talking to the incoming patients, taking special note of the success stories. She said she wanted me to find out what they did, how they did it, and what they thought. I knew she actually wanted me to discover for myself that cancer can be beaten.

My routine was quickly established. I would rise at 6:00 AM, read the Bible, bathe, eat breakfast, and then read some more. When time allowed, I would enter into prayerful meditation. Then I would begin my work at the clinic.

I used my life there as my testing ground, my retreat center, the laboratory in which to explore and develop a different self. I experimented with a new personality, one that was open to life, receptive to others, in touch with the spiritual dimension of existence. This self could function well in my new world, in exile, because there was little around me to support the thoughts and actions of the Mike Mahaffey I had been for the first forty-two years of my life.

When I went home, however, I got a rude awakening. Then I felt as if I were a hired hand in my own home. Kathy and the kids were leading a full life in Auburn and I had no part in it. The old manipulative, controlling patriarch came alive in full form. When one of these outbursts was over, I would wonder, *What have I done? What have I learned? What is the value of a God who is now in my life if I keep drowning while trying to implement what He has taught me?*

I was left with the naked truth: I had a lot of work to do on myself. I had to bring my spiritual purpose into every moment of my life.

Think about how you might bring your spiritual purpose into every moment of your life. For instance, at one time I was addicted to and dependent on alcohol. Now if I want to walk away from that, I have to depend on something or someone bigger than alcohol. So I switched my dependency from alcohol to God and let God filter everything. If my purpose is big enough (and because it is God, it is), then it's bigger than my present circumstances.

At first this heightened my desperation because I saw how my mind directed my life. Think about this analogy. We desire to lose weight. We even imagine what we will look like thinner, but when it comes to putting this purpose into motion (running every morning about 7:00), we don't do well. About 6:00 AM our mind begins thinking of all the reasons we can't run that morning: It's too cold. It's too hot. We're too tired. That's part of human nature.

We want to be thin, but we don't want to stop eating. We want our blood pressure to go down, but we don't want to watch our coffee intake. Our actions are not matching our purpose. There is no rhythm between the two.

The apostle Paul confessed this war within himself in his letter to the Roman Christians: "For what I am doing, I do not understand. For what I will to do, that I do not practice; but what I hate, that I do" (Rom. 7:15).

Most of us don't think about taking our challenge to the level of a power greater than ourselves. Once I brought my purpose into every moment of my life, I began looking at my desires and urges. I found a very selfish person who used alcohol to cloak his selfishness. When I drank, I would reach a certain state where I would give myself permission to do anything I wanted. Selfishness was the root of my disease. That same selfishness played itself out in my eating, in my relationships with my business partner whom I bullied, and my family.

Richard, the intern who was with me the night I almost died, later told me, "You're trying with all your might to stand on your own two feet, to make life happen through your personal exertions. Although the effort is heroic, it's just unnecessary. If you let go a bit, take your hands off life's jugular vein and let life happen, you will trust more. Trusting in Him will give you the ability to continue when things seem hopeless."

Think about how you can bring your spiritual purpose into every moment of your life. Write those thoughts on that piece of paper.

Part of my spiritual purpose was to find my unique purpose. I believe each one of us is specifically and uniquely a part of God's creation. How do we find this unique purpose?

FIND YOUR UNIQUE PURPOSE

If we use our spiritual purpose as our filter, God begins to reside in our heart through the Holy Spirit. He completes His creation in us—the uniqueness in us—by coming alive in us.

In October of 1984, a brief conversation with a patient produced an invitation to take a sabbatical at a nearby nunnery. Here the spoken word was acceptable for just forty-five minutes a day. The balance of the twenty-four hours was spent silently working, reading, praying, and reflecting on one's life. It was required that I read John 15:1–17 many times each day throughout my entire stay of seventeen days.

Group sessions were the only times when talking was encouraged. During these sessions, I was drawn to a small, frail-looking nun who was fighting with the dreaded cancer disease. I drew upon the new skills I had acquired in my work at the clinic to ask questions and listen, not only to what was said, but to those hidden thoughts that were not easily said or heard. After a few weeks of these sessions, the nun suggested that my calling might be to work with cancer patients and the terminally ill. As she said so beautifully, "You seem to have the ability to assist people to go to the places behind their words, those places that need to be cleansed so that they might seek healing."

As I listened to her words, I knew I had found my unique purpose in life: I could be an instrument of God by serving other cancer patients and those who were seeking God.

Stop a moment now to think about your own unique purpose. If one comes to mind, write it down. If not, continue to ponder this question in the weeks and months to come.

EXAMINE YOUR TRUST IN YOUR SPIRITUAL PURPOSE

You need to trust your spiritual purpose to assist you when you are tempted to revert to your old personality flaws. It took me several years of working with my purpose to keep my old character at bay. I would find myself telling a lie or thinking about someone sexually. All the various traits of my old personality haunted me.

I struggled with how I would learn to trust that no matter what I did, I could take it to God and He would deal with it. Either God was in every moment of my life or He was in and out—and I'd never know if He was there or not.

This struggle was difficult for me because my mind kept dealing with my unworthiness. How could I serve God when I was such a sinner? How could I be working toward an intimate relationship with God, trusting that He was part of every moment of my day? If I believed that, He was also there with every drink I had taken. With every thought I had and every immoral act I ever did. It was bad enough that I had to carry these memories, but it was even worse that God had to see all of this, too. He had been there all along, and I had been so spiritually ignorant, I didn't realize it.

I began to bring the Spirit of Christ into my struggle with my old desires. I would say to myself, "Wait a minute. My purpose is to be part of the Holy Spirit right now in this moment. So if this is not of God, why am I doing it?" Then I would say an instant prayer, "Lord, take this away. Take this thought from me now. I'm going to know that You have done so when I feel Your peace."

Spiritual purpose was a way for God to give me a whole new moral standard to live by. He was rebuilding my character from the inside out. Before I got cancer, I had lived my life as if I were God. I unconsciously said to myself, *I know what to do. I know how to do it. I know what's best for me so I'll just follow myself.*

Now I began to realize that if my life was out of tilt, or I was anxious, I hadn't prayed or gone to my spiritual purpose for weeks. I wasn't choosing between good and bad. Or right and wrong. I wasn't even choosing between good and evil. My purpose was so important that it was the only choice I had. It was just a choice for God. Period. My spiritual purpose was now a part of my life. I could trust this purpose to guide me.

You also have to be able to trust your spiritual purpose when your life may seem to be falling apart. One summer during my time at the Bio Med

Clinic, I asked Kathy to spend the summer with me in San Diego. For the first month Kathy and I had a wonderful time. We ate and laughed until our sides hurt. We played like children. Together we walked the beach. Each weekday morning I left to work with the clinic patients. Each night I returned to our beach house. I became very tanned, with sun-bleached, blonde hair. I was off all medications except the herbal tonics. My stomach was as hard and as flat as a teenager's. Kathy, too, was golden all over, and I watched as her blonde, blonde hair was tousled by the soft ocean breezes.

We've begun to understand that to have a truly integrated medical approach to cancer care, a patient's values and beliefs must be taken into account.

—Dr. Kenneth Bakken, Health Vision International

While I was extremely anxious to restart our relationship, my wife began to let me know, in many subtle ways, that she was uncomfortable with the direction my life was taking. In the month of August, our differences arose to confront us and would not return to their hidden places. What I wanted from life and the kind of work I wanted to do differed greatly from the picture that Kathy had in her mind. And things that were important to me before the diagnosis no longer mattered. Functions that Kathy found fun and exciting no longer interested me. Before our summer was officially at an end, we had decided that Kathy would return to the Bay Area alone.

When she left, I was devastated. I tried to work, but couldn't focus. I returned to the familiar role of hermit and recluse. I sat on the deserted beach and looked over the water. At the same time, however, I was grateful to be alive. When depression overwhelmed me, I took a trip through Bio Med to remind me how lucky I really was. I was no longer in treatment. In fact, my work at the clinic had evolved to counseling patients on a one-to-one basis. Long hours of helping others see how their dysfunctional relationships contributed to their illnesses often blurred the distinction between them and me. When I would receive a letter or a phone call from patients I had counseled, telling me of their successes, I was thankful for the opportunity to be part of their progress.

I saw God walking with me through my struggles with my former addictions and my losses. I saw Him helping me to find peace and grow through my problems, and I began to trust my spiritual purpose.

In the next months and years you will want to examine your trust in your spiritual purpose. For instance, in the months and years after I got out of the hospital, I would remind myself, *Michael, you had thirty days to live when you started this. Now three-and-a-half years later, you're still alive, so the Lord is right there with you. And He's blessing you for one more day. You have to be grateful for that.* In those years I learned to trust my spiritual purpose.

Finally, you will find that your spiritual purpose evolves over time.

YOUR SPIRITUAL PURPOSE WILL EVOLVE

As you continue in your spiritual journey, the bar will rise, and so will the purpose. There's the first "A-ha!" when you find salvation and receive forgiveness. But then you and I get to work out our sanctification, living our spiritual purpose every day of our lives. God's done what He promised, but He asks us to clear away anything that blocks us from loving Him.

In the hospital my spiritual purpose was to override my mind by focusing on the Twenty-third Psalm. Then I realized that I was unable to do this myself, so my purpose changed to *How do I take my fear to God? How do I rely on Him to get me through this period?* The vision that was part of this purpose was to see myself alive with healthy, cancer-free cells. But I soon realized I couldn't influence my cells on my own. I had to allow God to be part of that. I had to learn to trust Him. The truth was: I could not will my way through anything in my life. Without God, I was stuck.

That's when I surrendered. My spiritual purpose became to allow God to be in my life and then to find the Lord in every circumstance and in every moment. In doing so, I realized that I was created to be an instrument of God. At that retreat at the nunnery I discovered my unique purpose: I could be God's instrument by serving other cancer patients and those who were seeking Him. As I endeavored to do this in the next years, my spiritual purpose became to train myself to allow the Spirit of God to filter through me into the world. And I'm still working there. I've found it's a lifetime occupation.

In 1987 I moved to Seattle, Washington, to work in an alcohol and drug center. One day in 1987, I was out walking around Green Lake when I sensed a presence beside me. Immediately, I knew that the Holy

Spirit was walking alongside me! Stepping quickly and lightly, while praying and laughing, I broke off my walk and returned to the house. In a few minutes I had plane tickets to go to Sacramento.

I rushed from the airport to the hospital, the same hospital where I had been tested, poked, and chemically treated for cancer. I had spent long hours in contemplation of my life in the sterile rooms of this institution. Here I had begun to explore my relationship with God.

I immediately went to the lab and asked to have the normal testing performed. While I awaited the results, I prayerfully reviewed the last five years of my life. I looked at who I had been and who I had become. I examined my most intimate relationships. I consciously thanked every person who had assisted me, offered counsel, or just loved me during this time.

In just a short time, the lab technician came out and said to me, "Mr. Mahaffey, I know that you have been here a lot through the years, because I've seen you. But, sir, I really don't know what I'm supposed to be looking for in these tests."

The cancer was gone! I now knew that nothing would ever be able to separate me from God. He took away my cancer! He gave me back my life!

I was no longer separate and alone.

14

CELEBRATE LIFE!

I stay near the door, I neither go too far in, nor stay too far out. That is the most important door in the world . . . The most tremendous thing in the world is for men to find that door—the door to God.

—Sam Shoemaker,
Cofounder of Alcoholics Anonymous

It is my belief that miracles happen more often than we are willing to acknowledge. Instead of accepting the presence of a loving God, most of us reach into our human reasoning as to the why or why nots of a miracle: "an event that appears inexplicable by the laws of nature and so is held to be supernatural in origin or an act of God."[1]

For most of us, if we cannot explain "it," then "it" isn't real. My experiences in the last twenty years of my life have redefined what's real for me. I now believe in miracles. The leukemia has completely disappeared from my body. I haven't had one desire to drink or to smoke a cigarette in over twenty years. On top of that the Lord has given me an opportunity to do work with cancer patients and people who are searching for significance in their lives and to speak in front of major groups of people, neither of which I'm trained for.

And I could not even fantasize being on the shores of Big Lake in Northern Washington in September of 1993, celebrating my son's wedding with my family. After Kathy and I divorced I felt my relationship with her and my children would no longer include such festive occasions. Yet at that celebration I welcomed each and every member of my ex-wife's family and my children into my home and into my new life.

I looked down from my deck to the sixty-plus folks milling around in my front yard and was aware that only a host of angels could have arranged this party. My gratitude is chiefly to God, who through so many people and circumstances led me here. He directed me to a life that by myself I would not have chosen and to a style of living that is full of love, compassion, and forgiveness.

The outcome of my journey [with cancer] is that I'm a wiser soul, and there is a deeper knowing. I have a deeper sense of joy, and for the first time in my life, I understand how deeply people love me, and how deeply I love people.

—Jennifer, A survivor[2]

I never could have received this peace if I hadn't made a PurposeFull Living journey with Him.

PURPOSEFULL LIVING

An important step in this journey is a commitment to be your word.

BE YOUR WORD

When I was at the Bio Med Clinic in Mexico, I felt saddened as I watched the forty-five or fifty patients who arrived at the clinic per day, who had spent time and money to be there to learn about the medications and diet plan. I knew most of them wouldn't stay on the medications or the diet plan when they returned home, because many of their predecessors hadn't. The patients just didn't seem to realize the importance of the program that was given to them.

I thought, *I can't do that.* So I began to search for ways to remain committed to a new lifestyle. Believe it or not, I found my answer in the Bible. As I continued to meditate on the book of John, I saw that he, more than any other gospel writer, described a love story between himself and Jesus and between Jesus and the world, even though John showed that Jesus came into this world to incite a riot, if you will. He was trying to show us the way, the truth, and the life that would lead us home. This Jesus could make people squirm. If this Man called Jesus looked at you and said something, you knew it was going to happen—and you had no control over what He was going to say. Yet at the same time you knew He was the living Presence of love from His Father, God.

Somehow I needed to elevate my will, my thinking, and my desires to the level that Jesus was expecting. *Maybe if I do that,* I thought, *I can step into the regime of changing my eating habits and exercising to heal my body.*

In the next months and years I worked on the concepts that would become the Be Your Word philosophy. Then I moved to Orcas Island, Washington, in 1988, where I roomed in the home of a young couple. David witnessed the changes taking place in me and asked, "What concept do you live by?"

I told him, "I try to be my word in everything I do."

He relayed this to his pastor, who soon asked me to give a talk on this concept, then hired me to do a class we called "Be Your Word," which was based on the gospel of John, the book that made a mark on my life.

One of my favorite verses in the Bible is "In the beginning was the Word, and the Word was with God, and the Word was God," the first verse in the book of John. The Greek word for *word* is *logos*, which means "the self revealing thought and will of God."

I challenged the Be Your Word class, "What if the words you say and your thoughts and actions are Godlike? If that's so, what happens when you tell your wife you'll be home at 5:00 and you don't get there until 6:30? Is that being your word?"

"Oh, but you don't understand," one of the members of the class said.

"Just stay with me for a moment," I replied. "I do understand. Do you want your wife to be able to depend upon you? Do you want God to be able to depend upon you? What if you could be an instrument of God?" I asked. "After all, that's what most of you in this building have surrendered yourself to."

I suggested that the class would be set up around participants verbally making commitments that caused them to stretch beyond their comfort zones. "But we aren't here to be judgmental," I said. "We're just here to track the thoughts that go off in our heads, the ones that give us an excuse not to fulfill our word." I explained that it would be necessary for members of the class to question each other in a nonjudgmental way (the art of true dialogue); otherwise, people would not be willing to speak the truth. The words of Rumi, a poet who lived between 1875 and 1928, became the bedrock of the class: "Out beyond ideas of wrongdoing and rightdoing, there is a field. I will meet you there."[3]

During that first meeting people's commitments ranged from not eating sugar to running every day to praying and meditating first thing each morning. The next week we shared the commitments we kept and the ones we didn't. The guy who wanted to run every morning before 7:00 found that he woke up about 6:00 AM, with many excuses running through his head. And the excuses won. Participants were able to see the rationalizations that stopped them from being their word, to sit with the truth of their actions, and to be held accountable. It was a new experience for all of us.

As the weeks went by, I began to see how most people could not keep their word to themselves or anyone else. Like me, they would make agreements to do something and usually put it off or rationalize why they didn't do it. So I challenged them, "What if you held every word you said and every thought you had as being God-inspired? What if the things we say and think are God's thoughts coming through us? Wouldn't that be an interesting concept?"

I went on to explain, "When we ask Jesus to manage our lives, we are in essence giving our word to love Him with our all and to love our neighbor as ourselves. From that moment in time He will not let go. He is relentless! He uses every circumstance and decision we make to draw us closer and closer to Him. In short, this raises our living from the littleness of our self-made world to the business of God. He asks that we love Him and our neighbors as ourselves. That's the 'work it out' part. Being our word puts us on the track—He knows it, we know it, and the cells in our body know it."

Some people shared that they had been stuck in a religious box most of their lives. They could recite Scripture and verses, but their only experience of God was through *doctrines* of religion. They didn't seem to have an intimate relationship with God or His Word. They wanted more. And they wanted to find the strength to quit blaming others for their own shortcomings.

I told them that I had needed to make a distinction between religion and God. I also needed to make a distinction between the mind of God flowing through me and my wanting my own way. "Jesus is not interested in partial surrender," I said. "He wants full surrender, as in *all* of me."

The Be Your Word classes offered all of us a vehicle to see and experience the ways we said no to God in our lives. Together we learned to move beyond "right and wrong" thinking, to let go of judgments of ourselves and others, and to support one another in *being* our word.

Soon other churches began asking me to teach this concept. One April in 1991, I was teaching in a church in Mount Vernon, Washington. Nan Monk, a young woman in the class, was especially interested in the "Be Your Word" concept. She said, "I've lied to people and people have lied to me all my life. Now you are encouraging me to always speak the truth. I'm fascinated."

About seven weeks into the twelve-week session I challenged the single people in the class, "If you don't have a relationship with a person of the opposite sex that is fulfilling, make a list of what you want in a husband or wife. Then expect God to read your list and fulfill your desire."

When Nan Monk showed me her list I was surprised. Twenty items were on that list, three of which were "a person who could keep his word, a person who trusted God, a person who would love me and my two children, Braden and Bonnie." After I read through the list, I said, "I know some people in Seattle who would fit this list. Do you know anybody?"

"I think *you* might," Nan replied.

I quickly gave the list to her, turned, and went back into the church. I was attracted to this woman who was eleven years younger than I. She had addictions that were similar to mine, and I knew she had been fascinated by the Be Your Word concept. But I had spent several years alone—just me and God. I had hours and hours to be quiet with myself and to read Scripture and other inspiring books.

Eugene Peterson describes the way I felt in *The Message*, his paraphrase of the Bible: "The Word became flesh and blood, and moved into the neighborhood" (John 1:14). I knew God was living in my neighborhood and was grappling for all my heart, not just part. And I truly believed that the peace I felt came from loving Jesus Christ, and that is what turned the cells in my body around. I was afraid I might lose that. Could I be a loving husband? A father? The thought petrified me. I was so frightened by the idea of an intimate relationship, I didn't act on my feelings for five weeks.

Then a friend of mine, a sponsor in Alcoholics Anonymous, said, "The Lord is trying to answer one of your questions. You said you wanted to have a loving, nurturing partner. Someone to share in your work. Maybe Nan's the person."

And a woman I was counseling also challenged me. "You told me I didn't raise the bar high enough. When are you going to raise it?" she asked. She knew that I was trying to love God completely; now she wondered why I wouldn't try to love a wife and children.

Finally I told Nan, "I don't know much about emotional intimacy. I do know a little about intimacy with God because that's the path I'm on. Do you want to sign up for that?"

"Absolutely," she said. "Because you're on the same path I'm on."

In the next twelve years Nan and I worked together to found Cedar Springs Renewal Center. I needed a woman who was strong enough within herself to stand up to me, because I have to admit that I'm very bold and direct. At the same time I needed a woman who was loving enough to invite me out of my shell, so I could learn how to love and be compassionate. Nan was one of God's gifts to me.

A second important step of my journey was taking an honest look at my fears.

AN HONEST LOOK AT FEAR

In our sessions at the Cedar Springs Renewal Center, we ask participants to take a piece of paper and list their fears in the left-hand column and the root of each fear in the right. (For instance, one participant may fear rejection. When he thinks about it, he decides that the root of this fear is that he is afraid of being unworthy. Another participant might fear being alone and decide that she is really afraid of not being loved.) Take a moment now to make two columns on a piece of paper and list your fears in the left-hand column and what you are really afraid of in the right-hand column.

Once participants have identified their fears, I ask them to note the fear that is most prevalent. Let's say the person ended up with the fear of being alone as the main fear. Then I will ask that person, "So, what about being alone makes you really afraid?"

"I've always been alone," the person might say. "I've always had to make all my decisions and they haven't worked out well."

"What would happen if you were totally alone?"

The answer is usually "I would be depressed," or "Well, I might eventually die from loneliness." I've even had some people mention suicide.

"So is death what you are really afraid of?" I ask.

When the person admits that yes, this is so, I say, "So let's imagine you are dead. What are you really afraid of about death?"

Most people will usually get to the fundamental fear that drives their fear of death: what if there is no God? And if there is no God, there is no life after death.

To me the way to answer this question is to look for God's steps in your life. I ask people, "Have you ever spent any time adding up the benevolent events in your life? The events that there is no explanation for?"

Most of us haven't ever done this, because we usually take life for granted. But once cancer patients list two or three such events, they quickly add numerous others. They'll say, "And there was this and this and . . ."

Then I tell them that I know there is a God because I've seen His presence in my life. And I give them my list of benevolent events, starting with the healing of my cancer. But that's just the beginning. Nan and I started the original retreat center with just five hundred dollars. Then a man offered us a piece of land and said, "You pay me as you can."

> **Even if the statistics say it's only a million-to-one chance, what matters is if that "one's" name is "Nona" or "George." What matters is who that "one" is. We can't live or die by statistics.**
>
> **—Nona, A survivor[4]**

One day we were so broke we couldn't figure out what to do next, and two women with cancer were arriving that day. That morning we received a blue envelope from Santa Fe, New Mexico, with a one-thousand-dollar cashier's check. Identical envelopes showed up three times in the next six weeks.

Now Cedar Springs is located on property that is worth one million dollars. But I still don't have much money. God used other people's money and graciousness to provide this facility. When people say, "But you don't own this place," I admit no, I don't. But who cares?

God's footprints are all over my life.

Take a moment now to write your own benevolence list on a piece of paper.

Do you see God's footprints there? Then believe that He is beside you now. Jesus said, "I will never leave you nor forsake you" (Heb. 13:5).

Each day of our lives we either choose fear or faith. In my case I made a deal with God years ago when I said, "If You will take over my life, then I'll let You manage it." That also means life after death. I've never known what events lie around the corner in my life, but when I've trusted them to the Lord, He's taken care of them. In the same way, I choose to trust Him with life after death.

Until then I want to celebrate life.

CELEBRATE LIFE

I believe that gratitude and appreciation open the door to a healthy life. During my walk with cancer I learned that I needed to be thankful. I did not take for granted that I just went on a five-mile walk or rode my horse each morning for three days. I began to celebrate just being alive as a functioning person.

When cancer patients show me their benevolence lists, I ask them, "What do you have to celebrate here?"

Many answer as I did: "Being alive," or "Being at peace."

I encourage them to celebrate the things the Lord does for them on a daily basis. I celebrate my relationship with Nan. I celebrate having people in my life. If I had died in 1983, you'd have had to pay people to come to my funeral. Now I know people who would actually miss me.

I also celebrate life by looking for anything that keeps me healthy.

LOOK FOR WAYS TO KEEP YOURSELF HEALTHY

Every doctor I meet asks me the same question: "How long has it been since you've had a blood test?" The doctors think I'm in remission. They don't consider a complete healing.

Instead of trying to figure out when the disease is coming back, I constantly ask myself, "What message am I sending the cells in my body?" If I'm an orchestra leader and I'm telling the cells in my body to play the song, "The Cancer's Going to Be Back Any Day," then my cells begin to sing that song. Instead I think, *The cancer's not coming back. I'm going to find peace here and I'm going to live a long life.* I want my cells to sing that song of hope—hum it, if that's all they can do.

> **There are times when getting cancer can be the beginning of living. The search for one's being, the discovery of the life one needs to live, can be one of the strongest weapons against disease. Nothing can be more important for cancer patients to discover than their *particular song* and *learn to project it loudly and clearly.***
>
> **—DR. LAWRENCE LESHAN, *You Can Fight for Your Life***

That day in Green Lake when I knew I was healed, I felt it in my body. It was as if the majority of my cells swung into the rhythm of hope.

Candace Pert, author of the book *Molecules of Emotion*, clearly states that our state of mind absolutely influences all the cells in our body. If we're singing a song of woe, our cells are dancing to a song of woe, rather than a song of joy. We have a choice. But I believe we must have God in our life to do this; otherwise we are just hoping in our own human ingenuity. That doesn't last long. Believe me, I know. I believe in celebrating God in every moment.

I've also looked for many ways to keep myself healthy. Diet change. Juicing. Exercise. Reading uplifting books. Spending time with loving people and attending positive meetings. In AA I attended meetings called "The Design for Living," which talked about resolution—solving problems rather than dwelling on them. I've gone to thousands of AA resolution meetings where participants spend very little time talking about how it was and a whole lot of time discussing how it is now that they are sober. I'm now in a group that has about five hundred years of collective sobriety. Those guys don't go backward anymore. Those folks invited God to move into their neighborhoods.

Over twenty years after I was diagnosed with cancer, I am still learning to surrender to God. My life is easier, and I am happier than I ever dreamed. Am I there? All I know is that I am alive by Grace, and in God's time I will go home. Right now my days are full of learning more about the simple act of surrender.

EPILOGUE

In 2002, my wife and I were gifted a beautiful fifty-acre farm that houses our center called Cedar Springs. We do several programs every month. Our cleansing weeks focus on detoxing the colon and liver and offer participants a spiritual and physical renewing experience. We bring together a cleansing diet, purposeful living classes, education on whole foods, and a very pastoral setting for resting and reflecting.

Another program that we offer each month is called Dia-Theos. Dia-Theos means "through God." This contemplative program provides more focus on prayer, silence, Taize singing (for more information, visit www.taize.fr), and a discipline known as "lectio divina," in which we meditate on scripture and then share its personal message with the group.

Dia-Theos describes the prevailing attitude of our programs and the Cedar Springs community. At the center, guests are encouraged to look at beliefs that hold power over them, and to use the dialogue process to seek clarity regarding which beliefs are false.

Because our beliefs influence our biology, the more aware we are of them, the better chance we have of staying healthy. In order to fully embrace God, it is sometimes necessary to give up things that we treasure. We sometimes treasure our beliefs while not really knowing why. Through the center's programs, participants seek insight as to what it is they genuinely value, and then look at what beliefs may be blocking them from attaining their highest goals.

The rich young ruler story in the gospel of Mark is a good example of false beliefs. The young ruler had done everything to follow Jesus yet when Jesus told him, "One thing you lack: Go your way, sell whatever you have and give to the poor, and you will have treasure in heaven; and come, take up the cross and follow me" (Mark 10:21). The young man trusted the security his wealth offered more than his relationship with Jesus. So, consequently, he chose what he believed to be his highest good and turned from God to the world. As the young man went away disconsolate, Jesus said, "Children, how hard is it for those who trust in riches to enter the kingdom of God" (Mark 10:24).

In my own spiritual journey, I am reminded of the crippled man at the pool (John 5). When Jesus asked him, "Do you want to be made well?" the man must have experienced turmoil and doubt. The possibility of being healed challenged him both mentally and spiritually. If he said yes, his life would change and his dreams would become his future. If he said no, his fate would be sealed and his story would not change. To experience the unknown, he would have to surrender what was familiar and learn to trust. As the man internalized the question, Jesus said to him, "Rise, take up your bed and walk."

In stepping into our highest goals, many of us experience the same attitude of uncertainty. But if we slow down and learn to be patient for what God is trying to tell us, then God does come through and we do find peace. This peace comes with a quality of life that influences each cell in our body. Our old beliefs stop running the show and we feel ourselves come alive in different ways. We find relationships are different because we are changed. New things are made possible through God.

It has been twenty-five years since my diagnosis of cancer, and I have been truly blessed. My life through God has been transformed. I know that saying yes to God is just the beginning. There are times when I am tempted to settle by the pool and be content with how "my life is," versus choosing to be in the turbulent, uncharted waters. But my highest goal is to trust God with all my heart and to trust that the promises He made are just as real today as they were the day they were written.

I invite you to come to Cedar Springs and explore your beliefs as a path to wellness and ultimately to God.

Michael Mahaffey
www.cedarsprings.org
www.diatheos.com

ACKNOWLEDGMENTS

I wish to express my deep and lasting appreciation to all the people who have assisted me with this book, especially our friend and coauthor Michael Mahaffey, who was my inspiration to write *The Complete Cancer Cleanse.* To Vicki Chelf, friend and coauthor of *Cooking for Life,* who assisted me in researching and writing several chapters; as always, you're the best! A very special thanks to my literary agent, Pamela Harty, who believed in this project from the start and never gave up until we found our publishing home. You're one of God's gifts to me, and I'm so glad I found you. To my editor Janet Thoma, thank you for making a dream become reality. For your expertise, endless hours of work and input, and creative organization, I am so very grateful. Also, I want to thank Rachel Jones for making sense out of all my editing notes and scribbles. And to Jenny Baumgartner, Carol Martin, and all the staff at Thomas Nelson Publishers who helped to make this book a reality, thank you for your help. Many thanks to Dr. Myron Wentz and Brian Shillavy for reading our manuscript and offering very valuable comments. My gratitude also goes to the Bastyr University faculty who helped me begin my research on nutrition and cancer over a decade ago. To John, my husband, friend, and for the first time, my coauthor—well-done, buddy! And most of all to God, who answered our prayers concerning this project, I give my eternal gratitude. You have never, ever failed—and never will.

—CHERIE CALBOM

I join with my wife, Cherie, in expressing my gratitude to Michael Mahaffey, Pamela Harty, Janet Thoma, and all the staff at Thomas Nelson Publishers who have helped me with *The Complete Cancer Cleanse.* In addition I want to thank Rosie Lovejoy for her endless hours of research and the help she provided me with my chapters. To my dearest friend, Dr. Ken Bakken, who was the catalyst to my work with cancer patients at St. Luke Medical Center, my appreciation for all the years of friendship and heart-level sharing. To my lovely wife, Cherie, whose passion for helping people beat cancer inspired me to join her and Michael to make this book a complete approach to The Cancer Cleanse. And most of all to the Holy Trinity in whose image we are made, I am very grateful that You have called us to wholeness through love.

—FR. JOHN CALBOM

I am grateful for the assistance I received from many people during the course of writing this book. I do not have enough words to thank Darlene Mindrum for her tenacity and determination. And Jan Duke who brought wisdom and patience to the project. Then there is Janet Thoma, who stayed with me and helped to communicate God's intent in my heart to words. Then there is Nan. What can I say to describe your humor, your compassion, and your overwhelming love. You encouraged me to tell the story. Tell the people about Jesus' love. Let the people know that healing cannot happen without love and truth. Nan, thank you for having faith in me and loving me the way you do. Thanks for making it all worthwhile.

—MICHAEL WILBA MAHAFFEY

APPENDIX

Sources of Information and Products

The first part of this appendix, the Resource Guide, contains information that can help you in the cleansing and healing process, and the second part, Products and Information, lists products that are recommended for the various detoxification programs.

RESOURCE GUIDE

HEALTH CENTERS

The following centers offer a raw foods/juice detoxification program. Most of them offer nutritional classes and some offer other health classes that address the emotional, mental, and spiritual aspects of healing and renewal. Most of the centers also offer massage and colonics. It is best to contact the various centers to find out which one best fits your needs.

Cedar Springs Renewal Center
Dia-Theos Program
Michael Mahaffey and Nan Monk, Dirs.
31459 Barben Road
Sedro Woolley, WA 98284
Phone: (360) 826-3599
Fax: (360) 826-3599
Web site: www.cedarsprings.org

Health*Quarters* Ministries
David Frahm, N.D., Director
3620 W. Colorado Ave.
Colorado Springs, CO 80904
Phone: (719) 593-8694
Fax: (719) 531-7884
E-mail : healthqu@healthquarters.org
Web site: www.healthquarters.org

Hippocrates Institute
Brian and Anna Maria Clement, Dirs.
1443 Palmdale Ct.
West Palm Beach, FL 33411
Phone: (800) 842-2125
Fax: (561) 471-9464
E-mail: hippocrates@worldnet.att.net
Web site: www.hippocratesinstitute.org

Oasis of Hope Hospital
Paseo Playas #19
Playas de Tijuana
Mexico
Director: Dr. Contraras
Phone: (888) 500-Hope
E-mail: phillips@oasisofhope.com
Web site: www.oasisofhope.com

Optimum Health Institute of Austin
265 Cedar Lane
Cedar Creek, TX 78612
Phone: (512) 303-4817
Fax: (512) 303-1239
E-mail: austin@optimumhealth.org
Web site: www.optimumhealth.org

Optimum Health Institute of San Diego
6970 Central Ave.
Lemon Grove, CA 91945-2198
Phone: (800) 993-4325
Fax: (619) 589-4098
E-mail: optimum@optimumhealth.org
Web site: www.optimumhealth.org

Sanoviv Medical Institute
Dr. Myron Wentz, Director
Playa de Rosarito, Km 39
Baja, California, Mexico 22712
Phone: (800) 726-6848
Fax: (801) 954-7477
Web site: www.sanoviv.com

We Care
Susana and Susan Lombardi, Directors
18000 Long Canyon Rd.
Desert Hot Springs, CA 92241
Phone: (800) 888-2523
Fax: (760) 251-5399
E-mail: info@wecarespa.com
Web site: www.wecarespa.com

PRAYER CENTER (SOAKING PRAYER)

Christian Healing Ministries
Francis and Judith MacNutt, Directors
P. O. Box 9520
Jacksonville, FL 32208
Phone: (904) 765-3332
Fax: (904) 765-4224

BOOKS AND OTHER RESOURCES

Healing Retreats and Spas Magazine
5036 Carpinteria Ave.
Carpinteria, CA 93013
(805) 74505413
www.healingretreats.com

CANCER BOOKS

A Gift of Hope with Michael Mahaffey, DVD and VHS (Sedro Wooley, WA: Cedar Springs Renewal Center). Call to order (360) 826-3599.

Anne E. Frähm with David J. Frähm, *A Cancer Battle Plan* (Colorado Springs, CO: Piñon Press, 1992).

Michael Mahaffey and Nan Monk, *The Hope for Life Manual: The Purposeful Living Program Workbook* with audio CD. (Sedro Wooley, WA: Cedar Springs Renewal Center). Call to order (360) 826-3599.

Michael Murray, Tim Birdsall, Joseph Pizzorno, and Paul Reilly, *How to Prevent and Treat Cancer with Natural Medicine* (New York: Riverhead Books, 2002).

Patrick Quillin with Noreen Quillin, *Beating Cancer with Nutrition,* rev. ed. (Carlsbad, CA: Nutrition Times Press, Inc., 2001).

JUICE AND SMOOTHIE BOOKS

Cherie Calbom, *The Juice Lady's Guide to Juicing for Health* (New York: Avery, 1999).

Cherie Calbom, *The Juice Lady's Juicing for High-Level Wellness and Vibrant Good Looks* (New York: Three Rivers Press, 1999).

Cherie Calbom, *The Ultimate Smoothie Book* (New York: Warner Books, 2001).

HEALTHY OILS

Jade Butler, *Flax for Life.* At health food stores or order from Barlean's Organic Oils at (800) 445-FLAX

Cherie Calbom with John Calbom, *The Coconut Diet* (New York: Warner Books, 2005).

VEGAN AND RAW FOODS COOKBOOKS

Vicki Chelf, *The Arrowhead Mills Cookbook* (New York: Avery, 1992).

Paul Pritchford, *Healing with Whole Foods,* rev. ed. (Berkeley, CA: North Atlantic Books, 1993). This has about two hundred vegan [macrobiotic] recipes and information on cooking with sea vegetables.

Nomi Shannon, *The Raw Gourmet* (Vancouver, B.C.: Alive Books, 1999).

ORGANIC PRODUCE INFORMATION

Campaign for Sustainable Agriculture
12 North Church Street
Goshen, NY 10924
Phone: (914) 294-0633

Environmental Working Group
1718 Connecticut Avenue N.W.
Suite 600
Washington, D.C. 20009
Phone: (202) 667-6982

Mothers & Others for a Livable Planet
40 West 20th Street
New York, NY 10011
Phone: (212) 242-0010

PRODUCTS AND INFORMATION

PRODUCTS FOR THE CLEANSING PROGRAMS

Many of the products we recommend can be ordered through Trinity Wellness Shoppe (866) 8GetWell or (866) 843-8935 and www.tropicaltraditions.net and gococonuts.com.

Intestinal Cleanse

Barlean's Forti-Flax (fiber with trace minerals, omega-3, and lignans), phone: (800) 445-3529

Dr. Schulze's Intestinal Formula #1 and #2, phone: (866) 843-8935

Cleanse Thyself Program by Arise & Shine (Includes psyllium husk, bentonite clay, Herbal Nutrition, and Chomper), phone: (800) 688-2444

Liver Cleanse

Liver Life I and II by Arise & Shine, phone: (800) 688-2444 or (866) 843-8935

Dr. Schulze's Liver Cleanse, phone: (866) 843-8935

Milk thistle is available at most health food stores.

Kidney Cleanse

Kidney Life Tea and Kidney Life herbal supplement by Arise & Shine, phone: (800) 688-2444

Parasite Cleanse

Fungal Defense by Garden of Life (candida and yeast cleanse)

Green/black walnut hull tincture (parasite cleanse) by Arise & Shine, phone: (800) 688-2444

Wormsquirm I and II by Arise & Shine, phone: (800) 688-2444

Heavy Metal Detox

Dentox by Arise & Shine, phone: (800) 688-2444

FOOD PRODUCTS

Coconut Oil

See gococonuts.com, or call (866) 843-8935

Flax Oil

You may order the following products by calling (800) 445-3529 or by visiting this Web site: www.barleans.com.

Barlean's Organic Flaxseed Oil (excellent for salad dressing; also in capsules as a nutritional supplement)

Barlean's Organic Lignan Flaxseed Oil (also in capsules)

Barlean's Omega Twin (flaxseed and borage oil)

Barlean's Lignan Omega Twin (flaxseed and borage oil)

The Essential Woman, oil and capsules (organic primrose and flaxseed oils, lignans, and phytonutrients)

Barlean's Borage Oil (also in capsules)

Barlean's Organic Evening Primrose Oil (only in capsules)

Flax Fiber

Barlean's Forti-Flax (fiber with trace minerals, omega-3, and lignans), phone (800) 445-3529
www.barleans.com or (866) 843-8935

NUTRITIONAL SUPPLEMENTS

Enzymes

Digestive and Systemic Enzymes (vegetarian formula) by The Ness Formulas, phone: (866) 843-8935

Whey Protein and Other Protein Powders

Perfect Protein—Vanilla (whey protein) by Metagenics, phone: (866) 843-8935

UltraClear* (rice protein) by Metagenics, phone: (866) 843-8935

UltraClear Plus** (rice protein) by Metagenics, phone: (866) 843-8935

*UltraClear supplies vitamins, minerals, and accessory nutrients to support both Phase I and II of detoxification.

**UltraClear Plus has all the basics of UltraClear and has added nutritional support for "imbalanced detoxifiers"—people with low Phase II activites.

Probiotics

Ultra Flora Plus DF by Metagenics (dairy-free, *Lactobacillus acidophilus* and *Bifidobacterium lactis*)

Exercise and Lymph Cleansing Equipment

"Walk Away the Pounds" video with weights
Unlimited Energy
P.O. Box 939
Hicksville, NY 11802

Lymphasizer (Swing machine), phone: (866) 843-8935

Health Products

Rebounder by Needak

Juiceman® Juicer by Salton, phone: (866) 843-8935

Complete Health Center (Power Blender) by Salton, phone: (866) 843-8935

Dehydrator by Excalibur

Water Alkalizer and Ionizer, phone: (866) 843-8935

Non-toxic water bottles by Nalgene (available at sports stores and health food stores)

DONATIONS FOR CANCER RESEARCH UTILIZING NATURAL MEDICINE

If you wish to support the advancement of cancer research using natural medicine, you may donate to the Research Department of Bastyr University, earmarked *Cancer Research*. If you wish to support the education of doctors who use natural medicine or nutritionists trained in whole foods education, you may donate to the Scholarship Fund of Bastyr University. All donations may be sent to:

Bastyr University
14500 Juanita Drive N.E.
Kenmore, Washington 98028
(425) 823-1300
www.bastyr.edu

NOTES

CHAPTER 1

1. Michio Kushi, *The Cancer Prevention Diet* (New York: St. Martin's Press, 1983).
2. J. C. Bailar and E. M. Smith, "Progress Against Cancer?" *New England Journal of Medicine*, 3114 (18 May 1986), 1225-32.
3. Otto Warburg, "On the Origin of Cancer Cells," *Science* 123 (1956), 309-14.
4. M. V. Krause and L. K. Mahan, *Food, Nutrition and Diet Therapy*, 7th ed. (Philadelphia: W.B. Saunders Co., 1984).

CHAPTER 2

1. H. Sheldon, *Boyd's Introduction to the Study of Disease*, 10th ed. (Philadelphia: Lea and Febiger, 1988).
2. C. Bailar III, "The Case for Cancer Prevention." *J.N.C.I.* 62 (1979), 727-31.
3. Candace Pert, *Molecules of Emotion: Why You Feel the Way You Feel* (New York: Scribner, 1997).
4. Don Colbert, *Toxic Relief* (Lake Mary, FL: Siloan Press, 2001).
5. Anne Frähm and David Frähm, *The Cancer Battle Plan* (Colorado Springs, CO: Piñon Press, 1992).
6. Carol Morley and Liz Wilde, *Detox* (London: MQ Publications, 2001).
7. Michael Murray and Joseph Pizzorno, *Encyclopedia of Natural Medicine*, 2d ed. (Rocklin, CA: Prima Publishing, 1998).
8. Rachael Carson, *Silent Spring* (Boston: Houghton Mifflin, 1962), in Sandra Steingraber, *Living Downstream* (New York: Addison-Wesley, 1997).
9. *Toxic Release Inventory of 1993*, EPA Office of Environmental Protection, www.epa.gov/triexplorer/chemical.htm.
10. Murray and Pizzorno, *Encyclopedia.*
11. Linda Page, *Detoxification* (Carmel Valley, CA: Healthy Healing Publications, 1999).
12. Kenneth L. Bakken and Kathleen H. Hofeller, *A Journey Toward Wholeness* (New York: Crossroad, 1988).
13. Richard Anderson, *Cleanse & Purify Thyself, Book 1.5* (Mt. Shasta, CA: Triumph, 1998).
14. Anderson, *Cleanse & Purify Thyself.*
15. Colbert, *Toxic Relief.*
16. Frähm, *Cancer Battle Plan.*
17. Ginger Chalford, "Understanding the Healing Crisis," http://www.upwardquest.com/healing-crisis.html.
18. Ibid.
19. Ibid.

CHAPTER 3

1. Bernard Jensen, *Dr. Jensen's Guide to Better Bowel Care* (New York: Avery, 1999).
2. Bernard Jensen, *Food Healing for Man* (Escondido, CA: 1983).
3. T. L. Vaughan, P. A. Stewart, et al., "Occupational Exposure to Formaldehyde and Wood Dust and Nasopharyngeal Carcinoma," *Occup Enviro Med* 57 (2000), 376-84; C. Y. Yang, et al., "Female Lung Cancer and Petrochemical Air Pollution in

Taiwan," *Arch Environ Health* 54(3) (May/June 1999), 180-85; S. M. Enger, et al., "Alcohol Consumption and Breast Cancer Oestrogen and Progesterone Receptor Status," *Br J Cancer* 79(7/8) (1999), 1308-14; W. D. King, et al., "Case-Control Study of Colon and Rectal Cancers and Chlorination By-Products in Treated Water," *Cancer Epidemiol Biomarkers Prev* 9 (August 2000), 813-18; R. Chen and A. Seaton, "A Meta-Analysis of Painting Exposure and Cancer Mortality," *Cancer Detect Prev* 22(6) (1998), 533-39; G. G. Swartz, et al., "Solid Waste and Pancreatic Cancer: An Ecologic Study in Florida, USA," *Int J Epidemiol* 27 (1998), 781-87; B. Hunter, "Some Food Additives as Neuroexcitors and Neurotoxins," *Clinical Ecology*, 2 (1984), 83-89; L.T. Stayner, et al., "A Retrospective Cohort Mortality Study of Workers Exposed to Formaldehyde in the Garment Industry," *Am J Ind Med* 13 (1988), 667-81; T. D. Sterling, et al., "Health Effects of Phenoxy Herbicides," *Scan J Work Environ Health*, 12 (1986), 161–73.

4. Richard Anderson, *The Liver: Cleansing & Rejuvenating the Vital Organ* (Mt. Shasta, CA: Cristobe Publishing, 1999).
5. Lars Johansson and Lene Frost Anderson, "Who Eats 5 a Day? Intake of Fruits and Vegetables Among Norwegians in Relation to Gender and Lifestyle," *Journal of the American Dietetic Association* 98(6) (June 1998), 689-91; Tufts University, *Health and Nutrition Newsletter* 18(5) (July 2000), 3.
6. Tufts, *Newsletter.*
7. Murray and Pizzorno, *Encyclopedia.*
8. Sandra Cabot, *The Liver Cleansing Diet* (Scottsdale, AZ: S.C.B. International, 1997).
9. Ibid.
10. Brenda Watson, *Renew Your Life* (Clearwater, FL: Renew Life Press, 2002).
11. Donna Gates with Linda Swartz, *The Body Ecology Diet: Recovering Your Health & Rebuilding Your Immunity*, 6th ed. (Atlanta, GA: B.E.D. Publications, 1996).
12. Sidney MacDonald Baker, *Detoxification & Healing: The Key to Optimal Health* (New Canaan, CT: Keats Publishing, Inc., 1997).
13. G. Talska, et al., "Genetically Based n-Acetyltransferase Metabolic Polymorphism and Low-Level Environmental Exposure to Carcinogens," *Nature* 396 (1994), 154-56, in Murray and Pizzorno, *Encyclopedia.*
14. Michael Murray, Tim Birdsall, Joseph Pizzorno, and Paul Reilly, *How to Prevent and Treat Cancer with Natural Medicine* (New York: Riverhead Books, 2002).
15. Murray and Pizzorno, *Encyclopedia.*
16. Michael Murray, *Encyclopedia of Nutritional Supplements* (Rocklin, CA: Prima Publishing, 1996).
17. Michael Murray, *The Healing Power of Herbs* (Rocklin, CA: Prima Publishing, 1991).
18. D. Schuppan, J. D. Jia, B. Brinkhaus, and E. G. Hahn, "Herbal Products for Liver Diseases: A Therapeutic Challenge for the New Millennium," *Hepatology* 30(4) (1999), 1099-1104.
19. A. Valenzuela, et al., "Selectivity of Silymarin on the Increase of Glutathione Content in Different Tissues of the Rat," *Planta Med* 55 (1989), 420-22, in Murray and Pizzorno, *Encyclopedia.*
20. Elaine Feldman, "How Grapefruit Juice Potentiates Drug Bioavailability," *Nutrition Review* 55(11) (1998), 398-400; Barbara Ameer and Randy Weintraub, "Drug Interaction with Grapefruit Juice," *Clinical Pharmacokineticsv* 33(2) (August 1997), 103-21.
21. Jensen, *Dr. Jensen's Guide.*
22. Ibid.
23. Ibid.
24. Anderson, *Cleanse & Purify.*

25. Ibid.
26. Jensen, *Dr. Jensen's Guide.*
27. Gerald Tortora and Nicholas Anagnostakos, *Principles of Anatomy and Physiology*, 5th ed. (New York: Harper & Row, 1987).
28. Paul Pritchford, *Healing with Whole Foods: Oriental Traditions and Modern Nutrition* (Berkeley, CA: North Atlantic Books, 1993).
29. Ibid.
30. H. Sarles and A. Gerolami, "Diet and Cholesterol Gallstones: A Multicenter Study," *Digestion* 17 (1978), 121-27.
31. Anderson, *The Liver.*
32. Pritchford, *Healing with Whole Foods.*
33. J. Toouli, et al., "Gallstone Dissolution in Man Using Cholic Acid and Lecithin," *Lancet* 6 December 1975, 1124-26.
34. S. M. Johnston, et al., "Iron Deficiency Enhances Cholesterol Gallstone Formation," *Surgery* 122(2) (August 1997), 354-62.
35. G. Nassuato, et al., "Effect of Silibinin on Billiary Lipid Composition Experimental and Clinical Study," *J Hepatol* 12 (1991), 290-95.
36. C. J. Moerman, et al., "Dietary Sugar Intake in the Etiology of Biliary Tract Cancer," *Int J Epidem* 22 (1993), 207-13, in Murray and Pizzorno, *Encyclopedia.*
37. Ibid.

CHAPTER 4

1. Cancer Treatment Centers of America, *CTCA News.*
2. "Foods for Cancer Prevention," Physicians Committee for Responsible Medicine, www.pcrm.org.
3. Pritchford, *Healing with Whole Foods.*
4. Ibid.
5. Center for Science in the Public Interest, "Chemical Cuisine CSPI's Guide to Food Additives," www.cspinet.org.
6. Ibid.
7. Marion Nestle, *Food Politics: How the Food Industry Influences Nutrition and Health* (Berkley and Los Angeles: University of California Press, Ltd., 2002).
8. Ibid.
9. Pritchford, *Healing with Whole Foods.*
10. Ibid.
11. *You Are In: Health,* BBC News, Thursday, 8 June 2000.
12. "Cancer, Diet, and Lifestyle," *Nutrition Week* 30(19) (12 May 2000), 351-52.
13. American Medical Association, *Nutritional Basics: How Does My Diet Affect My Health?*
14. Physicians Committee for Responsible Medicine, *Nutrition Education Curriculum, Section Two: Cancer Prevention.*
15. *Health Plus,* Vanderbilt University, 2001.
16. *Food, Nutrition and the Prevention of Cancer: A Global Perspective,* World Cancer Research Fund in association with the American Institute for Cancer Research, 1997.
17. P. Appleby, *Diet and Cancer: A Summary of the World Cancer Research Fund Report* (4), 1997.
18. M. Gerber and D. Corpet, "Energy Balance and Cancers," *Eur J Cancer Prev* 8 (1999), 77-89.
19. Dean Ornish, "Good Morning America—Battling Cancer with Veggies," The Preventative Medicine Research Institute, 15 April 2002, www.pmri.org/wsj.

20. CBC News: *High-Fiber, Vegan Diet Key to Battling Prostate Cancer: 2002 Study.*
21. Physicians Committee, *Nutrition Education.*
22. "rBGH and US Feedlots—This is the Real Mad Cow Disease," *Daily Mail* (UK), 12 June 1999.
23. L. Felton, Ph.D., "Linking a Dietary Carcinogen to Breast Cancer Susceptibility," 1998.
24. Neal D. Barnard, M.D., et al., "Chicken: Run Away," Physicians Committee for Responsible Medicine, www.pcrm.org/health/Commentary/commentary 0009.html.
25. "Seafood Selector," Environmental Defense, www.environmentaldefense.org.
26. "Vegetarian Diets—Position of ADA," American Dietetic Association, www.eatright.org.
27. Susan M. Lark and James A. Richards, *The Chemistry of Success* (San Francisco, CA: Bay Books, 2000).
28. Maud Tresillian Fere, *Does Diet Cure Cancer?* (Northhamptonshire, England: Thorsons, 1971), 18-21, in Michio Kushi, *The Cancer Prevention Diet* (New York: St. Martin's Press, 1983), 193-94.
29. Lark and Richards, *The Chemistry of Success.*
30. Ibid.
31. Dominique LaPierre and Javier Moro, *Five Past Midnight in Bhopal* (New York: Warner Books, 2002).
32. "Health Hazards of Pesticides," Natural Resources Defense Council, www.nrdc.org.
33. Theo Colburn, Dianne Dumanoski, and John Peterson Myers, *Our Stolen Future* (New York: Plume, 1996).
34. "NYCAP Alternatives to Pesticides," *Health Effects of Pesticides,* 1996.
35. "Banned Pesticide, Others Found on Washington State Apples," The Environmental Working Group, www.ewg.org.
36. Cynthia L. Curl, et al., "Organophosphorus Pesticide Exposure of Urban and Suburban Pre-School Children with Organic and Conventional Diet," Health Hazards of Pesticides, 2002 Natural Resource Defense Council, www.nrdc.org.
37. *Journal of Complementary and Alternative Medicine,* 2001.
38. Pritchford, *Healing with Whole Foods.*
39. Steingraber, *Living Downstream.*
40. David Suzuki, *Science Matters,* 2002.

CHAPTER 5

1. Iowa Lifestyle Education Assessment Program; S. Kleiner, "Defense Plants: Foods that Fight Disease," *The Physician and Sportsmedicine* 25(12) (December 1997), 89-90; A. M. Wolf, "Phytochemicals: The Newest Frontier in Disease Prevention," *Hospital Medicine,* August 1998, 55-6; W. J. Craig "Phytochemicals: Guardians of Our Health," *Journal of the American Dietetic Association* 97 (10, supplement 2) (October 1997), S199-204.
2. Sharon Begley, "Beyond Vitamins," *Newsweek,* 23 April 1994, 45-46.
3. J. D. Potter, "Your Mother Was Right: Eat Your Vegetables," *Asia Pacific J Clin Nutr* 9(supplement), S10-12.
4. Murray, *How to Prevent and Treat Cancer.*
5. K. Johnson, "Dairy Products Linked to Ovarian Cancer Risk," *Family Practice News,* 15 June 2000, 8, in Murray, et al., *How to Prevent.*
6. R. Jevning, et al., "Cruciferous Vegetables and Human Breast Cancer: An Important Interdisciplinary Hypothesis in the Field of Diet and Cancer," Los

Angeles International University, Irvine, CA., www.usda.gov/cnpp/FENR/Fenrv/12n2/Ferv12n2p26.pdf.

7. The Cancer Project, The Physicians Committee for Responsible Medicine, Washington, D.C., www.cancerproject.org.
8. C.W.W. Beecher, "Cancer Preventative Properties of Varieties of *Brassica oleracea:* a Review," *Am J Clin Nutr* 59 (supplement) (1994), S1166-70, in Murray and Pizzorno, *Encyclopedia*.
9. "Tomatoes and Cancer," www.holistic-online.com; S. Agarwal and A.V. Rao, "Tomato Lycopene and Its Role in Human Health and Chronic Disease," *CMAJ* 163(6) (19 September 2000); 739-44.
10. Begley, "Beyond Vitamins."
11. Ibid.
12. Lisa Sheppard, "UI Research Continues Search for Evidence Linking Tomatoes and Cancer Risk," University of Illinois, March 1999.
13. Benjamin Lau, *Garlic and You: The Modern Medicine* (Richmond, B.C.: Apple Publishing, 1999).
14. Ibid.
15. Ibid.
16. Dr. Lenore Arab, et al., University of North Carolina at Chapel Hill 10; Victoria Renoux, *For the Love of Garlic* (New York: Square One Publishing, 2002).
17. L. Torres-Sanchez, L. Lopez-Carrillo, et al., "Food Sources of Phytoestrogens and Breast Cancer Risk in Mexican Women," *Nutr Cancer* 37(2) (2000), 134-39.
18. Pritchford, *Healing with Whole Foods.*
19. Ginger Webb, "Medicine from the Sea—Medicinal Qualities of Sea Plants," *Vegetarian Times*, April 1997.
20. C. E. Borgeson, et al., "Effects of Dietary Fish Oil on Human Mammary Carcinoma and on Lipid Metabolizing Enzymes," *Lipids* 24 (1989), 290-95.
21. J. Cortiss, "Seafood Fatty Acids May Lower Cancer Risk," *J Amer Cancer Inst* 81(20) (1989), 152-53.
22. R. W. Moss, "Flax Seed Muffins Fight Breast Cancer," *The Cancer Chronicles #14; BBC News,* 9 December 2000.
23. P. Bougnoux, S. Koscielny, V. Chajes, et al., "Alpha-Linolenic Acid Content of Adipose Breast Tissue: A Host Determinant of the Risk of Early Metastisis in Breast Cancer," *Br J Cancer* 70 (1994), 330-34, in Michael Murray, et al., *How to Prevent and Treat Cancer.*
24. Murray, et al., *How to Prevent and Treat Cancer.*
25. James Meschino, "Flaxseed and Breast Cancer Prevention," www.nutratherapeutics.com.
26. "Preventative Medicine and Nutrition: Cancer Foods," Physicians Committee for Responsible Medicine, http://www.pcrm.org/.
27. B. R. Goldin, H. Adlercreutz, S. L. Gorbach, et al., "Estrogen Excretion Patterns and Plasma Levels in Vegetarian and Omnivorous Women," *New England Journal of Medicine* 307 (1982), 1542-47.
28. D. Kritchevsky, "Diet, Nutrition, and Cancer: The Role of Fiber," *Cancer* 58 (1986), 1830-36.
29. L. A. McKeown, "Diet High in Fruits and Vegetables Linked to Lower Breast Cancer Risk," *Medical Tribune,* 9 July 1992, 14.
30. Murray and Pizzorno, *Encyclopedia.*
31. N. Nagabhushan and S. V. Bhide, "Curcumin as an Inhibitor of Cancer," *J Am Coll Nutr,* 1992, 192-98, in Murray and Pizzorno, *Encyclopedia.*

32. "How Well Do You Know Your Herbs?" The American Institute for Cancer Research, November 2002, www.aicr.org.
33. Ibid.
34. Ibid.
35. Ibid.
36. Ibid.
37. Ibid.
38. Cherie Calbom, *The Juice Lady's Guide to Juicing for Health* (New York: Avery, 1999).
39. Jeanne Brand-Miller, Thomas M. S. Wolever, et al., *The Glucose Revolution* (New York: Marlowe & Co., 1999).
40. Ann Wigmore, *The Wheatgrass Book* (New York: Avery, 1985).
41. Alan Gaby, "Wheat Grass Juice Effective Against Ulcerative Colitis," www.pcc-naturalmarkets.com.
42. F. Batmanghelidj, *Your Body's Many Cries for Water: You Are Not Sick, You Are Thirsty* (Falls Church, VA: Global Health Solutions, Inc., 1995).
43. G. Mathe, "Red Wine, Green Tea and Vitamins: Do Their Antioxidants Play a Role in Immunologic Protection Against Cancer or Even AIDS?" *Biomed Pharmacother* 53 (1999), 165-67; Y. Cao and R. Cao, "Angiogenesis Inhibited by Drinking Tea," *Nature* 398 (1 April 1999), 381; J. L. Bushman, "Green Tea and Cancer in Humans: A Review of the Literature," *Nutr Cancer* 31(3) (1998), 151-59.
44. A. S. Truswell, "Glycemic Index of Foods," *Eur J Clin Nutr* 46 (supplement 2) (1992), S91-101, in Murray and Pizzorno, *Encyclopedia;* Jennie Brand-Miller, Thomas M. S. Wolever, Stephen Colagiuri, and Kay Foster-Powell in Stephen Sinatra, M.D., *The Sinatra Health Report, Dr. Sinatra's Protocol, Eating the Mediterranean Way* (New York: Marlowe & Co., 1999), 5.
45. D. J. A. Jenkins, T. M. S. Wolever, R. H. Taylor, et al., "Glycemic Index of Foods: A Physiological Basis for Carbohydrate Exchange," *Am. J. Clin Nutr* 24 (1981), 362-66, in Murray and Pizzorno, *Encyclopedia*, 415.
46. J. M. Argiles and F. J. Lopez-Soriano, "Insulin and Cancer (Review)" *Int J Oncol* 18 (2001), 683-87, in Murray, et al., *How to Prevent and Treat Cancer.*
47. Murray, et al., *How to Prevent and Treat Cancer.*
48. Y. Donden, *Health Through Balance* (Ithaca, NY: Snow Lion Publications, 1986), 186, 198, in Pritchford, *Healing with Whole Foods.*
49. Pritchford, *Healing with Whole Foods.*
50. H. J. Roberts, "Does Aspartame Cause Human Brain Cancer?" *Journal of Advancement of Medicine* 4(4) (Winter 1991), 231-41.
51. S.A. Bingham, "High Meat Diets and Cancer Risk," *Proc Nutr Soc* 58 (1999), 243-48.
52. R. N. Maric and K. K. Cheng, "Meat Intake, Heterocyclic Amines, and Colon Cancer," *Am J. Geriatr* 95(12) (2000), 3683-84.
53. "Colon Cancer and NDMA," *Nutrition Week* 29(12) (26 March 1999), 7.
54. John D. Potter, et al., "Alcohol, Beer, and Lung Cancer in Postmenopausal Women: The Iowa Women's Health Study," *Annals of Epidemiology* 2 (1992), 587-95.
55. William J. Blot, "Alcohol and Cancer," *Cancer Research* 52 (supplement) (1 April 1992), S2119-23; J. L. Fruedenheim, "Diet, Smoking and Alcohol and Cancer of the Larynx: A Case-Controlled Study," *Nutrition and Cancer,* 17 (1992), 33-45; C. L. Vecchia, "Differences in Dietary Intake with Smoking, Alcohol, and Education," *Journal of Nutrition and Cancer* 17 (1992), 297-304.
56. Lark and Richards, *Chemistry of Success.*
57. K. Watabe, et al., "Lifestyle and Gastric Cancer," *Oncol Rep.* 5 (1998), 1191-94.

CHAPTER 6

1. Murray, et al., *How to Prevent and Treat Cancer.*
2. Lark and Richards, *The Chemistry of Success.*
3. Ibid.
4. Jensen, *Dr. Jensen's Guide.*
5. Catherine Rodgers, "Health & Fitness," *Arkansas Democrat Gazette,* 24 June 2002, p. 1e, 6e.
6. Lark and Richards, *Chemistry of Success.*
7. Anderson, *The Liver.*
8. Richard Mabey, *The New Age Herbalist* (New York: Collier Books, 1988).
9. John Heinerman, *Heinerman's Encyclopedia of Healing Juices* (New Jersey: Prentice Hall, 1994).
10. Linda Page, *Detoxification* (Carmel Valley, CA: Healthy Healing Publications, 1999).
11. Brenda Watson, *Renew Your Life* (Clearwater, FL: Renew Life Press, 2002).
12. "A Link Between Bras and Breast Cancer?" www.drdavidwilliams.com.
13. Watson, *Renew.*
14. Ann Louise Gittleman, *Natural Healing for Parasites* (New York: Healing Wisdom Publications, 1995).
15. Lark and Richards, *Chemistry of Success.*
16. Anderson, *Cleanse & Purify Thyself.*
17. Ibid.
18. Hulda R. Clark, *The Cure for All Cancers* (Vista, CA: New Century Press, 1993).
19. Gittleman, *Natural Healing.*
20. Ibid.
21. Anderson, *Cleanse & Purify.*
22. Murray and Pizzorno, *Encyclopedia.*
23. R. A. Passwater and E. M. Cranton, *Trace Elements, Hair Analysis, and Nutrition* (New Canaan, CT: Keats, 1983), in Murray and Pizzorno, *Encyclopedia.*
24. C.W. Cha, "A Study on the Effect of Garlic to Heavy Metal Poisoning of Rat," *J Korean Med Sci* 2 (1987), 213-23, in Murray and Pizzorno, *Encyclopedia.*
25. T. W. Clarkson, et al., "The Prediction of Intake of Mercury Vapor from Amalgam," *Biological Monitoring of Toxic Metals* (New York: Pleum Press, 1988), 247-64, in Sam Ziff, Michael Ziff, and Mats Hanson, *Dental Mercury Detox Revised Edition* (Orlando, FL: Bio Probe, Inc., 1988).
26. *Environmental Health Criteria 118:* "Inorganic Mercury," World Health Organization, International Programme on Chemical Sefety (PCS), 1991, Geneva, Switzerland, in *Biological Monitoring, Dental Mercury Detox.*
27. L. Redwood, L. Bernard, and D. Brown, "Predicted Mercury Concentrations in Hair From Infant Immunizations: Cause for Concern," *Neurotoxicology* 22 (2001), 691-97.

CHAPTER 7

1. F. B. Bass, et al., "The Need for Dietary Counseling of Cancer Patients as Indicated by Nutrient and Supplement Intake," *Journal of the American Dietetic Association,* 1995, 1319-21.
2. Frähm, *Cancer Battle Plan.*
3. J. H. Kim, et al., "The Use of High-Dose Vitamins as an Adjunct to Conventional Cancer Treatment," *Cancer and Nutrition,* 1998, 205-12.
4. Dan Hurley, "Beta-Carotene May Detoxify Carcinogens," *Medical Tribune* 20 August 1992, 24.
5. Vishwa N. Singh, "Role of B-Carotene in Disease Prevention with Special

Reference to Cancer," *Lipid-Soluble Antioxidants: Biochemistry of Clinical Applications,* 1992, 208-27.

6. C. L. Rock, "Nutritional Factors in Cancer Prevention," *Hematol Oncol Clin North Am* 12(5) (October 1998), 975-91.
7. Kim, et al., "Use of High-Dose Vitamins."
8. S. Mobarhan, "Calcium and the Colon: Recent Findings," *Nutr Rev* 57(4) (April 1999), 124-29.
9. "Colon Cancer Protection in Low-Fat Dairy Foods," *Emergency Medicine,* May 1999, 78-79.
10. P. H. Gann, "Diet and Prostate Cancer Risk: The Embarrassment of Riches," *Cancer Causes Control* 9 (1998), 541-43; J. M. Chan, et al., "Dairy Products, Calcium, Phosphorus, Vitamin D and Risk of Prostate Cancer," *Cancer Causes Control* 9 (1998), 559-66.
11. K. Johnson, "Dairy Products Linked to Ovarian Cancer Risk," *Family Practice News,* 15 June 2000, 8.
12. Murray, et al., *How to Prevent and Treat Cancer.*
13. M. W. Pariza, et al., "Conjugated Linoleic Acid and the Control of Cancer and Obesity," *Toxicol. Science* 52(supplement) (1999), 107-10.
14. Ibid.
15. Ibid.
16. Ibid.
17. "Cancer and Hesperetin," *Nutrition Week* 30(39) (13 October 2000), 31-38.
18. M. G. L. Hertog and M. B. Katon, "Querceitin in Foods, Cardiovascular Disease, and Cancer," *Flavonoids in Health and Disease* 20 (1998), 447-67.
19. Murray, *Encyclopedia of Nutritional Supplements.*
20. Patrick Quillin, *Beating Cancer with Nutrition* (Carlsbad, CA: Nutrition Times Press, Inc., 2001), 82, 114.
21. "Folate Intake and Colon Cancer Risk in Women," *Women's Health and Primary Care* 2(2) (February 1999), 98.
22. Ibid.
23. I. S. Dokal, et al., 300 (1990), 1263, in Quillin, *Beating Cancer,* 249.
24. Quillin, *Beating Cancer,* 250.
25. C. B. Simone, et al., "Nutritional and Lifestyle Modification to Augment Oncology Care: An Overview," *Journal of Orthomolecular Medicine* 12(4) (1997), 197-206.
26. Murray, et al., *How to Prevent and Treat Cancer,* 64-65.
27. Hirota Fujiki, "Cancer Inhibition by Green Tea," *Mutation Research* 402 (1998), 307-10.
28. Ibid.
29. G. Mathe, "Red Wine, Green Tea and Vitamins: Do Their Antioxidants Play a Role in Immunologic Protection Against Cancer or Even AIDS?" *Biomed Pharmacother* 53 (1999), 165-67.
30. A. R. Waladkhani and M. R. Clemens, "Effect of Dietary Phytochemicals on Cancer Development," *International Journal of Molecular Medicine* 1 (1998), 747-53.
31. I. Yip, et al., "Nutrition and Prostate Cancer," *Urologic Clinics of North America* 26(2) (May 1999), 403-11.
32. Murray, et al., *How to Prevent and Treat Cancer,* 91-92.
33. M. L . Zoler, "Lycopene May Reduce Prostate Cancer Tumor Grade," *Family Practice News,* 15 May 1999, 28.

34. Murray, et al., *How to Prevent and Treat Cancer,* 91-92; P. M. Bramley, "Is Lycopene Beneficial to Human Health?" *Phytochemistry* 54 (2000), 233-36.
35. R. R. Watson and T. K. Leonard, "Selenium and Vitamins A, E, and C: Nutrients with Cancer Prevention Properties," *J Am Diet Assoc* 86(4) (1986), 505-10.
36. National Research Council Committee on Diet, Nutrition, and Cancer, *Diet, Nutrition and Cancer* (Washington D.C.: Assembly of Life Sciences, National Academy Press, 1982).
37. L. C. Clark, "The Epidemiology of Selenium and Cancer," *Fed. Proc.* 44 (1985), 2584-89.
38. L.N. Vernie, et al., "Selenium Levels in Blood and Plasma, and Glutathione Peroxidase Activity in Blood of Breast Cancer Patients During Adjuvant Treatment and Cyclophsophamide, Methotrexate and 5-Fluorouracil," *Cancer Letter,* 18 (1983), 283-89; J. T. Salonen, et al., "Risk of Cancer in Relation to Serum Concentrations of Selenium and Vitamins A and E. Matching Case-Control Analysis of Prospective Data," *Br Med J,* 290 (1985), 417-20.
39. D. Albanes, O. P. Heinonen, et al., "Effects of Alpha-Tocopherol and Beta-Carotene Supplements on Cancer Incidence in the Alpha-Tocopherol, Beta-Carotene Cancer Prevention Study," *Am J Clin Nutr* 62 (1996), S1427-30, in Murray, et al., *How to Prevent and Treat Cancer,* 54.
40. L. Kiremidjian-Schumacher, et al., "Supplementation with Selenium and Human Immune Cell Functions. II. Effect on Cytotoxic Lymphocytes and Natural Killer Cells," *Bio Trace Elem Res* 41(1-2) (1994), 115-27, in Murray, et al., *How to Prevent and Treat Cancer,* 57.
41. G. N. Schrauzer, "Selenium: Role in Nutritional Cancer Prophylaxis Reaffirmed," *Anabolism: Journal of Preventative Medicine,* January 1983, 5-6.
42. Shari Lieberman and Nancy Bruning, *The Real Vitamin & Mineral Book* (New York: Avery, 1990), 115-16; Murray and Pizzorno, *Encyclopedia.*
43. H. H. Draper and R. P. Bird, "Micronutrients and Cancer Prevention: Are the RDAs Adequate?" *Free Radical Biology and Medicine,* 3 (1987), 203-07.
44. Watson and Leonard, "Selenium."
45. L. Pauling and C. Moertel, "Special Report. A Proposition: Megadoses of Vitamin C are Valuable in the Treatment of Cancer," *Nutr Rev* 44(1) (January 1989); E. Cameron and L. Pauling, "Supplemental Ascorbate in the Supportive Treatment of Cancer: Prolongation of Survival Times in Terminal Human Cancer," *Proc Natl Acad Sci USA* 73 (1976) 3685-89; E. Cameron and L. Pauling, *Cancer and Vitamin C* (Menlo Park: CA: The Linus Pauling Institute of Science and Medicine, 1979).
46. N. Gottlieb, "Cancer and Vitamin C: The Debate Lingers," *J Natl Cancer Inst* 91(24) (15 December 1999), 2073-75.
47. Draper and Bird, "Micronutrients."
48. Watson and Leonard, "Selenium."
49. J. P. Perchellet, et al., "Effects of Combined Treatments with Selenium, Glutathione, and Vitamin E on Glutathione Peroxidase Activity, Ornithine Decarboxylase Induction, and Complete and Multi-Stage Carcinogenesis in Mouse Skin," *Cancer Research* 47(2) (15 January 1987), 477-85.
50. E. P. Whitlock, "Selenium, Vitamin E and Vitamin A: Nutritional and Physiologic Findings," *Laboratory Management,* May 1987; N. J. Wald, et al., "Plasma Retinol, Beta Carotene and Vitamin E Levels in Relation to the Future Risk of Breast Cancer," *British J Cancer* 49:32 (1984), 1-4.
51. C. B. Simone, et al., "Nutritional and Lifestyle Modification to Augment Oncology

Care: An Overview," *Journal of Orthomolecular Medicine* 12(4) (1997), 197-206.

52. Ibid.
53. L. Wood, "Possible Prevention of Adriamycin-Induced Alopecia by Tocopherol," *New England Journal of Medicine* 312 (1985), 60.
54. "Scientists Find Key to Wasting Syndrome Seen in Cancer, AIDS," *UCSD School of Medicine News,* 3 December 2001.
55. Michael Janson, "Supplements Against Cancer," *Dr. Michael Janson's Healthy Living* 4 (December 2002), 12.
56. Sylvia Escott-Stump, *Nutrition and Diagnosis-Related Care,* 2d ed. (Philadelphia: Lea & Febiger, 1988), 358.
57. Maurice E. Shills and Vernon R. Young, *Modern Nutrition in Health and Disease,* 7th ed. (Philadelphia: Lea & Febiger, 1988), 1401.
58. Marie V. Krause and L. Kathleen Mahan, *Food, Nutrition & Diet Therapy,* 7th ed. (Philadelphia: W.B. Saunders Co., 1984), 743.
59. Ibid.
60. "Eating Hints," *National Cancer Institute Publication,* August 1986.
61. R. S. Kennedy, G. P. Konok, et al., "The Use of Whey Protein Concentrate in the Treatment of Patients with Metastic Carcinoma: A Phase I-II Clinical Study," *Anticancer Res* 15(6B) (November-December 1995), 2643-49.
62. G. Bounous, F. Gervais, et al., "The Influence of Dietary Whey Protein on Tissue Glutathione and the Diseases of Aging," *Clin Invest Med* 12 (1989), 343-49.
63. R. S. Kennedy, et al., "Use of Whey Protein"; S. Baruchel and G. Viau, "In Vitro Selected Modulation of Cellular Glutathione by a Humanized Milk Protein Isolate in Normal Cells and Rat Mammary Carcinoma Model," *Anticancer Res* 16(3A) (May-June 1996), 1095-99.
64. Murray, et al., *How to Prevent and Treat Cancer,* 154.

CHAPTER 8

1. *Toxicology Information Briefs*, Extension Toxicology Network; a Cooperative Extension Effort of the University California, Davis, Oregon State University, Michigan State University, Cornell University, and University of Idaho; files maintained at Oregon State University; EXTONET.
2. "Clean Water Fund's Home-Safe-Home Guide 2000," www.cleanwaterfund.org.
3. Steingraber, *Living Downstream.*
4. Samuel Epstein, M.D., *The Politics of Cancer Revised* (Fremont Center, NY: East Ridge Press, 1998).
5. "Cancer on the Rise in Children," www.epa.gov/OGWDW/ccl/ccl/fr.html.
6. Peter Montague, "*Living Downstream*: A Review," *Rachel's Environment and Health Weekly,* 565 (25 September 1997).
7. John Bower, *The Healthy House,* 4th ed. (Bloomington, IN: Healthy House Institute, 2001).
8. Elizabeth Flynn, M.D., et al., *Indoor Air Pollutants Affecting Child Health,* a project of the American College of Medical Toxicology, 2000.
9. S. M. Grundy, "Health Articles—Dietary Hazards, Processed Fats, 2002," www.amazingdiscoveries.org.
10. Lenore Kohlmeier, University of North Carolina At Chapel Hill, www.sciencedaily.com/releases/1997/09.
11. Rudolph Ballentine, *Radical Healing: Integrating the World's Great Therapeutic Traditions to Create a New Transformative Medicine* (New York: Three Rivers Press, 1999).

12. Grundy, "Health Articles."
13. "High Insulin Levels Hinder Cancer Recovery," *Good Medicine,* vol. XI, no. 3, 2002 (to be published in the American Chemical Society's *Journal for Agriculture and Food Chemistry).*
14. Pritchford, *Healing with Whole Foods.*
15. Karen Collins, MS., R.D., C.D.N., "Insulin Resistance Poses Many Health Risks," American Institute for Cancer Research, www.vegsource.com
16. Robert A. Wascher, M.D., F.A.C.S., "Health Briefs, 2002," www.mensnewsdaily.com.
17. Charles Fuchs, M.D., "News and Publications, 2002," www.dfci.harvard.edu/abo/news/press/090402.asp.
18. "Fried Foods, Figure, and Cancer Development," *Good Medicine.*
19. Hulda Regehr Clark, Ph.D., N.D., *The Cure for All Diseases* (Chula Vista, CA: New Century Press, 1995).
20. Bill Lambrecht, *Dinner at the New Gene Café: How Genetic Engineering Is Changing What We Eat, How We Live, and the Global Politics of Food* (NY: St. Martin's Press, 2001).
21. Clark, *The Cure for all Diseases.*
22. Pritchford, *Healing with Whole Foods.*
23. "Reducing Potential Cancer Risks from Drinking Water Part I: Contaminant Sources and Drinking Water Standards," Program on Breast Cancer and Environmental Risk Factors in New York State, Cornell University, 1998.
24. "Clean Water and Oceans: Drinking Water; in Brief: FAQ Arsenic in Drinking Water," Natural Resources Defense Council, 2000.
25. "The Real Cost of Bottled Water—Right to Water," 2001, twri.edu/watertalk/archive/2001-/May-05.l.html.
26. I. H. (Mel) Suffet, Ph.D., "Bottled Water," www.ioe.ucla.edu.
27. Ibid.
28. Bower, *Healthy House.*
29. Ibid.
30. Ibid.
31. Samuel Epstein and David Steinman, *The Safe Shopper's Bible: A Consumer's Guide to Nontoxic Household Products, Cosmetics and Food* (New York: Macmillan, 1995).
32. Aubrey Hampton and Susan Hussey, *The Take Charge Beauty Book* (Tampa, FL: Organic Press, 2000), 6.
33. Samuel S. Epstein, M.D., "Perfume: Cupid's Arrow or Poison Dart" (joint release issued by the Cancer Prevention Coalition and Environmental Health Network), updated February 2000.
34. Debbie Orozco, "Shoppers Beware: University of Texas-Houston Toxicologist Warns of Potential Cancer-Causing Agent in Cosmetics," University of Texas-Houston Health Science Center, 1996.
35. Samuel S. Epstein, M.D., "Major Cosmetic and Toiletry Ingredient Poses Avoidable Cancer Risks, Warns Professor of Environmental Medicine at University of Illinois, School of Public Medicine," 1998, www.nutrition4health.org/NOHAnews/NNS98CosmeticsCancer.htm.
36. *HSC Weekly,* University of Southern California, 19 April 2002.
37. Clark, *Cure for All Cancers,* 151; Hampton and Hussey, *Take Charge Beauty Book,* 215-20.
38. Bower, *Healthy House.*
39. Jean Renoux, "Building and Designing the Healthy Home," CEU www.ecolo-green.com.

40. Sherry A. Rogers, M.D., "Cancer and Diet," The Northeast Center for Environmental Medicine, Syracuse, NY, www.nzhealth.net.
41. Bower, *Healthy House.*
42. Gary Null, "Clearer, Cleaner, Safer, Greener," Installment 1: Introduction: *Where We Live and Work,* 1990, www.garynull.com.
43. Bower, *Healthy House.*
44. *Fact Sheet #49,* Environmental Health Science Information for the Berkeley Campus; University of California, Berkeley.
45. "Combustion Pollutants in Your Home—Indoor Air-Quality Guideline," no. 2, California Environmental Protection Agency Air Resources Board, March 1994, www.arb.ca.gov/research/indoor/combustf.htm.
46. "An Ounce of Prevention, Prevention 101; Recognizing Your Risks," UC Davis Cancer Center, wellness.ucdavis.edu.
47. "Addressing Indoor Environmental Concerns During Remodeling," U.S. Environmental Protection Agency, www.epa.gov/iag/home.
48. Dr. Joyce M. Woods, "Create a Safe and Healthy Home: Know Your A.B.C's," www.workingathomeparents.com.
49. Ralph W. Moss, Ph.D., "The Moss Report," www.cancerdecisions.com.
50. Clark, *Cure for All Diseases.*
51. Eliot Spitzer, Attorney General of New York State, "Home and Garden Pesticides: Questions and Answers About Safety and Alternatives," Environmental Protection Bureau, April 1999.
52. "More Kids Are Getting Brain Cancer. Why?" Center for Children's Health and the Environment, Mount Sinai School of Medicine, www.chem-tox.com/pesticides/pesticides.htm#leukemia.
53. Ibid.
54. "New Study Links Monsanto's Roundup to Cancer," June 1999, www.biotech-info.net.
55. Stephen Prata, *The EMF Handbook: Understanding and Controlling Electromagnetic Fields in Your Life* (Emeryville, CA: The Wait Group, Inc., 1993).
56. "Are Electromagnetic Fields and Cancer an Issue of Worthy Study?" *Cancer,* 69(2) (15 January 1992), 603-605.

CHAPTER 9

1. Institute of HeartMath, *HeartMath Freeze Framer Software/Hardware program* (Boulder Creek, CA).
2. Burton Goldberg Group, *Alternative Medicine—The Definitive Guide* (Puyallup, WA: Future Medicine Publishing, Inc., 1993).
3. Doc Childre, et al., *The HeartMath Solution* (New York: HarperSanFrancisco, 2000).
4. Christiane Northrup, M.D., *Women's Bodies, Women's Wisdom—Completely Revised and Updated* (New York: Bantam Books, 1998), 24.
5. John Diamond, M.D., et al, *Alternative Medicine Guide's Cancer Diagnosis—What to Do Next, 2000,* http://www.articleindex.com/Health/emotions_cancer.htm.
6. Diamond et al., *Alternative Medicine's Guide.*
7. Candace B. Pert, Ph.D., *Molecules of Emotion: Why You Feel the Way You Feel* (New York: Scribner, 1998).
8. Ibid.
9. Ibid.
10. Linda Marks, M.S.M., "Neglect Trauma," *Spirit of Change,* September/October 1999, 39-40.
11. Linda Marks, M.S.M., "Healing Trauma with Body Centered Psychotherapy,"

Spirit of Change, Spring 1994, 22.
12. Hillary Stokes and Kim Ward, "The Art of Forgiveness," *Sanoviv Health Retreat Healing Journal,* 191.
13. Dale Dwoskin and Sedona Training Associates, *The Sedona Method Course Workbook—Your Keys to Lasting Happiness, Abundance and Well Being* (Sedona, AR: Sedona Training Associates, 1991-2000).
14. Dale Dwoskin and Sedona Training Associates, *The Sedona Method Course Workbook—Your Keys to Lasting Happiness, Abundance and Well Being* (Sedona, AR: Sedona Training Associates, 1991-2000).
15. Ibid.
16. Sedona Training Associates, 60 Tortilla Drive, Suite 2, Sedona, AZ 86336. Telephone: 928-282-3522, release@sedona.com, www.sedona.com.
17. Michael Hutchison, *Mega Brain Power: Transform Your Life with Mind Machines and Brain Nutrients* (New York: Hyperion, 1994).
18. Murray, *How to Prevent and Treat Cancer* .
19. Norman Cousins, *Anatomy of an Illness as Perceived by the Patient: Reflections on Healing and Regeneration* (New York: Norton, 1979).
20. Murray, *How to Prevent and Treat Cancer.*
21. Steingraber, *Living Downstream.*

CHAPTER 10

1. M. Watson, et al., "Influence of Psychological Response on Survival in Breast Cancer: A Population-Based Cohort Study," *Lancet* 354 (16 October 1999), 1331-36; "Conquer Cancer with a Fighting Spirit," *Women's Health in Primary Care* 3(2) (February 2000), 131, 34460.
2. Ibid.
3. Barbara Hoberman Levine, *Your Body Believes Every Word You Say* (Boulder Creek, CA: Aslan Publishing, 1991).
4. John and Paula Sanford, *The Transformation of the Inner Man* (S. Plainfield, NJ: Bridge Publishing, Inc., 1982).
5. Ibid.
6. Rollin McCraty, et al., *Science of the Heart: Research Overview and Summaries* (Boulder Creek, CA: HeartMath Research Center, 2001).
7. Ibid.
8. Ibid.
9. Ibid.
10. "Attitudinal Breathing, A Tool from HeartMath," 2001 HeartMath, LLC.
11. Adapted from *Handbook to Higher Consciousness* by Ken Keyes, Jr., 5th ed., 1975 by the Living Love Center.

CHAPTER 11

1. Jeff Van Vonderen, "Interview," *Steps Magazine,* a publication of the National Association for Christian Recovery, 2000, http://www.spiritualabuse.com/dox/interview.htm.
2. Les Carter, Ph.D., and Frank Minirth, M.D., *The Choosing to Forgive Workbook* (Nashville, TN: Thomas Nelson, 1997).
3. Larry Dossey, M.D., *Prayer Is Good Medicine* (San Francisco, CA: HarperSanFrancisco, 1997).
4. Ibid.
5. Ibid.
6. "Relaxation/Music Therapy and Cancer Pain," http://www.internethealthlibrary.com/Therapies/MusicTherapy-Research.htm.

7. Peter Pettersson, translated by Yarrow Cleaves, *Cymatics—The Science of the Future* http://www.mysticalsun.com/cymatics.html.
8. Masara Emoto, Doctor of Medicine Alternative, *The Message from Water: The Message from Water Is Telling Us to Look at Ourselves* (Tokyo, Japan: HADO Publishing B.V., 1999).
9. Ibid.
10. Hutchison, *Mega Brain Power.*
11. "Dr. Tomatis," http://www.tomatis.com/English/Articles/Drtomatis.html.
12. Hutchison, *Mega Brain Power.*
13. Emoto, *Message.*
14. Hutchison, *Mega Brain Power.*
15. D. Carl Simonton, M.D., Stephanie Matthews-Simonton, James L. Creighton, *Getting Well Again* (New York, Toronto: Bantam Books, 1978).
16. Ibid.
17. Lynea Corson, Ph.D., et al, *The Secrets of Super Selling: How to Program Your Subconscious for Success* (New York: A Berkley Book, 1991).
18. Ibid.

CHAPTER 12

1. John Calbom recently told me that my prayer at this moment was an abbreviated version of an ancient prayer of the early church, the Jesus Prayer: "Lord Jesus Christ . . . have mercy on me." He then referred me to *The Bible of Orthodox Spirituality* and the following paragraph:

> St. Theophan explains how the mind and the heart can be united through the Jesus Prayer: "Lord Jesus Christ, Son of God, have mercy upon me." This prayer . . . when it becomes grafted to the heart, will lead you to the end, which you desire: it will unite your mind and heart, it will quell the turbulence of your thoughts, and it will give you power to govern the movements of your soul.

Taken from Anthony M. Coniaris Philokalia, *The Bible of Orthodox Spirituality* (Minneapolis, MN: Light and Life Publishing Co., 1998), 255.

CHAPTER 14

1. Michael Mahaffey and Nan Monk Mahaffey, *The Hope for Life Manual: The Development of the Total Human Being* (Cedar Springs: Cedar Springs Renewal Center, 2002).
2. Ibid.
3. John Moyne and Coleman Barks, *Open Secret Versions of Rumi* (Threshold Books, 1984).
4. Mahaffey and Mahaffey, *Hope for Life.*

INDEX

CPSIA information can be obtained at www.ICGtesting.com
Printed in the USA
LVOW092307190911

246944LV00019B/2/P